CANCER ETIOLOGY, DIAGNOSIS AND TREATMENTS

RENAL CELL CARCINOMA

CANCER ETIOLOGY, DIAGNOSIS AND TREATMENTS

Additional books in this series can be found on Nova's website under the Series tab.

Additional e-books in this series can be found on Nova's website under the e-book tab.

CANCER ETIOLOGY, DIAGNOSIS AND TREATMENTS

RENAL CELL CARCINOMA

JESUS M. FERNÁNDEZ-GOMEZ
AND
JORGE GARCÍA-RODRÍGUEZ
EDITORS

New York

Additional color graphics may be available in the e-book version of this book.

Library of Congress Cataloging-in-Publication Data

ISBN: 978-1-63482-495-8
Library of Congress Control Number: 2015935510

Published by Nova Science Publishers, Inc. † New York

Contents

Preface

Renal cell carcinoma (RCC) represents 90% of all kidney malignancies and 2-3% of all malignant diseases in adults. Although the RCC incidence has been increasing until recently, in the last years a tendency to decrease of rates has been demonstrated. However, mortality rates still continue to be high, especially in developed countries. Cigarette smoking, obesity and high blood pressure are the most important risk factors for RCC. On the other hand, approximately, 2-3% of RCC can be directly attributed to inherited genetic defects.

Clear Cell Renal Cell Carcinoma, composed of cell with clear or eosinophilic cytoplasm, is the most common type of RCC. In recent years, the advances in the understanding of molecular pathology, have allowed the recognition of numerous genetic alterations associated with the known renal carcinomas as well as the identification of new entities.

With the widespread use of abdominal imaging modalities such as ultrasound (US), computed tomography (CT) and magnetic resonance imaging (MRI) performed for unrelated indications as many as one-half of such carcinomas are discovered incidentally with a median tumor size of less than 5cm and in early-stage lesion. CT is considered the modality of choice for detection and diagnosis of renal carcinoma. The advent of Multidetector CT (MDCT) has helped to refine the diagnostic work-up of renal masses by allowing image acquisition in various phases of renal enhancement after intravenous administration of contrast material. Other modalities including ultrasound and the Positron-emission Tomography (PET) can also be utilized complimentarily.

Although radical nephrectomy is the standard of care for renal carcinoma in recent years minimally invasive surgery (laparoscopic nephrectomy and laparoscopic partial nephrectomy) has become an established surgical procedure worldwide as an alternative to open surgery which has demonstrated safety, feasibility and equivalent oncologic outcomes. In many cases the patients with RCC are elderly and have comorbidities that call into question the efficacy and cost-effectiveness of surgically treating them and active surveillance (AS) may a growing alternative to surgery. In these patients, percutaneous renal biopsy has an important role in determining the tumour characteristics and aggressiveness. Since currently there are no reliable data beyond the increase in tumour size, an increase in lesion diameter is the decisive factor that changes the approach to treating the patient.

Despite the advances in diagnosis staging and treatment a third of patients who undergo surgery with curative intent, will present recurrence. Although numerous studies have demonstrated that certain clinical, pathological and molecular factors can improve the prediction of tumour recurrence, new prognostic factors should be introduced to provide a rational approach to identify treatable recurrences and progression. As has been commented previously, the understanding of tumor biology gleaned from molecular biomarker research will be critical to the future treatment and prognosis determination of patients with RCC.

Renal cell carcinoma is a radioresistant tumor. Preoperative radiation therapy yields no survival advantage. Controversies exist concerning postoperative radiation therapy, but it may be considered in patients with perinephric fat extension, adrenal invasion, or involved margins. Furthermore, palliative radiation therapy is often used for local or symptomatic metastatic disease, such as painful osseous lesions or brain metastasis, to preclude potential neurologic progression. Stereotactic body radiotherapy is an excellent alternative to metastasectomy for treatment of not operable extracranial metastases.

For advanced disease the therapeutic options had been based on a non-specific systemic immunological treatment with cytokines (interleukin-2 and/or interferon-alfa) associated or not with primary cyto-reductive surgery. The identification of the genes involved in the process of renal carcinogenesis, as well as their expression pattern has allowed know different tumor types and their mechanisms of action. The best known are the changes related to the inactivation of the von Hippel Lindau (VHL) gene, which occur associated with both sporadic and hereditary carcinomas, mainly in CCRCC but also in papillary, playing an important role in the process of angiogenesis through the induction of the expression of vascular endothelial growth factor (VEGF). In this way, currently new agents targeting vascular growth factor and mammalian target of rapamycin signalling pathways have been developed. These drugs have shown an improvement in terms of survival and represent the present standard first- and second-line treatment options in advanced RCC.

In: Renal Cell Carcinoma
Editors: J. M. Fernández-Gomez, J. García-Rodríguez
ISBN: 978-1-63482-495-8

Chapter 1

Epidemiology and Hereditary Kidney Cancer Syndromes

P. Pellejero-Pérez, MD[1], J. Garcia-Rodriguez, PhD[1,*] and J. Fernandez-Gomez, PhD[1,2]

[1]Department of Urology, Hospital Universitario, Central de Asturias, Oviedo, Spain
[2]Department of Surgery, University of Oviedo, Oviedo, Spain

Abstract

Renal cell carcinoma (RCC) is the commonest type of kidney cancer in adults. It represents almost 90% of all kidney malignancies and 2–3% of all malignant diseases in adults. Incidence rates of kidney cancer are higher in Europe, North America, and Australia, whereas rates are lower in India, Japan, Africa, and China. Although the RCC incidence has been increasing until recently (2% every year), in the last years a tendency to decrease of rates has been demonstrated. The high incidence rates could be attributable to the use of more efficient diagnostic methods which yielda higher proportion of incidental findings consistent in small, localized tumors. However, mortality rates still continue to be high, especially in North America, Australia, New Zealand and Europe.

Numerous researches have established a role of some lifestyle-associated risk factors in the etiology of this cancer. Thus, cigarette smoking, obesity and high blood pressure are the most important and modifiable risk factors for RCC with a high prevalence in the general population. Recognizing the modifiable risk factors may open up perspectives for the primary prevention of RCC. On the other hand, approximately, 2–3% of RCC can be directly attributed to inherited genetic defects. Moreover, sporadic renal cell cancers have been shown to have a familial predisposition

Keywords: Renal cell carcinoma. Etiology. Risk factors. Incidence. Mortality

* Corresponding author: Jorge Garcia-Rodriguez. Department of Urology. Hospital Universitario Central de Asturias. Avda. de Roma sn. 33011. Oviedo. Asturias. Spain. E-mail: jgrmed@hotmail.com.

Introduction

Renal cell carcinoma (RCC) is the commonest type of kidney cancer in adults which is originated in the proximal convolutes tubules. RCC represents 90% of all kidney malignancies and 2-3% of all malignant diseases in adults. It is the 13th most common malignancy, with approximately 271 000 new cases diagnosed in 2008 [1]. Its incidence has been increasing over time to stabilize in recent years, with a substantial variation of incidence according to different geographic regions. Conversely, mortality rates continue to be high especially in North America, Australia, New Zealand and Europe (Figure 1).

There are different RCC types with specific histopathological and genetic characteristics. Historically, cancers of the renal pelvis have been grouped with RCCs when referring to kidney cancer. However, cancer of the renal pelvis is now recognized as urothelial cancers. Thus, it has been traditionally difficult to obtain clear patterns of incidence and mortality from RCC since mixed data of urothelial cancer and RCC have been reported.

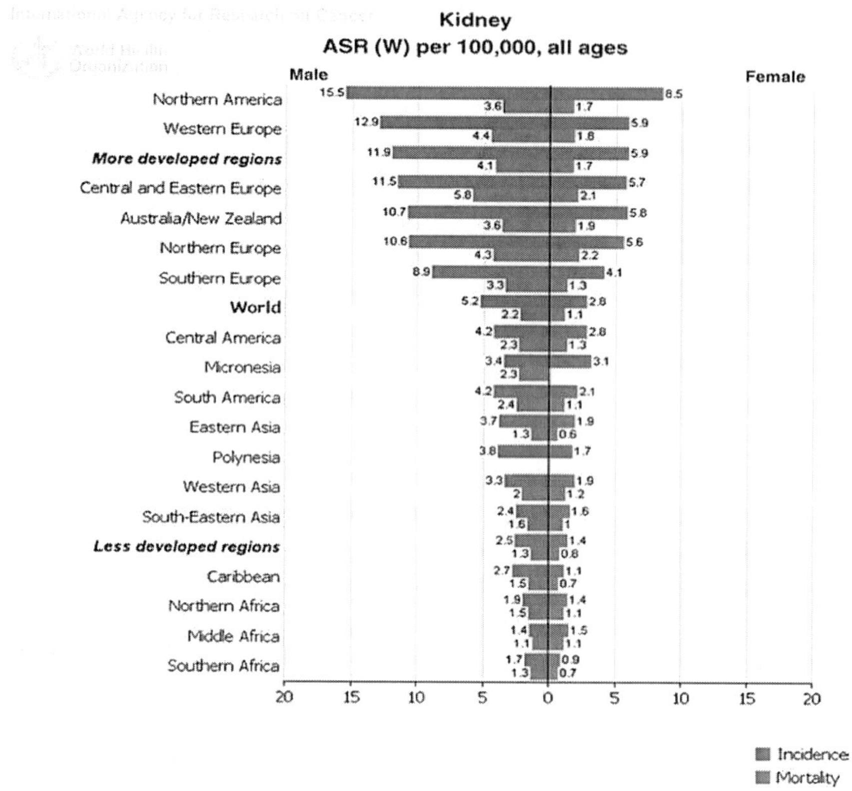

GLOBOCAN 2008 (LARC) (17.6.2011).

Reproduced from the public domain of the International Agency for Research on Cancer, GLOBOCAN database 2008, Cancer Incidence and Mortality Worldwide: IARC Cancer Base No. 10, Lyon, France (3), available at: http://www-dep.iarc.fr.

Figure 1. Age-standardised incidence and mortality rates for kidney cancer by gender on different continents [1].

Overall, the incidence of kidney cancer varies more than 10-fold between populations and geographic areas [1]. Currently the incidence rates are higher in developed countries than in the developing world [2]. The highest rates have been registered in Europe, North America and Australia, whereas the lowest rates have been recorded in India, Japan, Africa, and China. For example, in 2008, about 88,400 new cases of kidney cancer occurred in Europe [3]. The Surveillance, Epidemiology and results program (SEER) has been estimated that the number of new cases of kidney and renal pelvis cancer in the United States is 15.5 per 100,000 men and women per year [4]. In this way, in 2011 there were 358,603 people living with a kidney or renal pelvis cancer in the United States, with 63,920 new cancer cases in 2014.

Based on 2009-2011 data, approximately 1.6 percent of men and women will be diagnosed with kidney and renal pelvis cancer during their lifetime [4].

Until recently, the worldwide incidence of RCC has increased by approximately 2% every year, however, based on an analysis of SEER data a continued rise in incidence rates was confirmed in all age groups and for all tumor sizes in the US [5].

This incidence increase could be attributable to more efficient diagnostic methods which causes a rise of incidental diagnosis of small, localized tumors. Better detection techniques cannot explain the continued high number of advanced tumors and the increase in tumor size-specific mortality among kidney cancer patients [6]. Currently, about 20-30% of all patients are diagnosed with metastatic disease [7, 8, 9, 10, 11]. Although the global incidence of kidney cancer has increased from the 1970s to 1990s, now it has leveled out or decreased in many countries [12]. This phenomenon may be due to several reasons. Firstly the incidence decrease of some cancers [13] but also the reduction in the use of imaging studies between 2006 and 2010 [14]. In this way, a recent European study which analysed the change of the kidney cancer incidence pattern from 1980 to 2004 indicates a tendency towards stabilization or decrease of incidence in recent years in both sexes [15]. In conclusion, general data indicate that the incidence and mortality of renal malignancies have increased worldwide over the last 30 years, particularly in the Western world where kidney cancer has been classified among the tumors with the highest upward trend in incidence [12].

Epidemiology

Gender

According to most reports, an annual incidence rate increase of 2% in men and women in all regions and ethnic groups has been observed [15, 16]. RCC is the seventh commonest cancer in men and the ninth commonest in women [7].

RCC is more frequent in men with a male to female ratio between 1.5:1 and 2.5:1, according to different geographical regions. The highest incidence rates are found in the sixth and seventh decades [17], being higher in men, as has already been mentioned. This pattern is consistently observed throughout the world with the exception of Western Africa where reported incidence rates seem to be higher in women [2].

In the developed countries, kidney cancer represents approximately 2-4 % of all new cancers, with incidence rates ranging from 7 to 22 per 100,000 in males and 4 to 13 per 100,000 in females [11, 15, 18].

A recent analysis of the SEER database has also revealed that men present significantly larger (6.1 cm vs. 5.9 cm) as well as higher grade tumors than women [2]. Respect to mortality, in 2008 there were 116,000 deaths because of kidney cancer being twice as high more frequent in men than in women [1] (Figure 1).

Age

Age is an important factor to consider when analysing the incidence of RCC. In Europe and the United States, this incidence increases with age. Kidney and renal pelvis cancer is most frequently diagnosed among people aged 55-64. A study based on data from the "Cancer Incidence in Five Continents" database at the International Agency for Research on Cancer (IARC) and the US Surveillance, Epidemiology, and End Results (SEER) Program demonstrated that RCC rates in Europe and the US consistently increase with the age, with a plateau around the age group of 70–75 years and older [15].

Age-standardised incidences from developed regions of the world, suggest that men are at an increased risk of developing RCC, which probably is related to differences in associated risk factors such as cigarette smoking [19]. Approximately 90 % of all kidney cancers in Canadian adults occurs in individuals older than 45 [20].

Race

Regarding the racial factor, reported differences of incidence rates in the literature may be attributable to variations in frequency of diagnostic imaging tests, genetic background, access to health system and differences of lifestyle, as well as environmental risk factors, being almost impossible to distinguish the real cause.

Therefore, it is difficult to draw conclusions about an independent association between race and RCC risk [19].

The incidence appears to be lower among the Asian race, both in most Asian countries and in the United States. Moreover, the lowest incidences have been reported in African countries.

However, probably due to the previously mentioned differences in risk factors, incidence in African Americans in the United States is very high [5].

Thus, in the US, where the RCC incidence is higher among African Americans than in whites, the RCC incidence has risen more rapidly among African Americans than in whites in recent decades [1]. Based on data from the US Surveillance, Epidemiology, and End Results (SEER) program for the years 2002–2005, the age-adjusted RCC incidence rates among black men, white men, black women, and white women were 17.0, 14.3, 7.5 and 7.2 per 100,000 person-years, respectively. For white Hispanics in the United States the incidence are much higher than rates reported in Latin America, suggesting again the potential role of environmental exposures [5].

In conclusion, probably the differences in RCC incidence rates may be due to different factors and can differ according to various racial/ethnic populations [21].

Tumor Stage

Currently, 64.1% of kidney and renal pelvis cancers are diagnosed at the earliest stage of the disease. The changes in the use of certain diagnostic imaging tests, as ultrasonography and computed tomography (CT), have produced an increase in the early stages diagnosis of the disease. The incidence of metastasis tumors is now stable oreven decreases over time, although the diagnosis of tumors with regional spread remains unchanged [17].

Recently, the SEER current data base has shown the percentages of localized or confined tumors (64%), regional or spread to regional lymph nodes (17%) and distant or metastasized RCC (16%) [4]. According to these data, the percentage of RCC diagnosed in the localized stage ranges between 59 and 73% depending on race and gender [5].

Traditionally, stage-specific analyses show that the incidence rates of localized kidney cancer increased by 4.55% between 1975 and 2009, and by 4.42% between 2000 and 2009. The percentage of regional disease increased by 0.88% from 1975 to 2009 and then stabilized (0.56%). The incidence rates of distant disease have remained stable, in the short- and long-term trends (1975-2009: from 1.90 to 2.32 per 100,000 person-years).

RCC is currently diagnosed at earlier stages and therefore lower size lesions are detected [22, 23]. The marked increase in incidence has been noted for localized and very small tumors (<2.0 cm), because of the use of diagnostic techniques. Thus, in the United States a trend toward diagnosing very small tumor masses (< 2 cm) followed by tumors of 2.0-4.0 cm in size has been observed [5]. Moreover, an increase in the incidence rates of larger tumors has also been demonstrated although with a moderate rise. Additionally, 30% of renal cancer is still identified with distant disease at first diagnosis [24].

In conclusion, it seems clear that the diagnoses of renal cell cancer at earlier stages with smaller masses could have contributed to the recent stabilization of kidney cancer mortality rates in the United States. Likewise, in Europe the survival of patients diagnosed with tumors has also improved over time [11]. In respect to the continuous increase of large size cancers in younger patients, it could be related to the changing patterns of several risk factors [5].

Country Differences

Some authors have reported that incidence rates have increased at least until mid-1990, when rates stabilized or even fell in many records in Europe, Oceania, Asia, and Canada [25]. In a few countries, such as Hong Kong, and among men in Canada, the decline started earlier. In the United States, overall RCC incidence rates augmented consistently over time, with a rapid growth specially among African Americans [11, 26]. The highest rates are found in North America, Europe and Australia, and the lowest in Asia and African countries. In the Asian population, incidence rates seem to be substantially lower, both in most Asian countries and in the US. The lowest rates have been reported in African countries, although the incidence is higher among African Americans in the US, as has been commented [6].

- Europe. There were 88,400 new cases of RCC and 39,300 kidney cancer–related deaths in the European Union in 2008 [27]. There were approximately 84,400 new cases of RCC and 34,700 kidney cancer-related deaths within the European Union in

2012 [28]. These data show a stabilization or even decline of RCC incidence recently, between 1980 and 2004 [15]. Although the highest rates are found in several countries of the central and eastern Europe, globally the highest age standardized incidence has been demonstrated in the Western countries with an estimation of 5.8 new cases per 100,000 and mortality rates of 1.4 per 100,000 [29].

Over the last decades there has been a reduction of rates in Sweden, being stable in Denmark. Conversely, the United Kingdom represents an exception because of their increasing RCC rates [17]. The lowest rates have been reported in the southern Europe. However, an important variability is reported in different regions and even in the same country. This may be related to several factors which include the specific characteristics of data collection. In this way, the reported rates in males vary more than five-fold, from 2.9 per 100,000 in Serbia to 15.2 per 100,000 in the Czech Republic. Respect to regional variations, the incidence in Salerno was 3.6 per 100,000 and in the North East region of Italy 9.0 per 100,000 [11]. Analyzing the 27 European Union (EU) countries, the highest rates found in The Czech Republic, with a maximal incidence of 18.8 and 21.7 per 100,000 men in 1990–1994 and 2000–2004, respectively; 10.1 and 10.3 per 100 000 women in 1990–1994 and 2000–2004, respectively. Similarly, in Slovakia the corresponding incidence were 11.9 and 13.5 per 100 000 men, and 6.2 and 6.7 per 100,000 women. Likewise, Lithuania, Latvia, Estonia, and Iceland, had high rates while the lowest incidences have been reported in Romania, Cyprus and Portugal [15].

In recent years, RCC incidence is declining in some European countries, such as Sweden, where there has been a substantial drop of incidence in both sexes for 25 years, as well as in Poland, Finland and the Netherlands. Nevertheless, in England and Scotland or in Eastern Europe the rates are still increased (except for women in the early 2000s) [2].

- US. In United States RCC incidence is growing. It has been estimated that 64,770 new cases of kidney cancer were diagnosed in 2012 in the United States, with about 13,570 new deaths [30]. The highest incidence has been registered among American Indians and Alaskan Natives, which can be related to the high prevalence of obesity and smoking in this population [31].

Mortality

Equivalent mortality evolution of the rates has been shown over time in the past decades. The worldwide mortality rates of kidney cancer were estimated to be 116,000 in 2008, which represents 1.5% of all cancer deaths. Similarly to incidence, mortality varies considerably between regions [1] (Figure 1).

In Europe, until early 1990 there was an important increase in mortality rates with a later stabilization or even reduction in recent years. This decrease in mortality was higher among middle-aged men, particularly in the Western regions of the European Union. Thus, significant differences have been reported in mortality, with highest rates in the Czech Republic and Baltic countries and the lowest in Greece, Spain, Portugal, and Romania [15, 32]. This reduction of mortality rates has been demonstrated since the 1980s in Scandinavian countries and since the early 1990s in France, Germany, Austria, the Netherlands and in Italy.

However, in some European countries (Croatia, Estonia, Greece, Ireland, Slovakia), mortality rates still show an upward trend with increasing rates [15]. In the United States, between 1970 and mid-1990 the RCC became the tenth commonest cause of death from malignant tumors in men. There were 13,000 deaths from kidney cancer in 2010. The highest mortality rates have been reported among American Indians and Alaska Natives [8]. In recent years, the diagnosis of smaller renal tumors at earlier stages probably has contributed to the stabilization of the mortality seen in the United States and in many European countries [15]. Despite all these data the Surveillance Epidemiology and End Results (SEER), published their databases in relation to the registration of age-adjusted rates in tumors diagnosed from 1988-2006. These data show an increase of 0.78% annually, with mortality rates growths for localized of 3.16%, and conversely, a diminution of mortality rates for RCC with regional and distant disease of 0.46% and 0.53%, respectively.

Survival

Relative survival rates for kidney cancer are higher in the United States than in Europe. In an analysis published by Verdecchia et al., with data obtained from 47 European cancer registries (EUROCARE-4) between 2000 and 2002, these authors demonstrated that the mean 5-year relative survival for kidney cancer was 55.7% compared with 62.6% from 13 United States SEER registries [33].

In the United States, the 5-year relative survival rates increased from 1983 to 2002 across all stages [34]. The data obtained by the SEER concerning RCC diagnosed between 1998 and 2006, establish that 5-year relative survival for all stages increased from 63.7% in 1988 to 73.9% in 2002. In terms of survival, an increased survival rates from 91.7% in 1988 to 92.8% in 2002 is observed, although the survival rates remained unchanged for regional (63.7% to 64.2%) and metastatic disease (12.1 % to 11.9%) over time [10].

This clear improvement in survival data can be explained by an early diagnosis and treatment, although these results have not been reported by some authors and generate some controversy.

Etiological Risk Factors of Kidney Cancer

Numerous researches have established a role of some lifestyle-associated risk factors in the etiology of this cancer. Thus, cigarette smoking, obesity and high blood pressure are the most important and modifiable risk factors for RCC with a high prevalence in the general population. Recognizing the modifiable risk factors may open up perspectives for the primary prevention of RCC.

Smoking

Cigarette smoking is considered a causal risk factor for renal cell cancer by the International Agency for Research on Cancer (IARC) and the US Surgeon General [35, 36].

Moreover, cohort studies have also reported positive associations between smoking and kidney cancer incidence and mortality [37, 38]. The prevalence of cigarette smoking in industrialized countries generally has declined over time, while it has remained stable or increased in developing countries [39], such as the United States and Western Europe [11].

Etiopathogenic mechanisms involving cigarette smoking and renal cell cancer risk are hypothetically the chronic tissue hypoxia due to carbon monoxide exposure and smoking-related conditions such as chronic obstructive pulmonary disease [40, 41]. One study has demonstrated that chromosome 3p, a frequent site of genetic alterations in renal cell cancer, may be a specific molecular target of cigarette carcinogens and BPDE (benzo[alpha]pyrene diol epoxide), which is a major constituent of cigarette smoke, sensitivity in chromosome 3p may reflect the genetic susceptibility of an individual to renal cell carcinoma [42].

A meta-analysis including 19 case–control and 5 cohort studies confirmed that ever smoker, former smokers and current smokers, had an increased risk of RCC compared to those who never smoked (RR 1.38).

The increases in risk related to ever smoking were estimated to be 54% for men and 22% for women (RR 1.54 and 1.22 respectively). The association between smoking and RCC is relatively weak, but a clear dose–response relationship is evident with higher risk estimates with increasing amount of cigarettes smoked [43] and increasing duration of this habit in years. When compared with those smoking for less than 20 years, those who smoked for 20 years or longer experienced a 60% increase in RCC risk [44].

For cessation of smoking, it has been shown that reduces the risk of kidney cancer development, but only among long-term quitters of ten or more years [5, 43]. Ryan et al. reported the more conclusive findings in this issue, compared with others studies [45, 46, 47, 48]. They observed, among ex-smokers, a trend of decreasing risk across 10-year cessation intervals, with a 60% decrease in risk for those who had quit 11–20 years prior to interview.

While cigarette smoking is an established risk factor for RCC, little is known about the contribution of environmental tobacco smoke (ETS) to RCC incidence. Few studies have explored this association [45, 49], but they have established a potential etiologic role for ETS in kidney cancer risk, particularly in the home.

Hu et al. (2005) reported significant risk increases for 43 or more years of combined home and workplace ETS exposure (compared with those never exposed) among non-smoking men (OR = 3.9) and women (OR = 1.8) [49]. One of the first studies to observe associations between RCC and home ETS exposure among never smokers [50] reports that those with greater than 20 years of exposure were more than twice as likely to develop RCC compared with those reporting no home ETS exposure. Thus, individuals exposed to ETS in the workplace for 1 – 20 years were twice as likely to develop RCC as those never exposed, but, at the higher range (greater than 20 years), no association was observed.

Risk of RCC is known to increase with age, so associations between RCC and home ETS were particularly strong in the 70- to 79- year age group. These results showed that ETS exposure in the home may act as an independent risk factor for RCC, but it remains unclear why similar associations were not found for workplace or public ETS.

On the other hand, a history of smoking in patients with RCC was recently associated with worse pathologic features and survival outcomes and with an increased risk of having mutated p53 [51]. Both overall survival (OS) (62.37 months vs 43.64 months; P = .001) and cancer-specific survival (CSS) (87.43 months vs 56.57 months; P = .005) were significantly worse in patients who smoked.

Tobacco dosage classified by pack-years was retained as an independent predictor of CSS in patients with non-metastatic disease. Each pack-year was associated with a 1% increase in the risk of death from RCC. Finally, p53 expression was retained as an independent predictor of CSS for all patients (HR, 1.013; 95% CI, 1.005-1.022; P = .002) and it appears that a continuous influence of 1 key carcinogen of tobacco smoke and environmental pollution, benzo(a)pyrene diol epoxide (BPDE), can contribute to p53 mutations.

The prognostic value of immunohistochemically detectable (i.e., mutated) p53 expression in RCC has been demonstrated in 4 large studies [52], that showed the importance of p53 on the recurrence of localized and metastatic RCC [53, 54, 55], disease specific- survival [56] and disease progression [57] in patients with RCC.

Obesity

Recently, obesity has become accepted as a major risk factor for RCC, and its incidence has increased markedly not only in industrialized countries, but also in low- and middle income countries in recent decades. The global rise in obesity likely has also contributed to the upward RCC incidence trends [58]. Multiple studies have indicated that the increased incidence of RCC in Western countries can be partially attributed to local increases in obesity, with some reports suggesting that 40 % or more of RCC cases in the US and 30% in Europe are causally linked to excess body weight [59-61]. A meta-analysis of prospective studies [62] provided evidence for an association between body-mass index (BMI) and risk of RCC with risk estimates of 1.24 in men and 1.34 in women. Results suggested a somewhat stronger association in women than in men, but this difference was not significant. In contrast, a review published by Bergstrom et al. [63] identified equally strong associations in both sexes. Overall, evidence on sex-specific differences in the association between BMI and RCC risk is not conclusive. They determined that each unit of increased BMI was associated with a relative risk of RCC development of 1.07, which mean that for approximately every 3 kg of increased body weight, the risk of RCC is increased by about 7 %. Furthermore the UK million-woman study found that a 10-unit increase in BMI was associated with relative risk of developing RCC =1.53 [64]. Other study has demonstrated that as BMI increased linearly, the relative risk of RCC increased, with a relative risk of 1.8 for kidney cancer in obese patients [65]. Two current studies have also confirmed these trends [59, 66].

One is a meta-analysis of 21 reports, and found an overall relative risk for developing RCC of 1.77 in obese versus lean men and women [59].

It has been suggested that body fat distribution influences in the risk of kidney cancer development. An increased risk was observed with increasing waist-to-hip ratio [67, 68, 69], but evidence is too limited to conclude that abdominal obesity is a risk factor for RCC independently of BMI or body weight *per se*. The same occurs with weight cycling and weight gain during adulthood [5].

Although many studies have demonstrated the relationship between obesity and RCC, the effect of high body weight on tumor progression and cancer-specific survival remains unclear, with several contradictory conclusions among studies [70-73].

The causes of increased kidney cancer risk in obese adults remain unclear. Renal cell cancer is an immunogenic tumor, meaning that the immune system recognizes RCC-derived tumor antigens as foreign.

Taking this into account, current therapy for metastatic renal cell carcinoma is focused on immunebased therapies, targeted molecular therapies, and antiangiogenesis therapies, as Sunitinib [74]. It is suggested that obesity-mediated immune dysfunctions contribute to enhanced tumor progression and diminished responses to immune-based therapies, an idea that has not yet been tested clinically [75]. All this is related with the state of chronic inflammation secondary to the condition overweight [61, 76].

As chronic inflammation is known to inhibit protective immunity it is not surprising that in humans, obesity is associated with notable alterations to the immune system overall, and T cell immunity in particular. Decreased T cell responsiveness would likely impair the efficacy of many immunotherapies currently being used or developed for RCC. Presently, direct support of this idea is not available from human studies [75].

In addition to the state of chronic inflammation, obesity has been related with renal cell cancer development through the following mechanisms [77]: lipid peroxidation and oxidative stress, chronic tissue hypoxia, increased levels of insulin and insulin-like growth factor I [61], increased circulating estrogen levels, increased arterionephrosclerosis, increased glomerular filtration rate and increased renal plasma flow, which may render the kidney more susceptible to kidney damage and carcinogenesis [78]. On the other hand, few studies have examined obesity and hypertension together as risk factors for kidney cancer, since obesity is a risk factor for hypertension, they may represent a shared causal mechanism [66]. It has been identified a relative risk of 2.82 for kidney cancer in individuals who were both hypertensive and obese when compared with their lean normotensive counterparts [79]. Moreover, one large cohort study [66] analyzed this longitudinal relationships in almost 160,000 participants of The Women's Health Initiative (WHI) clinical trials and observational studies [80, 81] and showed that RCC incidence significantly increased with higher systolic and diastolic blood pressure (SBP, DBP), and higher BMI or waist circumference (WC) categories. However, consistently significant data were only found for women with a BMI≥30. Among obese women, increasing SBP showed a dose–response association with kidney cancer risk.

The biologic mechanisms underlying the association between hypertension and renal cell cancer are unclear, but are suggested to include oxidative stress [82] and lipid peroxidation [78, 83], which is hypothesized to play a role in kidney cancer pathogenesis.

Hypertension

Hypertension has also been established as another major risk factor for kidney cancer. Numerous large prospective studies have shown that high blood pressure levels are associated with elevated risk of RCC and several cohort studies demonstrated, moreover, a clear dose-response relationship [84, 85]. Weicker et al. reported that relative risks for the highest versus the lowest category of systolic (≥160 mmHg vs. <120 mmHg) and diastolic (≥100 mmHg vs. <80 mmHg) blood pressures were 2.48 and 2.34 respectively. Risk estimates did not significantly differ according to sex or use of antihypertensive medication [86].

Nowadays, the prevalence of this entity is rising and is estimated to affect about 20% to 40% of the world's population [87, 88]. Moreover, it was estimated that as of 2013, one in three US adults has uncontrolled blood pressure [89]. Thus, it is possible that the widespread prevalence of hypertension could be contributing to the increased rates of RCC.

There was speculation a possible role of the antihypertensive treatments use in the increase renal cell cancer risk. A large cohort of US women showed higher rates of kidney cancer among women with treated (versus untreated) hypertension and slightly lower point estimates of kidney cancer incidence among those without hypertension [66]. Furthermore, Setiawan et al. found that diuretic use increased women risk of CCR once corrected for hypertension [79], implying the possible impact of estrogens, which has been that increases in animal models the effect of diuretics in renal tubules cells. However, some researchers have concluded that this association may be due to confounding by severity or duration of hypertension rather than its medications. So, data from two cohort studies suggest that better control of blood pressure may lower RCC risk, suggesting a tumor-promoting effect for hypertension [84, 86], whereas use of antihypertensive medications including diuretics is probably not a causal risk factor [79, 90, 91]. As stated above, despite the high correlation between obesity and hypertension, their associations with renal cell cancer risk have been shown to be independent of each other [11].

The Women's Health Initiative (WHI) [80] and the Multiple Risk Factor Intervention Trial (MRFIT) [92] are the 2 largest studies on the relationship of blood pressure levels and risk of kidney cancer that include both the actual measurements of BP and the long-term follow-up to account. Kristen M Sanfilippo et al. [66] analyzed both studies and found, as mentioned, that both systolic blood pressure levels and body mass index (BMI) were predictors of kidney cancer. Women with systolic hypertension (≥140 mmHg) showed higher point estimates of kidney cancer risk when compared with levels of ≤120 mm Hg, and women with slight SBP (120.1 to 130.0 mmHg) had also a significant increase vs. those normotensive (HR, 1.33; 95% CI, 1.01-1.75).

However, elevated diastolic blood pressure and BMI were independently associated with kidney cancer. These authors also examined the effect of blood pressure on kidney cancer deaths for over 25 years among the 353,340 men screened for the MRFIT, and showed an increased risk in a dose-response fashion with increasing SBP (hazard ratio, 1.87 for SBP > 160 mmHg versus <120 mmHg; 95% confidence interval, 1.38-2.53).

The percentage dying of kidney cancer increased with higher BP levels even throughout the normotensive range. The relationship between baseline DBP and mortality from kidney cancer was weaker than for SBP. The biologic mechanisms underlying the association between hypertension and renal cell cancer are unclear, but are hypothesized to include chronic renal hypoxia and lipid peroxidation [93]. Gago-Dominguez et al. proposed that lipid peroxidation, which is increased in obese and hypertensive subjects, is one mechanism responsible for the increased risk of renal cell carcinoma. In experimental animals lipid peroxidation of the proximal renal tubules is a necessary mechanistic pathway in renal carcinogenesis induced by several different chemicals [82]. Chronic kidney disease could represent other likely alternative explanation for associations between hypertension and kidney cancer. Elevations of blood pressure is a strong independent risk factor for end-stage renal disease, which is an important risk factor for kidney cancer [94].

Dyslipidemia

Dysregulated metabolism is emerging as an important contributor to renal cell carcinoma pathogenesis [95] and sometimes it results difficult to discern a role independent from several conditions that usually appear together on these patients, such as obesity, hypertension, diabetes mellitus and abnormal serum lipid metabolism [79, 96]. We also must take into account that some cancers, included renal cell carcinoma, might, in turn, affect cholesterol metabolism or utilization [97]. There is evidence that high serum cholesterol may decrease the risk of kidney cancer development [98] and mortality [99].

However, others studies found cancer risk showed no relation at all [100]. Results of a recent case-control study [101] also indicate that serum lipid profile is associated with RCC. Compared with the controls, the renal cell carcinoma cases had higher triglyceride level, lower total cholesterol, LDL cholesterol and HDL cholesterol levels, and were more likely to smoke and to be hypertensive and diabetic. They suggest that the renal cell cancer hazard decreased by 25.5% as the LDL-C concentration increases by 1 mmol/L. This study also showed a greater hazard of renal cell carcinoma of 165% among low HDL-cholesterolemia patients. However, risk caused by high serum triglycerides showed no statistical significance. Biological mechanisms that might link low serum levels of HDL cholesterol with cancer are not well established [102] but the inflammation may play a role, since it is known to reduce HDL-cholesterol and likely increases risk of renal cell carcinoma.

As well as high levels of total cholesterol, LDL cholesterol and HDL cholesterol have an inverse relationship with RCC development. In contrast, increased serum triglyceride concentrations have shown a positive association with renal cancer in men in a cohort study in Austria [103]. The prognostic role of serum cholesterol in patients with RCC is uncertain although some evidence exists to suggest that higher levels of cholesterol before nephrectomy are associated with significantly better survival and a greater response to systemic treatment with temsirolimus. De Martino et al. [104] proposed the preoperative serum cholesterol as an independent prognostic factor for patients with RCC, with lower levels being associated with worse survival. Therefore, they assessed the inclusion of serum cholesterol in a multivariable prognostic model. As cholesterol is a broadly available routine marker, its use may provide a meaningful adjunct in clinical practice. On the other hand, several studies have shown that statin use may also modify the risk of kidney cancer, but yielding different results.

Some experimental studies have found that these drugs may inhibit tumor growth, invasion and angiogenesis in kidney cancer, as well as metastasis [105, 106]. However, clinical studies have provided contradictory results of the effect of statins on the kidney cancer risk. A large cohort study in Austria found that patients who were being treated with statins for control of dyslipidemia appeared to have a significantly reduced risk of kidney cancer [103]. Another which has shown a reduced risk is the case-control study performed by Khurana et al. [107]. They found that statin use was associated with a statistically significant risk reduction of renal cancer by 55%. Others have not found any effect [108-110] and there were also some studies describing an increased overall kidney cancer risk [111].

Alsheikh-Ali et al. reported an inverse and significant association between on-treatment LDL-C levels and cancer incidence in statin-treated patients enrolled in large randomized controlled trials [112, 113]. However, a similar relationship was noted between LDL cholesterol levels and incident cancer among control patients not treated with statins; so statin therapy, despite significantly reducing LDL-cholesterol levels, was not associated with an increased risk of cancer.

Zhang et al. developed a detailed meta-analysis of 12 published studies regarding these subjects [114]. They found no substantial evidence for reduction in kidney cancer risk among statin users, both men and women, as compared with non-users.

Pooled results indicated that statin use did not significantly affect the risk of kidney cancer (RR = 0.92, 95% CI 0.71, 1.19). The calculated combined RR for kidney cancer in long term statin use was found to be 1.01 (95% CI 0.83, 1.22). Despite experimental data which suggested that statins can suppress proliferation, induce apoptosis and inhibit metastasis of kidney cancer in a murine model [105, 106], results of this meta-analysis indicated that there is no conclusive preventive effect of statin use on kidney cancer risk. These findings were in line with the recent meta-analysis of statin use and overall cancer risk [115-118]. Because hypertension is a strong risk factor for kidney cancer and is strongly correlated with the use of statins, it is an important confounder of the association between statins and kidney cancer and needs to be taken into account in future studies.

Diabetes Mellitus (DM)

There is evidence that type 2 diabetes affects the risk of developing a variety of cancers, notably of breast, colorectal, pancreatic and endometrial cancer [119]. A history of diabetes mellitushas also been linked to renal cell cancer risk in several cohort studies. However controversial results exist [120], and its role independent of obesity and hypertension has not been demonstrated conclusively [79, 96, 121]. A recent meta-analysis including 24 studies conducted in North America, Europe and Asia from 1960 to 2012, suggests that DM may increase risk of kidney cancer by about 40% [122]. Nevertheless, it failed to detect that there was a significant association between diabetes and kidney cancer mortality (RR=1.12, 95% CI=0.99 to 1.20). Diabetes was significantly associated with increased risk of kidney cancer (RR=1.40, 95% CI=1.16 to 1.69), and it was independent of alcohol consumption, body mass index (BMI)/obesity and smoking. A slightly stronger positive relation was observed in women (RR=1.47, 95% CI=1.18 to 1.83) than in men (RR=1.28, 95% CI=1.10 to 1.48).

For specific kidney cancer, the summary association was stronger for total or unspecified kidney cancer than for renal cell carcinoma, indicating that diabetes may have different effects on parenchyma and renal pelvis. A significant elevated rate of kidney cancer among individuals with DM was observed in studies conducted in North America (RR=1.33, 95% CI=1.14 to 1.61) and in Asia (RR=1.34, 95% CI=1.10 to 1.63), but the association was not significant in Europe (RR=1.33, 95% CI=0.97 to 1.82). In contrast, type 1 DM, may not increase the risk of kidney cancer [123].

Recently, Sarah Psutka et al. further investigated this relationship in a large matched-cohort study, derived from a series of 1,964 consecutive patients who underwent nephrectomy for RCC [124]. 13% of patients had diabetes mellitus and they were significantly older and more likely to be obese, had higher Charlson scores (CCI), renal impairment and smoking rates, and worse performance status at surgery. Results suggest that diabetes mellitus is independently associated with decreased cancer specific and overall survival in patients with surgically treated clear cell renal cell carcinoma.

On multivariable analysis adjusting for CCI and BMI, patients with diabetes were at 55% and 32% increased risk of cancer-specific and all-cause mortality, respectively, than patients without diabetes. Several hypotheses on biological mechanisms have been proposed to explain the plausible causal association between DM and risk of cancer.

In additional to the increased risk of incident cancer, DM may also increase the risk of all-cause mortality among people with cancer [125].

The increased cancer risk is likely to be related to the interplay between obesity, diabetes and cancer, with hyperglycemia [126] and hyperinsulinemia playing a crucial role [127].

Insulin can influence tumorigenesis directly, acting on the insulin/insulin like growth factors receptors, or indirectly influencing other modulators such as sex hormones, insulin-like growth factors and adipokines [128].

Metformin, the drug of choice for the management of DM 2, was related with either an increased or reduced risk of cancer. Evidence from both in vitro and in vivo studies indicates that metformin may inhibit cancer cell growth and reduce cancer risk of some solid tumors. A comprehensive systematic review selected 12 randomized controlled trials and 41 observational studies from 1966 to 2012 [129]. Results suggest that metformin use might be associated with a significant reduction in the risk of several forms of cancers, but not be demonstrated significant association with other neoplasms such as kidney, prostate, breast, melanoma, uterus, ovarian, lung, and bladder cancer.

Renal Disease and Dialysis

End-stage renal disease, in particular related to acquired renal cystic disease (ARCD) is thought to increase the risk of RCC [130]. Moreover, patients were reported to have increased risk of renal cell cancer while undergoing long-term hemodialysis as well as after renal transplantation [131, 132]. Thus, in a recent study it has been observed a statistically significant increased risk of RCC in relation to history of chronic renal failure (OR 4.7, 95% CI 2.2–10.1) and among subjects with ESRD who received dialysis (OR 18.0, 95% CI 3.6–91) or a transplanted kidney [133]. Further, kidney transplant patients are more likely to have a subsequent RCC diagnosed in the native kidney than the graft kidney [134]. Autopsy studies in deceased dialysis patients demonstrated a point prevalence of 33% and 0.6% for acquired renal cystic disease and RCC, respectively [130]. So, the fact of having dyalisis-adquired renal cystic disease is a risk factor to develop RCC by itself [135]. In this context, it has been reported a standardized incidence ratio of kidney cancer in dialysis patients of 24.1 (P <.01) compared with general population [136] and increased incidence of invasive tumors in this patients [137]. Although more common, the histology and prognosis of RCC may differ in dialysis patients from the general population [138]. Moreover, one study found a major risk in those younger than 35 years, suggesting that the risk gradually decreased with increasing age [139]. Nevertheless, there is no clear consensus for screening in the long-term dialysis population. Current literature indicates that most patients will develop acquired renal cysts after 3 to 7 years on dialysis, associated with a 1.6-7.0% incidence of RCC [140].

However, a retrospective cohort analysis of the United States Renal Data System (USRDS) dialysis files [141] showed that most cases of RCC in long-term dialysis patients were diagnosed in those without documented acquired renal cystic disease, with only 12.1% diagnosed in patients with known cysts.

Results also found that RCC was independently associated with an increased risk of mortality for the entire dialysis population (AHR, 1.97; 95% CI, 1.90- 2.04-2.08). Risks were similar when stratified analysis were performed for age $\geq$65 or age <65. The incidence of RCC was most strongly associated with older age, male gender, acquired renal cysts, and ESRD caused by obstruction, tuberous sclerosis, and Focal Segmental Glomerulosclerosis (FSGS).

In return, was not found relationship with autosomal dominant polycystic kidney disease, dialysis modality, or smoking.

On the other hand, patients with polycystic kidney disease (PKD) seem to have a lower risk of developing cancer than do those with other kidney diseases. Autosomal Dominant Polycystic Kidney Disease (ADPKD) is the most common form of inherited cystic renal disease and the fourth most common cause of ESRD in the United States [142].

James Wetmore et al. [143] found that kidney transplant patients with polycystic kidney disease were less likely to develop cancer than were those with other kidney diseases (incidence rate ratio 0·87, 95% CI 0·80–0·95). Compared with the general population, overall cancer risk was increased 48% in PKD recipients, while in non-PKD recipients was increased 86%. Furthermore, ADPKD recipients are more likely to undergo nephrectomies than their non-PKD counterparts [144], and nephrectomy rates of 20%–30% could lead to a deficit of RCCs among ADPKD recipients. Moreover, PKD recipients underwent transplant after a shorter duration on dialysis compared with non-PKD recipients.

The relative protection in this entity from developing cancer was unexpected given that ADPKD is a multiorgan disease process with characteristics of neoplasia [145]. The causal mechanisms are also unexplained but may related to biologic characteristics of ADPKD or to cancer risk behaviors associated with ADPKD.

Hofmann et al. developed the first population-based case-control study to report differences in RCC risk in relation to history of chronic renal failure between blacks and whites [133]. They suggest that the association between chronic renal failure and RCC was considerably stronger among patients who were black, among subjects who did not report a history of diabetes, among those had chronic renal failure for an extended time period (≥10 years), and among subjects diagnosed with RCC before age 65.

However, they did not observe any notable difference by sex in the association between chronic renal failure and RCC risk. The reason for the stronger association between chronic renal failure and risk of RCC observed among blacks is unclear.

It may be due to racial differences in the prevalence of hypertension-related ESRD [146], which may be more strongly associated with RCC than diabetes-related ESRD [135]; access to care or aggressiveness of treatment for chronic renal failure [147]; modifiable risk factors related to both chronic renal failure and RCC (e.g., obesity, smoking) [148]; and/or genetic susceptibility.

It has been suggested that interactions between blood and hemodialysis membranes may have a carcinogenic effect, although this was not demonstrated later [149]. As noted by Stewart et al. [132], there is little evidence that dialysis itself is responsible for the increased risk of RCC among patients receiving this treatment.

Rather, the strong association between dialysis and RCC risk is likely due to pathologic changes related to loss of renal function; complications of chronic renal failure include development of acquired cystic kidney disease [135].

The association between kidney transplantation and risk of RCC in a native kidney is also likely to be attributable to pathologic changes in the kidney related to ESRD, although immunosuppressive therapy administered to prevent rejection of the transplanted kidney could potentially contribute to the excess risk of RCC [150].

In fact, it has been reported an incidence rate of kidney cancer between 9 and 25 times higher among patients with a worker kidney transplant versus general population [151].

Diet and Nutrient Factors

Different incidence and mortality rates in kidney cancer between Western and Eastern countries suggest that may exists a diet influence in addition to the known role of environmental in the etiology of RCC. In particular, dietary habits associated with a Western lifestyle have been proposed as potential risk factors of RCC.

In contrast, it has been suggested that high intake of fruit or vegetables may lower the risk, though results are inconclusive. Fruit and vegetables consumption was associated with a reduced risk of RCC in a recent pooled analysis of 13 cohort studies. Carotenoids, present in these foods, may partly contribute to this protection [152].

In this line, it has also reported a significant reduced risk of kidney cancer secondary the intake of cruciferous vegetables [153]. Another case-control study had already suggested the protective effect of vegetables, vitamin E and calcium in females, and vitamin E and iron in men [154], but this association with antioxidant nutrients, such as vitamins A, C, E, and carotenoids, is questioned in other current studies [155-157]. Furthermore, other large prospective cohort study failed to demonstrate such an association [86]. Cruciferous vegetables include cabbage, broccoli, cauliflower, Brussels sprouts and others, which are rich sources of glucosinolates (GLS) that may contribute to reduce risk of RCC [158].

The issue was corroborated in a meta-analysis developed in China [159] where it has been observed a significantly inverse association between CV intake and RCC risk (RR = 0.81, 95% CI [0.72, 0.91]). Interestingly, in subgroup analyses, CV intake was significantly associated with reduced RCC risk among studies conducted in America (RR = 0.77, 95% CI [0.70, 0.86]); but not in Europe (RR = 0.87, 95% CI [0.71, 1.07]).

The differences in genetic susceptibility, ethnic composition, culture, and lifestyles may explain part of the inconsistency of the results.

However, they did not find any substantial differences by adjustment for smoking status, alcohol intake, meat intake, total energy intake, or hypertension status, indicating that the influence of those adjusted confounders on the results might be small.

On the other hand, the consumption of red or processed meat was associated with increased risk of RCC in another meta-analysis of case–control studies [160]. Nevertheless, this association to risk was not confirmed in a pooled analysis of cohort studies [161].

Because of the strong association of obesity with the risk of develop RCC, and the general effect of calorie restriction on reduced tumor growth, as was commented before, it has been suggested that a high energy intake may be associated with an increased risk of renal cell carcinoma, a finding reported in several large case-control studies [162-164].

In this context, a large prospective European analysis [165] found no strong evidence that macronutrient intake during adulthood is related to subsequent risk of renal cell carcinoma. A non-significant positive association of total protein and animal protein intake with risk of RCC is consistent with results of other pooled analysis [161]. Moreover, an association with energy intake has not been found, which is in agreement with other prospective studies [166, 167]. Similarly, they found no evidence that a high intake of total or saturated fat, or a low polyunsaturated fat intake, as previously reported in some case-control studies [163, 164] are significantly positively associated with renal cell carcinoma risk.

It is known that high sodium intake may cause a rise on blood pressure and prolonged sodium excess may contribute directly to kidney damage, perhaps throughout its inflammatory properties [168, 169].

So, high sodium intake may be a risk factor for RCC, potentially through hypertension or end-stage renal disease. Because of their implication in this context, potassium intake and fluid intake may also individually influence RCC risk or modify potential effects of sodium on RCC development. A decreased risk of CRR for higher sodium intake was observed in men, but not in women [164]. However, it has not found any association with potassium intake. With regard to fluid intake, there are controversial results, since some prospective cohort studies have not found any influence to CCR risk [155, 165]. However, it has been showed an increased RCC risk for higher fluid intake in a case-control study [170]. The Netherlands Cohort Study, the first prospective study to investigate it [171], suggests that sodium intake is a potential risk factor for RCC, particularly if fluid consumption is low. Potassium, fluid intake and gender were not associated with RCC risk. In addition, they found no effect-modification by high blood pressure, suggesting that sodium intake may be associated with RCC risk independently of hypertension.

Other food groups including fish, poultry and dairy products could not be consistently linked to the risk of RCC development in previous studies. Interestingly, the risk of RCC was lower among women with high consumption of fatty fish in a Swedish cohort study [172], but this association needs confirmation in other studies. As a protective factor has been suggested the alcohol intake, which has recently linked, in moderate consumption, with decreased risk of kidney cancer development [79, 173], with an estimated 28% reduction among those who drank ≥15 gram/day [173]. This is applicable for all types of alcoholic drinks. In contrast, no association was found with other beverage, including coffee, tea, milk, juice and soda.

Occupation and Environment

Kidney cancer has been associated with several exposures factors though without a strong evidence [174] so, generally is not considered an occupational disease. The influence of asbestos exposure may be weak [175] and the exposure to other industrial agents, including cadmium and uranium, as well as some environmental exposures, such as nitrate and radon in drinking water has not been consistently linked to renal cell cancer risk [176, 177].

Acrylamide is a "probable" human carcinogen (Group 2A of IARC-International Agency for Research on Cancer), present in fried and baked foods [178]. However, epidemiologic studies assessing its relation with kidney cancer have reported contradictory results [179].

Inconsistent results have been also reported for occupational studies examining the relationship between RCC risk and workers who may have high levels of Polycyclic Aromatic Hydrocarbons (PAHs) exposure, such as asphalt workers, printers, machinists, and mechanics [180, 181]. A quantitative review of eight cohort studies revealed only limited evidence of such association [182]. However, an increased risk among heavily PAH-exposed aluminum plant workers was reported in a large, multicenter Norwegian study [183]. Several types of these chemicals that are emitting in significant amounts by numerous industries have been considered carcinogenic or probably carcinogenic to humans [182, 1842, 185].

A large, multicenter, case-control study [186] was carried out in Central and Eastern Europe, an area with historically heavy industrial exposures and one of the highest rates of RCC in the world [187], but significant associations between RCC risk and having ever been occupationally exposed to any agents estimated to contain PAHs or plastics were not found.

However, suggestive positive trends were observed for occupational cumulative exposure to styrene and acrylonitrile and RCC risk. These had been shown to negatively affect kidney function in human and animal studies, but with limited evidence of carcinogenicity [188, 189]. Two cohort studies have reported an increased risk for kidney cancer mortality among workers with high levels of styrene exposure, however, it has not been repeated in subsequent studies [190, 191]. Cumulative exposure to petroleum/gasoline engine emissions was inversely associated with risk, which was unexpected because of are known to contain benzene, a famed human carcinogen [192]. Moreover, some animal and human studies have reported a consistent relationship among gasoline exposure and kidney cancer risk [193].

The biological mechanism linked to kidney cancer development through PAH exposure depends on the specific chemical composition and implies Cytochrome P450 enzymes and GST genes. Within the kidneys, they influence on forming PAH-DNA adducts which can lead to DNA replication errors and thus renal carcinogenesis [194].

Trichloroethylene (TCE), which was recently reclassified by the IARC as carcinogenic to humans (group 1), is by far the most extensively examined chemical in relation to renal cell cancer risk. There is sufficient epidemiologic and animal evidence for kidney cancer and qualitative mechanistic similarities between humans and rodents [195]. It is a strong solvent of metal and organic materials and because of its widespread occupational use has become a common environmental contaminant [196]. Very high doses of TCE have been associated with a variety of cancers [197] andmost recent studies have reported a rising risk of RCC with increasing levels of exposure [198-200]. Three independent reviews reported similar results in this line [201] with a RR between 1.33 and 1.34 [202], and others a summary RR of 1.58 [203]. Hansen et al. developed an analysis of three Nordic Cohort Studies, including 5,553 workers with individual documented exposure to TCE [204] and, despite long-term follow-up, they did not observe an overall increased risk of kidney cancer [199, 200, 205, 206]. Data on arsenic in drinking water as a cause of kidney cancer are suggestive but inconclusive [207, 208]. There are few studies that had reviewed this association. Baastrup et al. found no evidence of risk at low exposures in Denmark [209], however, data from Cordoba (Argentina) and Taiwan, found a convincing excess of cases for both men and women in the high arsenic areas [210, 211]. Bangladesh has high rates of arsenic in tube wells water, and an overall increase in cancer mortality has been reported for one high exposure area [212]. However, there were not data of the relation with kidney cancer until 2013, when Mostafa et al. published their study [213] suggesting, once again, that arsenic is a causal factor in kidney cancer, both renal cell cancer and transitional cell cancer. Risk increased monotonically with arsenic concentration $\geq$50 mg/L for both cell types. Men had a higher proportion of malignant diagnoses (71.9%) than women (54.9%), with this difference most marked for RCC, with 65.8% of men but only 48.8% of women. Renal cancer is thought to have a lower but rising incidence in the Indian subcontinent than in Western Europe and North America [214], suggesting that with the continued use of highly contaminated sources of drinking water, the rate of renal cancer in rural areas of Bangladesh will greatly exceed.

Kidney Stones

Kidney stones have also been proposed to contribute the development of malignant neoplasms by chronic irritation of urinary tract [215].

The reported risks of renal cell carcinoma (RCC) and transitional cell carcinoma (TCC) in patients with a history of kidney stones, however, are still conflicting. Several studies have demonstrated that a history of kidney stones is associated with RCC [163, 216] and TCC [215]. Chung et al. found that TCC and RCC patients were 3.96 and 2.76 times, respectively, more likely to have been previously diagnosed with urinary calculi (UC) compared to controls. While in the case of TCC, the results were merely confirmatory, the association detected between RCC and UC refuted the results of the most powerful study until then, in which the authors failed to detect an increased risk of RCC among UC patients [215]. In addition, the magnitude of the observed associations was stronger among females (OR 3.59; 95% CI 2.87-4.48) vs. males (OR 2.93, 95% CI 2.42-3.55), maybe due to their higher frequency of urinary tract infections [217]. In a very recent meta-analysis [218] Cheungpasitporn et al. also confirmed a significant association between a history of kidney stones and the two most common kidney cancers, with an overall 1.76-fold increased risk of RCC (95% CI, 1.24–2.49) and a 2.14-fold increased risk of TCC. However, the increased risk of RCC was noted only in males (RR, 1.41 [95% CI, 1.11–1.80]) but not in female patients (RR, 1.13 [95% CI, 0.86–1.49]). This underlying pathophysiology is unclear but, interestingly, the prevalence of kidney stones [219] and kidney cancers, both RCC and TCC, is higher in males than females [220, 221]. Men with kidney stones may be exposed to dietary or environmental factors that could increase their risk of RCC (smoking, eating habits).

Thus, dietary habits may be a confounding factor in this association because some foods have been related to both the exposure (urinary calculi) and outcome (kidney cancer), i.e., red meat [222]. It is possible that the association between kidney stones and renal cancer resulted from irritation and infections secondary to lithiasis, which promoted proliferative urothelial changes and development of malignant neoplasms [215, 223].

Analgesics

Experimental and epidemiologic evidence, many years ago, had suggested that phenacetin use increased the risk of transitional cell cancers of the urinary tract. Later, a metabolite commonly used as analgesic and antipyretic, acetaminophen, was linked to an increased risk of renal cancer. However, a case-control study conducted from 1976 to 1996 in the United States suggested opposite data [224]. This drug ceased to be used for more than two decades, so there are not current data that allows its role as carcinogen on kidney cancer.

Aspirin has also been associated with an elevated risk of RCC in some epidemiologic studies [225-227], others reported a null association [225, 228-230], and recent meta-analyses suggest that aspirin may reduce incidence and mortality of several cancer sites [231, 232].

Several studies suggested a positive relationship among other non-steroidal anti-inflammatory drugs (NSAIDs) and RCC risk [226, 233], especially among those who used the drug for a long duration. Thus the HR for those who used $\geq$ 10 years was 2.92 (95 % CI 1.71–5.01) [229]. Moreover, one retrospective cohort study in Denmark found that ibuprofen prescription was associated with kidney cancer mortality [RR 1.72 (95 % CI 1.4–2.1)] [234].

Liu et al. reported the largest prospective cohort study of NSAID use and risk of RCC, following nearly 300,000 subjects in the United States for over a decade [235]. They found no overall association between aspirin use and risk of RCC, which is consistent with other US studies and one randomized controlled trial [236].

Frequency of use of NSAIDs was also not associated with RCC risk, but it had been showed some differences in association by age, suggesting an increased risk among NSAIDs users younger than 63 years and a reduced risk among those ≥63.

Physical Activity

Data linking physical activity to renal cell cancer risk are still limited, but most studies reported an inverse association [237, 238]. A systematic review and meta-analysis inclusive of 19 studies based on more than 2 million subjects has demonstrated a significantly inverse association between physical activity and renal cancer risk (relative risk = 0.88) [239].

Moreover, the noted reduction in renal cancer risk was not affected by the specific type of physical activity, the timing in life of physical activity, gender, or adjustments for smoking, obesity, hypertension, and diabetes. The postulated biological mechanisms underlying the findings are largely intuitive given the recognized risk factors for kidney cancer.

In this way, physical activity has been shown to reduce body weight and blood pressure, improve insulin sensitivity, and reduce chronic inflammation and oxidative stress [240, 241], changes that could contribute to reducing RCC risk.

Reproductive and Hormonal Factors

A role of hormonal or reproductive factors in kidney cancer etiology has been hypothesized [11]. High doses of exogenous estrogens have been shown in animals to promote and induce kidney cancer development [242, 243], and sex hormone receptor expression in renal tissue suggests that endocrine regulation could directly influence this [244, 245]. Some studies have linked the hysterectomy with kidney cancer development showing statistical significance [246-249]. This association, if real, represents a potentially important cause of this cancer, because hysterectomy is the second most common surgical procedure for women of reproductive age in the United States [250].

One of the most comprehensive investigation of reproductive factors and kidney cancer risk was conducted by Karami et al. in two prospective cohorts of 283,952 postmenopausal women [249]. Results showed an approximately 30%–40% increased risk of kidney cancer among women who had underwent a hysterectomy, independently to had also underwent oophorectomy or not and the age at surgery. However, an inverse association with increasing age at menarche was observed in one cohort. On the other hand, use of oral contraceptives and hormone replacement therapy (HRT) were associated with reduced kidney cancer risk. Typically, previous findings for oral contraceptive use and HRT linking to kidney cancer risk have been null. Only one study had shown HRT use to significantly increase kidney cancer risk [247], though no trend with duration of use was seen.

Likewise, a statistically significant inverse association between oral contraceptive use and kidney cancer risk had been reported in only one previous study [251]. The inverse association observed between kidney cancer risk and use of HRT and oral contraceptives could be related to estradiol, which has been shown to lower blood pressure levels and to inhibit oxidative stress and lipid peroxidation [83].

A history of endometriosis was also associated with kidney cancer risk (HR = 1.69, 95% CI: 1.09, 2.62), as correlates with the latest epidemiologic study on this topic, which showed a statistically significant 36% increase in risk [252]. Data were compared with another large study, in which a significantly increased risk of kidney cancer after hysterectomy was also observed [248]. In contrast, stronger associations were observed for earlier age at surgery.

Respect to the age at menarche, there are contradictory findings from previous case-control studies, which generally have found increasing age at menarche to be non-significantly associated with reduced cancer risk [246, 253].

Nevertheless, some cohort studies have shown trends in the opposite direction [254, 255]. The reason for which hysterectomy may be related to the risk of renal cancer development is unclear. It has been speculated that hormonal and iatrogenic factors might play a role in the etiology of this cancer. We have already seen that estrogen would promote carcinogenesis in animals [256, 257] and progesterone has been shown to alter the normal renal function [257]. Other hypotheses, directly related to surgery, are renal damage secondary obstruction as a result of unintentional ureteral injury, the twisting and constricting of the distal ureter secondary to pelvic anatomy changes, that could be associated with renal cell proliferation [248] and the increased lipid peroxidation after gynecological surgery [83].

Regarding parity as risk factor of kidney cancer, observational studies have reported conflicting results. The first meta-analysis that provides evidence of the association between parity and kidney cancer risk was published in 2013 [258]. This study indicated that ever parity increases the risk by 23%, and that increased parity numbers are associated with a rise of 8% for per one live birth (95% CI: 1.05–1.10; Q = 9.34; P = 0.500; $I^2 = 0\%$). Although the majority of the included studies showed positive association between parity and kidney cancer risk, not all of them [251, 254] showed statistical significance, which could be attributed to the limited statistical power.

In the subgroup analysis by geographic location, significantly positive associations were both observed in Europe and North America. Compared with the reports from Western countries, the study performed by Chiu et al. [259] was the only one to show a tendency for decreased kidney cancer risk with increased parity, but without statistical significance [11].

Although the exact biologic mechanisms underlying the association between parity and increased risk of kidney cancer are not fully understood, several potential mechanisms might have been proposed. Anatomical changes to the kidney during pregnancy might make nephrons more vulnerable to inflammation and oxidative stress [260] which has been hypothesized to be responsible for renal carcinogenesis [83, 260].

In addition, hormones, either directly or through growth factors, may act as promoters of malignant changes by stimulating renal cell proliferation.

On the other hand, obesity and hypertension [261] are known risk factor for kidney cancer and are often associated with pregnancy. Pregnancy-associated weight gain may contribute toward an increased risk of kidney cancer [262].

Hereditary Kidney Cancer Syndromes (Table 1)

The genetic background of RCC is illustrated by its association with family history [263]. Approximately, 2–3% of RCC can be directly attributed to inherited genetic defects.

Table 1. Hereditary kidney cancer syndromes

Hereditary Kidney Cancer Syndromes	Genetic Element	Clinical Manifestations
Von Hippel Lindau (VHL) disease	mutations in the *VHL* tumor-suppressor gene loss of chromosome 3p	*Angiomas of the retina, benign hemangioblastomas in brain and spine, renal cysts, pheochromocytomas, pancreatic cysts and tumors, cystadenomas of the epididymis, endolymphatic sac tumors in inner ear. Approximately 50% of patients develops clear cell kidney cancer.*
Hereditary Papillary Renal Cell Cancer (HPRCC)	c-MET proto-oncogene chromosome 7q31-34	*Papillary RCC: type 1*
Hereditary Leiomyomatosis and Kidney Cell Cancer (HLRCC)	fumarate hydratase	*Papillary RCC: type 2* *Uterine leiomyomas, cutaneous leiomyomas. Renal tumors, benign renal cysts, and cystic renal tumors*
Birt-Hogg-Dube Disease (BHD)	Folliculin Chromosome 17p11.2	*Chromophobe RCC* *Benign hair-follicle tumors, pulmonary cysts, spontaneous pneumothoraces*

Moreover, sporadic renal cell cancers have been shown to have a familial predisposition, according to a recent case–control study and systematic meta-analysis showing that having a first-degree relative with kidney cancer is associated with a 4.3-fold (95% CI, 1.6–11.9) increased risk of RCC [264]. A family history of kidney cancer had already been associated with a 2.8-fold (95% CI, 1.0–7.8) increased risk of RCC. Moreover, this meta-analysis further confirmed this association, with a 2.2-fold increased risk of RCC (95% CI, 1.6–2.9). The interplay of exposures to environmental risk factors and genetic susceptibility of exposed individuals is believed to influence the risk of developing sporadic renal cell cancer.

Some hereditary syndromes are currently associated with an inherited susceptibility of kidney cancer, and 12 genes have been identified. Over 2 decades ago, the first cancer gene responsible for an inherited renal cancer syndrome was identified (VHL) [265]. Subsequently, others hereditary syndromes were being described. Kidney cancer in this context appears at an earlier age; furthermore, the tumors can be multifocal, bilateral, and heterogeneous. Many of the genes identified through the study of familial renal cancer have also proven to be important in sporadic kidney cancers, with von Hippel Lindau (VHL) disease being the exemplar of this paradigm [266].

Von Hippel Lindau (VHL) Disease

This autosomal-dominant syndrome was the first described within the inherited syndromes associated with an increased risk of kidney cancer [265, 267]. These patients have inactivating mutations in the *VHL* tumor-suppressor gene [268, 269] characterized by the loss of chromosome 3p [270], which results in angiogenesis and proliferation and has important effects on energy metabolism [271]. Genetic testing for mutations in VHL, detects nearly 100% of individuals with VHL disease [272].

Patients with VHL may present angiomas of the retina (49-59%), benign hemangioblastomas in brain and spine (42-72%), renal cysts (22-59%), pheochromocytomas (18%), pancreatic cysts and tumors (21-72%) (12%), cystadenomas of the epididymis (10-26%) and endolymphatic sac tumors in inner ear (10%). Approximately 50% of patients develops clear cell kidney cancer, appearing in the third or fourth decade of life, presenting as bilateral and sometimes as hundreds of lesions within the kidney [266, 273].

Patients with type 2A missense mutations have a high risk of clear cell renal cell carcinoma (ccRCC), whereas other missense mutations, including types 2B and 2C, do not appear to be associated with kidney cancer [274]. These data implicate a biological difference accounting for the variable risk of kidney cancer associated with different types of kidney cancer. Notably, VHL is mutated not only in inherited ccRCC but also in 91% sporadic ccRCCs [275]. The management of VHL disease involves a familial genetic screening, routine imaging, and a surgical approach to kidney tumors in early-stage disease using nephron-sparing approaches in patients with disease limited to the kidneys. However, in patients with locally advanced disease, the likelihood of recurrent disease and ESRD is much higher; thus, bilateral resection of the kidneys followed by kidney transplantation is a more accepted approach [276]. Given the low reported rate of metastasis among patients with sporadic kidney cortical neoplasms smaller than 3 cm [277], it has been adopted a policy of initial observation for these tumors and immediate intervention for lesions greater than 3 cm in VHL patients [278].

Hereditary Papillary Renal Cell Cancer (HPRCC)

It is an autosomal-dominant syndrome characterized by multifocal, bilateral, type I papillary RCCs [279, 280]. The mean age of onset of the disease is 45 years, and the penetrance is 50% [273]. Activating mutations in the c-MET proto-oncogene on chromosome 7q31-34 [281] have been causally associated with this syndrome [282], however, MET is mutated in less than 10% of sporadic-type papillary kidney cancers. Families with inherited mutations in MET leading to multifocal papillary kidney cancer (type I) are rarest than most of the other described inherited kidney cancer syndromes [266].

Hereditary Leiomyomatosis and Kidney Cell Cancer (HLRCC)

HLRCC is another autosomal-dominant hereditary syndrome, which is caused by germline mutations in the *FH* gene that encodes one enzyme of Krebs cycle, the fumarate hydratase (FH) [283, 284]. These mutations have not been observed in sporadic RCC.

The most common manifestations of HLRCC are cutaneous leiomyomata, which occur in 76%–100% of patients [283]. Multiple and symptomatic uterine fibroids are also frequent, especially in young women (median 28–32 years) [285], and may result in early myomectomies or hysterectomies [286]. Patients with HLRCC are also at risk for the development of renal tumors, benign renal cysts, and cystic renal tumors.

Papillary type II kidney cancer is the pathological type most commonly associated and tends be of high grade, and to have an early age of onset (10–44 years), and an aggressive course [287], presenting even metastatic disease in the teens.

They may appear as solitary lesions [288]; however, they can also be bilateral and/or multifocal. Other types of kidney cancers can also occur, including collecting duct and clear cell cancers [288]. Additional manifestations have been reported to occur in patients affected with HLRCC such as adrenal cortical adenomas (10%) [289], Leydig cell tumors, gastrointestinal stromal tumors [290], ovarian cystadenomas and Wilm's tumor, which has even been reported in 2 pediatric patients with FH mutations, suggesting a possible associated predisposition [283, 291]. Germline mutations in the *FH* gene are diagnostic for HLRCC, so genetic counseling is extremely important for patients with a family history. Given the highly aggressiveness of renal tumors it is recommended that genetic testing be offered at the parents' discretion to children as young as 8–10 years of age. At-risk members of an HLRCC family who test positive for the familial germline *FH* mutation should undergo surveillance by annual magnetic resonance imaging from the age of 8 years.

Since HLRCC-associated renal tumors can be more aggressive than renal tumors in other hereditary renal cancer syndromes, immediate surgical intervention is recommended rather than active surveillance. A therapeutic approach for patients with advanced HLRCC-associated renal tumors has been developed utilizing bevacizumab, combined with erlotinib [284].

Birt-Hogg-Dube Disease (BHD)

Autosomal-dominant syndrome characterized by the development of benign hair-follicle tumors, pulmonary cysts, spontaneous pneumothoraces 13–16 and kidney cancer- early onset (50 years) [292, 293]. It is caused by mutation in the folliculin (FLCN) tumor-suppressor gene, and the most common type of tumor associated is an unusual hybrid oncocytic tumor (mixed oncocytoma and chromophobe). However, a wide spectrum of kidney cancers (papillary RCC, ccRCC) has been observed in these patients, even within the same kidney [294]. So, it appears frequently as a multifocal o bilateral lesions. Mutations in FLCN have been identified in sporadic chromophobe kidney cancers, although this is not common. Chromophobe tumors when diagnosed early are often curable with surgery.

Metastatic disease is difficult to treat due to the unusual presentation and the lack of defined therapeutic targets for chromophobe tumors. Sporadic chromophobe tumors can contain mutations in KIT but it is unknown if treatment with imatinib or sunitinib, which target KIT mutations, are active [295].

Other Syndromes

Other inherited syndromes with an increased risk of kidney cancer are: Tuberous Sclerosis Complex [296], PTEN Hamartoma Tumor Syndrome or Cowden Disease [297], Succinate-Dehydrogenase-associated paraganglioma and pheochromocytoma [298], BAP1 (BRCA-Associated Protein-1) Mutations and Familial Kidney Cancer [299] and chromosome 3 translocations [300].

Conclusion

The RCC incidence has been increasing until recently, although in the last years a tendency to decrease of rates has been demonstrated. However, mortality rates still continue to be high, especially in North America, Australia, New Zealand and Europe. Cigarette smoking, obesity and high blood pressure are the most important and modifiable risk factors for RCC. On the other hand, approximately, 2–3% of RCC can be directly attributed to inherited genetic defects. Moreover, sporadic renal cell cancers have been shown to have a familial predisposition.

References

[1] Ferlay, J., Shin, H. R., Bray, F., Forman, D., Mathers, C., Parkin, D. M. Estimates of worldwide burden of cancer in 2008: GLOBOCAN 2008. *Int. J. Cancer* 2010; 15: 2893–917.
[2] Weikert, S., Ljungberg, B. Contemporary epidemiology of renal cell carcinoma: perspectives of primary prevention. *World J. Urol.* 2010 28: 247–252.
[3] Ferlay, J., Parkin, D. M., Steliarova-Foucher, E. Estimates of cancer incidence and mortality in Europe in 2008. *Eur. J. Cancer* 2010; 46: 765–81.
[4] http://seer.cancer.gov/statfacts/html/kidrp.html.
[5] Chow, W. H., Devesa, S. S. (2008) Contemporary epidemiology of renal cell cancer. *Cancer J.* 2008; 14:288–301.
[6] Hollingsworth, J. M., Miller, D. C., Daignault, S., Hollenbeck, B. K. Rising incidence of small renal masses: a need to reassess treatment effect. *J. Natl. Cancer Inst.* 2006; 98:1331–1334.
[7] Gupta, K., Miller, J. D., Li, J. Z., Russell, M. W., Charbonneau, C. Epidemiologic and socioeconomic burden of metastatic renal cell carcinoma (mRCC): a literature review. *Cancer Treat. Rev.* 2008; 34: 193–205.
[8] Chow, W. H., Devesa, S. S., Warren, J. L., Fraumeni, J. F., Jr. Rising incidence of renal cell cancer in the United States. *JAMA* 1999; 281: 1628–31.
[9] Brian I. Rini, Steven C. Campbell, Bernard Escudier. Renal cell carcinoma. *Lancet* 2009; 373: 1119–32.
[10] Sun, M., Thuret, R., Abdollah, F., et al. Age-adjusted incidence, mortality, and survival rates of stage-specific renal cell carcinoma in North America: A trend analysis. *Eur. Urol.* 2011; 59:135-41.
[11] Chow, W.-H., Dong, L. M., Devesa, S. S. Epidemiology and risk factors for kidney cancer. *Nat. Rev. Urol.* 2010; 7:245-57.
[12] Mathew, A., Devesa, S. S., Fraumeni, J. F. Jr, et al. Global increases in kidney cancerincidence, 1973–1992. *Eur. J. Cancer Prev.* 2002;11:171–8.
[13] Jemal, A., Simard, E. P., Dorell, C., et al. Annual Report to the Nation on the Status of Cancer, 1975-2009, featuring the burden and trends in human papillomavirus (HPV)-associated cancers and HPV vaccinationcoverage levels. *J. Natl. Cancer Inst.* 2013;105: 175-201.

[14] Smith-Bindman, R., Miglioretti, D. L., Johnson, E., et al. Use of diagnostic imaging studies and associated radiation exposure for patients enrolled in large integrated health care systems, 1996-2010. *JAMA* 2012; 307:2400-9.

[15] Levi, F., Ferlay, J., Galeone, C., Lucchini, F., Negri, E., Boyle, P., et al. m() The changing pattern of kidney cancer incidence and mortality in Europe. *BJU Int.* 2008; 101:949–958.

[16] Lindblad, P. Epidemiology of renal cell carcinoma. *Scand. J. Surg.* 2004; 93: 88–96.

[17] Eunyoung Cho, Hans-Olov Adami, Per Lindblad. Epidemiology of Renal Cell Cancer. *Hematol. Oncol. Clin. N. Am.* 2011; 25: 651–665.

[18] Prithwish De Michael C. Otterstatter, Robert Semenciw, Larry F. Ellison, Loraine D. Marrett, Dagny Dryer. Trends in incidence, mortality, and survival for kidney cancerin Canada, 1986–2007. *Cancer Causes Control* 2014; 25:1271–1281.

[19] Borje Ljungberg a, Steven C. Campbell b, Han Yong Cho c, Didier Jacqmin d, Jung Eun Lee e, Steffen Weikert f, Lambertus A. Kiemeney g. Epidemiology of Renal Cell Carcinoma. *European urology* 2011; 60: 615–621.

[20] Canadian Cancer Society's Steering Committee (2010) *Canadian Cancer Statistics 2010*. Canadian Cancer Society, Toronto Study source Population-based data on cancer incidence were abstracted from the National Cancer Institute (NCI)'s Surveillance, Epidemiology, and End Results (SEER) program.http://seer.cancer.gov/popdata/methods.html.

[21] Curado, M. P., et al., editors. *IARC Scientific Publications No. 160*. Lyon: IARC; 2007. Cancer Incidence in Five Continents, Vol. IX.

[22] Kane, C. J., Mallin, K., Ritchey, J., Cooperberg, M. R., Carroll, P. R. Renal cell cancer stage migration:analysis of the National Cancer Data Base. *Cancer* 2008;113:78–83.

[23] Sánchez-Martín, F. M., Millán-Rodríguez, F., Urdaneta-Pignalosa, G., Rubio-Briones, J., Villavicencio-Mavrich, H. Small renal masses: incidental diagnosis, clinical symptoms, and prognostic factors. *Adv. Urol.* 2008: 310694 (online).

[24] National Cancer Institute. Surv*eillance Epidemiology and End Results (SEER) Program*. http://seer.cancer.gov/popdata/methods.html.

[25] Parkin, D. M., Whelan, S. L., Ferlay, J., Storm, H. IARC Cancer Base No. 7. Lyon: 2005. *Cancer Incidence in Five Continents*, Vol. I to VIII. Surveillance, Epidemiology, and End Results (SEER) Program (www.seer.cancer.gov/seerstat).

[26] Kovacs, G., Akhtar, M., Beckwith, B. J., Bugert, P., Cooper, C. S., Delahunt, B., et al. The Heidelberg classification of renal cell tumours. *J. Pathol.* 1997; 183: 131–133.

[27] Ferlay, J., Steliarova-Foucher, E., Lortet-Tieulent, J., et al. Cancer incidence and mortality patterns in Europe: estimates for 40 countries in 2012. *Eur. J. Cancer* 2013; 49:1374-403.

[28] Jemal, A., Bray, F., Center, M. M., Ferlay, J., Ward, E., Forman, D. Global cancer statistics. *CA Cancer J. Clin.* 2011; 61: 69–90.

[29] Siegel, R., Naishadham, D., Jemal, A. *Cancer statistics*, 2012. *CA Cancer J. Clin.* 2012; 62:10-29.

[30] Espey, D. K., Wu, X. C., Swan, J., et al. Annual report to the nation on the status of cancer, 1975-2004, featuring cancer in American Indians and Alaska natives. *Cancer*, 2007;110: 2119-2152.

[31] Levi, F., Lucchini, F., Negri, E., et al. Declining mortality from kidney cancer in Europe. *Ann. Oncol.* 2004; 15:11305.

[32] Verdecchia, A., Francisci, S., Brenner, H., et al. Recent cancer survival in Europe: a 2000–02 period analysis of EUROCARE-4 data. *Lancet Oncol.* 2007;8:784–96.

[33] Chow, W. H., Linehan, W. M., Devesa, S. S. Re: Rising incidence of small renal masses: a need to reassess treatment effect. *J. Natl. Cancer Inst.* 2007; 99:569–70.

[34] IARC Working Group on the Evaluation of Carcinogenic Risks to Humans. Tobacco Smoke and Involuntary smoking. *IARC Monogr. Eval. Carcinog. Risks Hum.* 2004; 83: 1-1438.

[35] Warren, G. W., Alberg, A. J., Kraft, A. S., Cummings, K. M. The 2014 Surgeon General's report: "" health consequences of smoking--50 years of progress": a paradigm shift in cancer care. *Cancer.* 2014; 120: 1914-6.

[36] Weir, J., Dunn, J. E. Jr: Smoking and Mortality: A Prospective Study. *Cancer* 1969, 25: 105-11.

[37] Coughlin, S. S., Neaton, J. D., Randall, B., Sengupta, A.: Predictors of mortality from kidney cancer in 332,547 men screened for the Multiple Risk Factor Intervention Trial. *Cancer* 1997, 79:2171-7.

[38] Thun, M. J., DeLancey, J. O., Center, M. M., Jemal, A., Ward, E. M. The global burden of cancer: priorities for prevention. *Carcinogenesis.* 2010; 31:100-10.

[39] Sharifi, N., Farrar, W. L. Perturbations in hypoxia detection: a shared link between hereditary and sporadic tumor formation? *Med. Hypotheses* 2006; 66:732–735.

[40] Clague, J., et al. Sensitivity to NNKOAc is associated with renal cancer risk. *Carcinogenesis* 2009; 30:706–10.

[41] Zhu, Y., Horikawa, Y., Yang, H., Wood, C. G., Habuchi, T., Wu, X. BPDE induced lymphocytic chromosome 3p deletions may predict renal cell carcinoma risk. *J. Urol.* 2008; 179:2416–2421.

[42] Hunt, J. D., van der Hel, O. L., McMillan, G. P., Boffetta, P., Brennan, P. Renal cell carcinoma in relation to cigarette smoking: meta-analysis of 24 studies. *Int. J. Cancer.* 2005; 114:101–8.

[43] Theis, R. P., Dolwick Grieb, S. M., Burr, D., Siddiqui, T., Asal, N. R. Smoking, environmental tobacco smoke, and risk of renal cell cancer: a population-based case-control study. *BMC Cancer* 2008, 8:387.

[44] Kreiger, N., Marrett, L. D., Dodds, L., Hilditch, S., and Darlington, G. A.: Risk factors for renal cell carcinoma: results of a population-based case-control study. *Cancer Causes Control* 1993, 4:101-110.

[45] Mellemgaard, A., Engholm, G., McLaughlin, J. K., Olsen, J. H.: Risk factors for renal cell carcinoma in Denmark. I. Role of socioeconomic status, tobacco use, beverages, and family history. *Cancer Causes Control* 1994, 5:105-113.

[46] La Vecchia, C., Negri, E., D'Avanzo, B., Franceschi, S.: Smoking and Renal Cell Carcinoma. *Cancer Res.* 1990, 50:5231-5233.

[47] Parker, A. S., Cerhan, J. R., Janney, C. A., Lynch, C. F., and Cantor, K. P.: Smoking cessation and renal cell carcinoma. *Ann. Epidemiol.* 2003, 13:245-251.

[48] Hu, J., Ugnat, A.-M.: Active and passive smoking and risk of renal cell carcinoma in Canada. *Eur. J. Cancer.* 2005; 41:770-8.

[49] Theis, R. P., Dolwick Grieb, S. M., Burr, D., Siddiqui, T., Asal, N. R. Smoking, environmental tobacco smoke, and risk of renal cell cancer: a population-based case-control study. *BMC Cancer* 2008, 8:387.

[50] Kroeger, N., Klatte, T., Birkhäuser, F. D., et al. Smoking negatively impacts renal cell carcinoma overall and cancer-specific survival. *Cancer*. 2012; 118:1795-802.

[51] Noon, A. P., Vlatkovic, N., Polanski, R., et al. p53 and MDM2 in renal cell carcinoma: biomarkers for disease progression and future therapeutic targets? *Cancer*. 2010; 116: 780-90.

[52] Shvarts, O., Seligson, D., Lam, J., et al. p53 is an independent predictor of tumor recurrence and progression after nephrectomy in patients with localized renal cell carcinoma. *J. Urol*. 2005; 173:725-8.

[53] Klatte, T., Seligson, D. B., LaRochelle, J., et al. Molecular signatures of localized clear cell renal cell carcinoma to predict disease-free survival after nephrectomy. *Cancer Epidemiol. Biomarkers Prev*. 2009; 18:894-900.

[54] Haitel, A., Wiener, H. G., Baethge, U., Marberger, M., Susani, M. mdm2 expression as a prognostic indicator in clear cell renal cell carcinoma: comparison with p53 overexpression and clinicopathological parameters. *Clin. Cancer Res*. 2000; 6:1840-4.

[55] Kim, H. L., Seligson, D., Liu, X., et al. Using protein expressions to predict survival in clear cell renal carcinoma. *Clin. Cancer Res*. 2004; 10:5464-5471.

[56] Zigeuner, R., Ratschek, M., Rehak, P., Schips, L., Langner, C. Value of p53 as a prognostic marker in histologic subtypes of renal cell carcinoma: a systematic analysis of primary and metastatic tumor tissue. *Urology*. 2004; 63:651-5.

[57] Wiseman, M. The second World Cancer Research Fund/American Institute for Cancer Research expert report. Food, nutrition, physical activity, and the prevention of cancer: a global perspective. *Proc. Nutr. Soc*. 2008; 67: 253-6.

[58] Wang, F., Xu, Y. Body mass index and risk of renal cell cancer: a dose–response meta-analysis of published cohort studies. *Int. J. Cancer*. 2014; 135:1673-86.

[59] Beebe-Dimmer, J. L., Colt, J. S., Ruterbusch, J. J., Keele, G. R., Purdue, M. P., Wacholder, S., Graubard, B. I., Davis, F., Chow, W. H., Schwartz, K. L. Body mass index and renal cell cancer: the influence of race and sex. *Epidemiology*. 2012; 23:821–8.

[60] Calle, E. E., Kaaks, R. Overweight, obesity and cancer. Epidemiological evidence and proposed mechanisms. *Nat. Rev. Cancer* 2004:579-91.

[61] Renehan, A. G., Tyson, M., Egger, M., Heller, R. F., Zwahlen, M. Body-mass index and incidence of cancer: a systematic review and meta-analysis of prospective observational studies. *Lancet*. 2008; 371:569-78.

[62] Bergstrom, A., Hsieh, C. C., Lindblad, P., Lu, C. M., Cook, N. R., Wolk, A. Obesity and renal cell cancer: a quantitative review. *Br. J. Cancer*. 2001; 85:984–90.

[63] Reeves, G. K., Pirie, K., Beral, V., Green, J., Spencer, E., Bull, D. Cancer incidence and mortality in relation to body mass index in the million women study: cohort study. *BMJ*. 2007; 335:1134.

[64] Samanic, C., Chow, W. H., Gridley, G., Jarvholm, B., Fraumeni, J. F. Jr. Relation of body mass index to cancer risk in 362,552 Swedish men. *Cancer Causes Control*. 2006; 17:901–9.

[65] Sanfilippo, K. M., McTigue, K. M., Fidler, C. J., Neaton, J. D., Chang, Y., Fried, L. F., Liu, S., Kuller, L. H. Hypertension and obesity and the risk of kidney cancer in 2 large cohorts of US men and women. *Hypertension*. 2014; 63:934–41.

[66] Adams, K. F., Leitzmann, M. F., Albanes, D., Kipnis, V., Moore, S. C., Schatzkin, A., et al. Body size and renal cell cancer incidence in a large US cohort study. *Am. J. Epidemiol.* 2008; 168:268–77.

[67] Luo, J., Margolis, K. L., Adami, H. O., Lopez, A. M., Lessin, L., Ye, W.; Women's Health Initiative Investigators. Body size, weight cycling, and risk of renal cell carcinoma among postmenopausal women: the Women's Health Initiative (United States). *Am. J. Epidemiol.* 2007; 166: 752–759.

[68] Pischon, T., Lahmann, P. H., Boeing, H., Tjonneland, A., Halkjaer, J., Overvad, K., et al. Body size and risk of renal cell carcinoma in the European Prospective Investigation into Cancer and Nutrition (EPIC). *Int. J. Cancer.* 2006; 118:728–738.

[69] Naya, Y., Zenbutsu, S., Araki, K., Nakamura, K., Kobayashi, M., Kamijima, S., Imamoto, T., Nihei, N., Suzuki, H., Ichikawa, T., et al. Influence of visceral obesity on oncologic outcome in patients with renal cell carcinoma. *Urol. Int.* 2010; 85:30–6.

[70] Zhu, Y., Wang, H. K., Zhang, H. L., Yao, X. D., Zhang, S. L., Dai, B., Shen, Y. J., Liu, X. H., Zhou, L. P., Ye, D. W. Visceral obesity and risk of high grade disease in clinical t1a renal cell carcinoma. *J. Urol.* 2013; 189:447–53.

[71] Waalkes, S., Merseburger, A. S., Kramer, M. W., Herrmann, T. R., Wegener, G., Rustemeier, J., Hofmann, R., Schrader, M., Kuczyk, M. A., Schrader, A. J. Obesity is associated with improved survival in patients with organ-confined clear-cell kidney cancer. *Cancer Causes Control.* 2010; 21:1905–10.

[72] Parker, A. S., Lohse, C. M., Cheville, J. C., Thiel, D. D., Leibovich, B. C., Blute, M. L. Greater body mass index is associated with better pathologic features and improved outcome among patients treated surgically for clear cell renal cell carcinoma. *Urology.* 2006; 68:741–6.

[73] Ko, J. S., Zea, A. H., Rini, B. I., Ireland, J. L., Elson, P., Cohen, P., Golshayan, A., Rayman, P. A., Wood, L., Garcia, J., et al. Sunitinib mediates reversal of myeloid-derived suppressor cell accumulation in renal cell carcinoma patients. *Clin. Cancer Res.* 2009; 15:2148–57.

[74] Chehval, V., Norian, L. A. Effects of obesity on immune responses to renal tumors. *Immunol. Res.* 2014; 59(1-3):211-9.

[75] Fontana, L., Eagon, J. C., Trujillo, M. E., Scherer, P. E., Klein, S. Visceral fat adipokine secretion is associated with systemic inflammation in obese humans. *Diabetes.* 2007; 56:1010–3.

[76] Klinghoffer, Z., Yang, B., Kapoor, A., Pinthus, J. H. Obesity and renal cell carcinoma: epidemiology, underlying mechanisms and management considerations. *Expert Rev. Anticancer Ther.* 2009; 9:975–87.

[77] Lipworth, L., Tarone, R. E., McLaughlin, J. K. The epidemiology of renal cell carcinoma. *J. Urol.* 2006; 176(6 Pt 1):2353–2358.

[78] Setiawan, V. W., Stram, D. O., Nomura, A. M., Kolonel, L. N., Henderson, B. E. Risk factors for renal cell cancer: the multiethnic cohort. *Am. J. Epidemiol.* 2007; 166:932–40.

[79] Design of the Women`s Health Initiative clinical trial and observational study. The Women`s Health Initiative Study Group. *Control Clin. Trials.* 1998; 19:61-109.

[80] Curb, J. D., McTiernan, A., Heckbert, S. R., Kooperberg, C., Stanford, J., Nevitt, M., Johnson, K. C., Proulx-Burns, L., Pastore, L., Criqui, M., Daugherty, S.; WHI

Morbidity and Mortality Committee. Outcomes ascertainment and adjudication methods in the Women's Health Initiative. *Ann. Epidemiol.* 2003; 13(9 Suppl.):S122-8.

[81] Gago-Dominguez, M., Castelao, J. E., Yuan, J. M., Ross, R. K., Yu, M. C. Lipid peroxidation: a novel and unifying concept of the etiology of renal cell carcinoma (United States). *Cancer Causes Control.* 2002; 13: 287–93.

[82] Gago-Dominguez, M., Castelao, J. E. Lipid peroxidation and renal cell carcinoma: further supportive evidence and new mechanistic insights. *Free Radic. Biol. Med.* 2006; 40:721–733.

[83] Chow, W. H., Gridley, G., Fraumeni, J. F. Jr, Järvholm, B. Obesity, hypertension and the risk of kidney cancer in men. *N. Engl. J. Med.* 2000 Nov. 2; 343(18):1305-11.

[84] Vatten, L. J. 1., Trichopoulos, D., Holmen, J., Nilsen, T. I. Blood pressuere and renal cancer risk: the HUNT Study in Norway. *Br. J. Cancer.* 2007; 97:112-4.

[85] Weikert, S. 1., Boeing, H., Pischon, T., et al. Blood pressure and risk of renal cell carcinoma in the European prospective investigation into cancer and nutrition. *Am. J. Epidemiol.* 2008 Feb. 15; 167(4):438-46.

[86] Kearney, P. M. 1., Whelton, M., Reynolds, K., Muntner, P., Whelton, P. K., He, J. Global Burden of hypertension: analysis of worldwide data. *Lancet.* 2005; 365(9455): 217-23.

[87] Mittal, B. V., Singh, A. K. Hypertension in the developing world: challenges and opportunities. *Am. J. Kidney Dis.* 2010 Mar; 55(3):590-8.

[88] Yoon, S. S. 1., Ostchega, Y., Louis, T. Recent trends in the prevalence on high blood pressure and its treatment and control, 1999-2008. *NCHS Data Brief.* 2010(48):1-8.

[89] Flaherty, K. T., Fuchs, C. S., Colditz, G. A., Stampfer, M. J., Speizer, F. E., Willett, W. C., Curhan, G. C. A prospective study of body mass index, hypertension, and smoking and the risk of renal cell carcinoma (United States). *Cancer Causes Control.* 2005 Nov; 16(9):1099-106.

[90] Fryzek, J. P., Poulsen, A. H., Johnsen, S. P., McLaughlin, J. K., Sørensen, H. T., Friis, S. A cohort study of antihypertensive treatments and risk of renal cell cancer. *Br. J. Cancer.* 2005 Apr. 11; 92(7):1302-6.

[91] Stamler, J. 1., Neaton, J. D. The Multiple Risk Factor Intervention Trial (MRFIT)--importance then and now. *JAMA.* 2008; 300: 1343-5.

[92] Sharifi, N., Farrar, W. L. Perturbations in hypoxia detection: a shared link between hereditary and sporadic tumor formation? *Med. Hypotheses* 2006; 66(4):732-5.

[93] Klag, M. J., Whelton, P. K., Randall, B. L., Neaton, J. D., Brancati, F. L., Ford, C. E., Shulman, N. B., Stamler, J. Blood pressure and end-stage renal disease in men. *N. Engl. J. Med.* 1996; 334:13-8.

[94] Linehan, W. M. 1., Srinivasan, R., Schmidt, L. S. The genetic basis of kidney cancer: a metabolic disease. *Nat. Rev. Urol.* 2010; 7: 277-85.

[95] Choi, M. Y., Jee, S. H., Sull, J. W., Nam, C. M. Kidney Int. The effect of hypertension on the risk for kidney cancer in Korean men. *Kidney Int.* 2005 Feb; 67(2):647-52.

[96] Vitols, S., Gahrton, G., Björkholm, M., Peterson, C. Hypocholesterolaemia in malignancy due to elevated low-density-lipoprotein-receptor activity in tumor cells: evidence from studies in patients with leukaemia. *Lancet.* 1985; 2(8465):1150-4.

[97] Asano, K. 1., Kubo, M., Yonemoto, K., Doi, Y., Ninomiya, T., Tanizaki, Y., Arima, H., Shirota, T., Matsumoto, T., Iida, M., Kiyohara, Y. Impact of serum total cholesterol on

the incidence os gastric cancer in a population-based prospective study: the Hisayama study. *Int. J. Cancer*. 2008 Feb. 15; 122(4):909-14.

[98] Panagiotakos, D. B. 1., Pitsavos, C., Polychronopoulos, E., Chrysohoou, C., Menotti, A., Dontas, A., Stefanadis, C. Total cholesterol and body mass index in relation to 40-year cancer mortality (the Corfu cohort of the seven countries study). *Cancer Epidemiol. Biomarkers Prev*. 2005 Jul; 14(7):1797-801.

[99] Stolzenberg-Solomon, R. Z., Pietinen, P., Taylor, P. R., Virtamo, J., Albanes, D. A prospective study of medical conditions, anthropometry, physical activity, and pancreatic cancer in male smokers (Finland). *Cancer Causes Control*. 2002 Jun; 13(5): 417–26.

[100] Zhang, C., Yu, L., Xu, T., Hao, Y., Zhang, X., Liu, Z., Xiao, Y., Wang, X., Zeng, Q. Association of Dyslipidemia with Renal Cell Carcinoma: A 1:2 Matched Case-Control Study. *PLoS One*. 2013; 8(3):e59796.

[101] Fiorenza, A. M., Branchi, A., Sommariva, D. Serum lipoprotein protein profile in patients with cancer. A comparison with non-cancer subjects. *Int. J. Clin. Lab. Res*. 2000; 30(3):141-5.

[102] Ulmer, H., Borena, W., Rapp, K., Klenk, J., Strasak, A., Diem, G., Concin, H., Nagel, G. Serum triglyceride concentrations and cancer risk in a large cohort study in Austria. *Br. J. Cancer*. 2009 Oct. 6; 101(7): 1202-6.

[103] de Martino, M., Leitner, C. V., Seemann, C., Hofbauer, S. L., Lucca, I., Haitel, A., Shariat, S. F., Klatte, T. Preoperative serum cholesterol is an independent prognostic factor for patients with renal cell carcinoma (RCC). *BJU Int*. 2014 Apr. 4.

[104] Horiguchi, A., Sumitomo, M., Asakuma, J., Asano, T., Asano, T., Hayakawa, M. 3-hydroxy-3-methylglutaryl-coenzyme a reductase inhibitor, fluvastatin, as a novel agent for prophylaxis of renal cancer metastasis. *Clin. Cancer Res*. 2004; 10:8648-55.

[105] Woodard, J., Sassano, A., Hay, N., Platanias, L. C. Statin-dependent suppression of the Akt/mammalian target of rapamycin signaling cascade and programmed cell death 4 up-regulation in renal cell carcinoma. *Clin. Cancer Res*. 2008 Jul. 15; 14(14):4640-9.

[106] Khurana, V., Caldito, G., Ankem, M. Statins might reduce risk of renal cell carcinoma in humans: case-control study of 500,000 veterans. *Urology* 2008. Jan; 71(1):118-22.

[107] Chiu, H. F., Kuo, C. C., Kuo, H. W., Lee, I. M., Lee, C. T., Yang, C. Y. Statin use and the risk of kidney cancer: a population-based case-control study. *Expert Opin. Drug Saf*. 2012 Jul; 11(4):543-9.

[108] Jacobs, E. J., Newton, C. C., Thun, M. J., Gapstur, S. M. Long-term use of cholesterol-lowering drugs and cancer incidence in a large United States cohort. *Cancer Res*. 2011 Mar. 1; 71(5):1763-71.

[109] Liu, W., Choueiri, T. K., Cho, E. Statin use and the risk of renal cell carcinoma in 2 prospectives US cohorts. *Cancer*. 2012 Feb. 1; 118(3): 797-803.

[110] Friedman, G. D., Flick, E. D., Udaltsova, N., Chan, J., Quesenberry, C. P. Jr, Habel, L. A. Screening statins for possible carcinogenic risk: up to 9 years of follow-up of 361,859 recipients. *Pharmacoepidemiol. Drug Saf*. 2008 Jan; 17(1):27-36.

[111] Alsheikh-Ali, A. A., Maddukuri, P. V., Han, H., Karas, R. H. Effect of the magnitude of lipid lowering on risk of elevated liver enzymes, rhabdomyolysis, and cancer: insights from large randomized statin trials. *J. Am. Coll. Cardiol*. 2007 Jul. 31; 50(5):409-18.

[112] Alsheikh-Ali, A. A., Trikalinos, T. A., Kent, D. M., Karas, R. H. Statins, low-density lipoprotein cholesterol, and risk of cancer. *J. Am. Coll. Cardiol.* 2008 Sep. 30; 52(14): 1141-7.

[113] Zhang, X. L., Liu, M., Qian, J., Zheng, J. H., Zhang, X. P., Guo, C. C., Geng, J., Peng, B., Che, J. P., Wu, Y. Statin use and risk of kidney cancer: a meta-analysis of observational studies and randomized trials. *Br. J. Clin. Pharmacol.* 2014 Mar; 77(3): 458-65.

[114] Browning, D. R., Martin, R. M. Statins and risk of cancer: a systematic review and metaanalysis. *Int. J. Cancer.* 2007; 120(4): 833–43.

[115] Dale, K. M., Coleman, C. I., Henyan, N. N., Kluger, J., White, C. M. Statins and cancer risk: a meta-analysis. *JAMA* 2006; 295: 74–80.

[116] Cholesterol Treatment Trialists' (CTT) Collaboration, Emberson, J. R., Kearney, P. M., Blackwell, L., Newman, C., Reith, C., Bhala, N., Holland, L., Peto, R., Keech, A., Collins, R., Simes, J., Baigent, C. Lack of effect of lowering LDL cholesterol on cancer: meta-analysis of individual data from 175,000 people in 27 randomised trials of statin therapy. *PLoS One* 2012; 7: e29849.

[117] Kuoppala, J., Lamminpää, A., Pukkala, E. Statins and cancer: a systematic review and meta-analysis. *Eur. J. Cancer* 2008; 44: 2122–32.

[118] Nicolucci, A. Epidemiological aspects of neoplasms in diabetes. *Acta Diabetol.* 2010 Jun. 47(2): 87-95.

[119] Lindblad, P., Chow, W. H., Chan, J., Bergström, A., Wolk, A., Gridley, G., McLaughlin, J. K., Nyrén, O., Adami, H. O. The role of diabetes mellitus in the aetiology of renal cell cancer. *Diabetologia.* 1999 Jan. 42(1):107–12.

[120] Inoue, M., Iwasaki, M., Otani, T., Sasazuki, S., Noda, M., Tsugane, S. Diabetes mellitus and the risk of cancer: results from a large-scale population-based cohort study in Japan. *Arch. Intern. Med.* 2006; 166: 1871–7.

[121] Bao, C., Yang, X., Xu, W., Luo, H., Xu, Z., Su, C., Qi, X. Diabetes mellitus and incidence and mortality of kidney cancer: A meta-analysis. *J. Diabetes Complications.* 2013 Jul.-Aug; 27(4):357-64.

[122] Zendehdel, K., Nyren, O., Ostenson, C. G., Adami, H. O., Ekbom, A., Ye, W. Cancer incidence in patients with type 1 diabetes mellitus: A population-based cohort study in Sweden. *J. Natl. Cancer Inst.* 2003 Dec. 3; 95(23):1797-800.

[123] Psutka, S. P., Stewart, S. B., Boorjian, S. A., Lohse, C. M., Tollefson, M. K., Cheville, J. C., Leibovich, B. C., Thompson, R. H. Diabetes Mellitus Is Independently Associated with an Increased Risk of Mortality in Patients with Clear Cell Renal Cell Carcinoma. *J. Urol.* 2014 Dec; 192(6):1620-7.

[124] Barone, B. B., Yeh, H. C., Snyder, C. F., Peairs, K. S., Stein, K. B., Derr, R. L. Longterm all-cause mortality in cancer patients with pre-existing diabetes mellitus: A systematic review and meta-analysis. *JAMA.* 2008 Dec. 17; 300(23):2754-64.

[125] Yang, X. L., Chan, J. C. Diabetes, insulin and cancer risk. *World J. Diabetes.* 2012 Apr. 15; 3(4), 60–4.

[126] Gunter, M. J., Hoover, D. R., Yu, H., et al. Insulin, insulin-like growth factor-I, and risk of breast cancer in postmenopausal women. *J. Natl. Cancer Inst.* 2009 Jan. 7; 101(1): 48-60.

[127] Pollak, M. N., Schernhammer, E. S., Hankinson, S. E. Insulin-like growth factors and neoplasia. *Nat. Rev. Cancer.* 2004 Jul; 4(7): 505-18.

[128] Franciosi, M., Lucisano, G., Lapice, E., Strippoli, G. F., Pellegrini, F., Nicolucci, A. Metformin Therapy and Risk of Cancer in Patients with Type 2 Diabetes: Systematic Review. *PLoS One.* 2013 Aug. 2; 8(8):e71583.

[129] Denton, M. D., Magee, C. C., Ovuworie, C., Mauiyyedi, S., Pascual, M., Colvin, R. B., Cosimi, A. B., Tolkoff-Rubin, N. Prevalence of renal cell carcinoma in patients with ESRD pre-transplantation: a pathologic analysis. *Kidney Int.* 2002 Jun; 61:2201–9.

[130] Vajdic, C. M., McDonald, S. P., McCredie, M. R., et al. Cancer incidence before and after kidney transplantation. *JAMA*. 2006 Dec. 20; 296(23):2823-31.

[131] Stewart, J. H., Vajdic, C. M., van Leeuwen, M. T., et al. The pattern of excess cancer in dialysis and transplantation. *Nephrol. Dial. Transplant.* 2009 Oct; 24(10):3225-31.

[132] Hofmann, J. N., Schwartz, K., Chow, W. H., et al. The association between chronic renal failure and renal cell carcinoma may differ between black and white Americans. *Cancer Causes Control*. 2013 Jan; 24(1):167-74.

[133] Klatte, T., Seitz, C., Waldert, M., de Martino, M., et al. Features and outcomes of renal cell carcinoma of native kidneys in renal transplant recipients. *BJU Int.* 2010 May; 105 (9):1260-5.

[134] Stewart, J. H., Buccianti, G., Agodoa, L., et al. Cancers of the Kidney and Urinary tract in patients on dialysis for end-stage renal disease: analysis of data from the United States, Europe and Australia and New Zealand. *J. Am. Soc. Nephrol.* 2003 Jan; 14(1): 197-207.

[135] Chen, K. S., Lai, M. K., Huang, C. C., Chu, S. H., Leu, M. L. Urologic cancers in uremic patients. *Am. J. Kidney Dis.* 1995; 25:694-700.

[136] Port, F. K., Ragheb, N. E., Schwartz, A. G., Hawthorne, V. M. Neoplasms in dialysis patients: a population-based study. *Am. J. Kidney Dis.* 1989 Aug; 14(2):119-23.

[137] Nouh, M. A., Kuroda, N., Yamashita, M., et al. Renal cell carcinoma in patients with end-stage renal disease: relationship between histological type and duration of dialysis. *BJU Int.* 2010 Mar; 105(5):620-7.

[138] Maisonneuve, P., Agodoa, L., Gellert, R., et al. Cancer in patients on dialysis for end-stage renal disease: an international collaborative study. *Lancet.* 1999; 354:93-99.

[139] Levine, E., Slusher, S. L., Grantham, J. J., Wetzel, L. H. Natural history of acquired renal cystic disease in dialysis patients: a prospective longitudinal CT study. *AJR Am. J. Roentgenol.* 1991; 156:501-506.

[140] Hurst, F. P., Jindal, R. M., Fletcher, J. J., Dharnidharka, V., Gorman, G., Lechner, B., Nee, R., Agodoa, L. Y., Abbott, K. C. Incidence, Predictors and Associated Outcomes of Renal Cell Carcinoma in Long-term Dialysis Patients. *Urology.* 2011 Jun; 77(6): 1271-6.

[141] Steinman, T. I. Polycystic kidney disease: A 2011 update. *Curr. Opin. Nephrol. Hypertens.* 2012 Mar; 21: 189–94.

[142] Wetmore, J. B., Calvet, J. P. 2, Yu, A. S. 3, Lynch, C. F. 4, Wang, C. J. 3, Kasiske, B. L. 5, Engels, E. A. 6. Polycystic Kidney Disease and Cancer after Renal Transplantation. *J. Am. Soc. Nephrol.* 2014 Oct; 25(10): 2335–41.

[143] Patel, P., Horsfield, C., Compton, F., Taylor, J., Koffman, G., Olsburgh, J. Native nephrectomy in transplant patients with autosomal dominant polycystic kidney disease. *Ann. R. Coll. Surg. Engl.* 2011 Jul; 93: 391–5.

[144] Grantham, J. J. Polycystic kidney disease: Neoplasia in disguise. *Am. J. Kidney Dis.* 1990; 15: 110–116.

[145] Martins, D., Tareen, N., Norris, K. C. The epidemiology of end-stage renal disease among African Americans. *Am. J. Med. Sci.* 2002; 323:65–71.
[146] Klein, J. B., Nguyen, C. T., Saffore, L., Modlin, C. 3rd, Modlin, C. S. Jr. Racial disparities in urologic health care. *J. Natl. Med. Assoc.* 2010; 102: 108–17.
[147] Lipworth, L., Tarone, R. E., McLaughlin, J. K. Renal cell cancer among African Americans: an epidemiologic review. *BMC Cancer.* 2011; 11: 133.
[148] Akizawa, T., Kinugasa, E., Koshikawa, S. Increased risk of malignancy and blood-membrane interactions in uraemic patients. *Nephrol. Dial. Transplant.* 1994; 9 Suppl. 2:162–4.
[149] Gutierrez-Dalmau, A., Campistol, J. M. Immunosuppressive therapy and malignancy in organ transplant recipients: a systematic review. *Drugs.* 2007; 67:1167–98.
[150] Gaya, S. B., Rees, A. J., Lechler, R. I., Williams, G., Mason, P. D. Malignant disease in patients with long term transplants. *Transplantation.* 1995; 59(12):1705-9.
[151] Lee, J. E., Mannisto, S., Spiegelman, D., Hunter, D. J., Bernstein, L., et al., Intakes of fruit, vegetables, and carotenoids and renal cell cancer risk: a pooled analysis of 13 prospective studies. *Cancer Epidemiol. Biomarkers Prev.* 2009; 18: 1730–9.
[152] Daniel, C. R., Park, Y., Chow, W. H., Graubard, B. I., Hollenbeck, A. R., et al. Intake of fiber and fiber-rich plant foods is associated with a lower risk of renal cell carcinoma in a large US cohort. *Am. J. Clin. Nutr.* 2013; 97: 1036–43.
[153] Hu, J., Mao, Y., White, K.; Canadian Cancer Registries Epidemiology Research Group. Diet and vitamin or mineral supplements and risk of renal carcinoma in Canada. *Cancer Causes Control.* 2003:14(8):705-14.
[154] Lee, J. E. 1., Giovannucci, E., Smith-Warner, S. A., Spiegelman, D., Willett, W. C., Curhan, G. C. Intakes of fruits, vegetables, vitamins A, C, and E, and carotenoids and risk of renal cell cancer. *Cancer Epidemiol. Biomarkers Prev.* 2006; 15:2445–52.
[155] Weikert, S. 1., Boeing, H., Pischon, T., et al. Fruits and vegetables and renal cell carcinoma: findings from the European Prospective Investigation into Cancer and Nutrition (EPIC). *Int. J. Cancer.* 2006 Jun. 15; 118(12):3133-9.
[156] Bertoia, M., Albanes, D., Mayne, S. T., Männistö, S., Virtamo, J., Wright, M. E. No association between fruit, vegetables, antioxidant nutrients and risk of renal cell carcinoma. *Int. J. Cancer.* 2010 Mar. 15; 126(6):1504-12.
[157] Hecht, S. S. Inhibition of carcinogenesis by isothiocyanates. *Drug Metab. Rev.* 2000; 32: 395–411.
[158] Zhao, J., Zhao, L. Cruciferous Vegetables Intake Is Associated with Lower Risk of Renal Cell Carcinoma: Evidence from a Meta-Analysis of Observational Studies. *PLoS One.* 2013 Oct. 28; 8(10):e75732.
[159] Faramawi, M. F., Johnson, E., Fry, M. W., Sall, M., Zhou, Y. Consumption of different types of meat and the risk of renal cancer: meta-analysis of case–control studies. *Cancer Causes Control.* 2007; 18: 125–33.
[160] Lee, J. E., Spiegelman, D., Hunter, D. J., Albanes, D., Bernstein, L., van den Brandt, P. A., et al. Fat, protein, and meat consumption and renal cell cancer risk: a pooled analysis of 13 prospective studies. *J. Natl. Cancer Inst.* 2008; 100:1695–1706.
[161] Chow, W. H., Gridley, G., McLaughlin, J. K., Mandel, J. S., Wacholder, S., Blot, W. J., Niwa, S., Fraumeni, J. F., Jr. Protein intake and risk of renal cell cancer. *J. Natl. Cancer Inst.* 1994; 86:1131–9.

[162] Maclure, M., Willett, W. A case-control study of diet and risk of renal adenocarcinoma. *Epidemiology* 1990; 1:430–40.

[163] Mellemgaard, A., McLaughlin, J. K., Overvad, K., Olsen, J. H. Dietary risk factors for renal cell carcinoma in Denmark. *Eur. J. Cancer* 1996; 32A: 673–82.

[164] Allen, N. E., Roddam, A. W., Sieri, S., Boeing, H., et al. A prospective analysis of the association between macronutrient intake and renal cell carcinoma in the European Prospective Investigation into Cancer and Nutrition. *Int. J. Cancer.* 2009;125(4):982-7.

[165] Prineas, R. J., Folsom, A. R., Zhang, Z. M., Sellers, T. A., Potter, J. Nutrition and other risk factors for renal cell carcinoma in postmenopausal women. *Epidemiology* 1997; 8: 31–6.

[166] van Dijk, B. A., Schouten, L. J., Kiemeney, L. A., Goldbohm, R. A., van den Brandt, P. A. Relation of height, body mass, energy intake, and physical activity to risk of renal cell carcinoma: results from The Netherlands Cohort Study. *Am. J. Epidemiol.* 2004; 160:1159–67.

[167] Kotchen, T. A., Cowley, Jr A. W., Frohlich, E. D. Salt in health and disease–a delicate balance. *N. Engl. J. Med.* 2013; 368: 1229–37.

[168] Fiore, M. C., Jimenez, P. M., Cremonezzi, D., Juncos, L. I., Garcia, N. H. Statins reverse renal inflammation and endothelial dysfunction induced by chronic high salt intake. *Am. J. Physiol. Renal Physiol.* 2011; 301: F263–70.

[169] Hu, J., Mao, Y., Desmeules, M., Csizmadi, I., Friedenreich, C., Mery, L. Total fluid and specific beverage intake and risk of renal cell carcinoma in Canada. *Cancer Epidemiol.* 2009; 33: 355–62.

[170] Deckers, I. A., van den Brandt, P. A., van Engeland, M., Soetekouw, P. M., Baldewijns, M. M., Goldbohm, R. A., Schouten, L. J. Long-term dietary sodium, potassium and fluid intake; exploring potential novel risk factors for renal cell cancer in the Netherlands Cohort Study on diet and cancer. *Br. J. Cancer.* 2014; 110, 797–801.

[171] Wolk, A., Larsson, S. C., Johansson, J. E., Ekman, P. Long-term fatty fish consumption and renal cell carcinoma incidence in women. *JAMA.* 2006; 296:1371–6.

[172] Lee, J. E., Hunter, D. J., Spiegelman, D., Adami, H. O., Albanes, D., Bernstein, L., et al. Alcohol intake and renal cell cancer in a pooled analysis of 12 prospective studies. *J. Natl. Cancer Inst.* 2007; 99:801–10.

[173] Siemiatycki, J., Richardson, L., Straif, K., et al. Listing occupational carcinogens. *Environ. Health Perspect.* 2004; 112:1447–59.

[174] Sali, D., Boffetta, P. Kidney cancer and occupational exposure to asbestos: a meta-analisis of occupational cohort studies. *Cancer Causes Control.* 2000; 11:37-47.

[175] Il'yasova, D., Schwartz, G. G. Cadmium and renal cancer. *Toxicol. Appl. Pharmacol.* 2005; 207:179–186.

[176] Canu, I. G., Ellis, E. D., Tirmarche, M. Cancer risk in nuclear workers occupationally exposed to uranium–emphasis on internal exposure. *Health Phys.* 2008; 94:1–17.

[177] Törnqvist, M. Acrylamide in food: the discovery and its implications: a historical perspective. *Adv. Exp. Med. Biol.* 2005; 561:1–19.

[178] Mucci, L. A., Adami, H.-O. The plight of the potato: Is dietary acrylamide a risk factor for human cancer?. *J. Natl. Cancer Inst.* 2009; 101:618–621.

[179] Parent, M. E., Hua, Y., Siemiatycki, J. Occupational risk factors for renal cell carcinoma in Montreal. *Am. J. Ind. Med.* 2000; 38:609–18.

[180] Zhao, Y., Krishnadasan, A., Kennedy, N., Morgenstern, H., Ritz, B. Estimated effects of solvents and mineral oils on cancer incidence and mortality in a cohort of aerospace workers. *Am. J. Ind. Med.* 2005; 48: 249–58.

[181] Bosetti, C., Boffetta, P., La Vecchia, C. Occupational exposures to polycyclic aromatic hydrocarbons, and respiratory and urinary tract cancers: a quantitative review to 2005. *Ann. Oncol.* 2007; 18:431–46.

[182] Romundstad, P., Andersen, A., Haldorsen, T. Cancer incidence among workers in six Norwegian aluminum plants. *Scand. J. Work Environ. Health.* 2000; 26:461–69.

[183] IARC Working Group on the Evaluation of Carcinogenic Risks to Humans. Some non-heterocyclic polycyclic aromatic hydrocarbons and some related exposures. *IARC Monogr. Eval. Carcinog. Risks Hum.* 2010; 92:1-853.

[184] Fustinoni, S., Campo, L., Cirla, A. M., et al. Biological monitoring in the molding of plastics and rubbers. *G. Ital. Med. Lav. Ergon.* 2007; 29 (suppl.):284–6.

[185] Karami, S., Boffetta, P., Brennan, P., Stewart, P. A., et al. Renal cancer risk and occupational exposure to polycyclic aromatic hydrocarbons and plastics. *J. Occup. Environ. Med.* 2011; 53: 218–23.

[186] International Agency for Research on Cancer. *GLOBACAN.* [October 7, 2010]. http://www-dep.iarc.fr.

[187] US Environmental Protection Agency. Acrylonitrile Fact Sheet: Support Document (CAS No 107--13-1). [October 7, 2010]. http://www.epa.gov/chemfact/acry-sd.txt.

[188] US Environmental Protection Agency. *Styrene.* [October 7, 2010]. http://www.epa.gov/ttn/atw/hlthef/styrene.html.

[189] Ruder, A. M., Ward, E. M., Dong, M., Okun, A. H., Davis-King, K. Mortality patterns among workers exposed to styrene in the reinforced plastic boatbuilding industry: an update. *Am. J. Ind. Med.* 2004; 45:165–76.

[190] Wong, O., Trent, L. S., Whorton, M. D. An updated cohort mortality study of workers exposed to styrene in the reinforced plastics and composites industry. *Occup. Environ. Med.* 1994; 51:386–96.

[191] Agency for Toxic Substances and Diseases Registry. *Benzene.* [October 7, 2010]. http://www.atsdr.cdc.gov/tfacts3.html.

[192] Dement, J. M., Hensley, L., Gitelman, A. Carcinogenicity of gasoline: a review of epidemiological evidence. *Ann. N Y Acad. Sci.* 1997; 837:53–76.

[193] Falahatpisheh, M., Kerzee, J., Metz, R., Donnelly, K., Ramos, K. Inducible cytochrome P450 activities in renal glomerular mesangial cells: biochemical basis for antagonistic interactions among nephrocarcinogenic polycyclic aromatic hydrocarbons. *J. Carcinog.* 2004; 3:12.

[194] Guha, N., Loomis, D., Grosse, Y., et al. Carcinogenicity of trichloroethylene, tetrachloroethylene, some other chlorinated solvents, and their metabolites. *Lancet Oncol.* 2012; 13:1192–3.

[195] Chiu, W. A., Caldwell, J. C., Keshava, N., Scott, C. S. Key scientific issues in the health risk assessment of trichloroethylene. *Environ. Health Perspect.* 2006; 114:1445–9.

[196] Jollow, D. J., Bruckner, J. V., McMillan, D. C., et al. Trichloroethylene risk assessment: a review and commentary. *Crit. Rev. Toxicol.* 2009; 39(9):782–797.

[197] Scott, C. S., Chiu, W. A. Trichloroethylene cancer epidemiology: a consideration of select issues. *Environ. Health Perspect.* 2006; 114: 1471–8.

[198] Charbotel, B., Fevotte, J., Hours, M., et al. Case–control study on renal cell cancer and occupational exposure to trichloroethylene. Part II: epidemiological aspects. *Ann. Occup. Hyg*. 2006; 50:777–87.

[199] Fevotte, J., Charbotel, B., Muller-Beaute, P., et al. Case–control study on renal cell cancer and occupational exposure to trichloroethylene. Part I: exposure assessment. *Ann. Occup. Hyg*. 2006; 50:765–75.

[200] Karami, S., Lan, Q., Rothman, N., et al. Occupational trichloroethylene exposure and kidney cancer risk: a meta-analysis. *Occup. Environ. Med.* 2012; 69:858–867.

[201] Kelsh, M. A., Alexander, D. D., Mink, P. J., et al. Occupational trichloroethylene exposure and kidney cancer: a meta-analysis. *Epidemiology*. 2010; 21:95–102.

[202] Scott, C. S., Jinot, J. Trichloroethylene and cancer: systematic and quantitative review of epidemiologic evidence for identifying hazards. *Int. J. Environ. Res. Public Health*. 2011; 8: 4238–72.

[203] Hansen, J., Sallmén, M., Seldén, A. I., et al. Risk of Cancer Among Workers Exposed to Trichloroethylene: Analysis of Three Nordic Cohort Studies. *J. Natl. Cancer Inst*. 2013; 105:869-77.

[204] Ulander, A., Selden, A., Ahlborg, G. Jr. Assessment of intermittent trichloroethylene exposure in vapor degreasing. *Am. Ind. Hyg. Assoc. J*. 1992; 53:742–3.

[205] Jollow, D. J., Bruckner, J. V., McMillan, D. C., et al. Trichloroethylene risk assessment: a review and commentary. *Crit. Rev. Toxicol*. 2009; 39: 782–97.

[206] Yang, C. Y., Chiu, H. F., Wu, T. N., et al. Reduction in kidney cancer mortality following installation of a tap water supply system in an arsenic-endemic area of Taiwan. *Arch. Environ. Health* 2004; 59:484–88.

[207] Yuan, Y., Marshall, G., Ferreccia, C., et al. Kidney cancer mortality: fifty-year latency patterns related to arsenic exposure. *Epidemiology* 2010; 21:103–08.

[208] Baastrup, R., Sorensen, M., Balstrom, T., et al. Arsenic in drinking-water and risk for cancer in Denmark. *Environ. Health Perspect*. 2008; 116:231–7.

[209] Hopenhayn-Rich, C., Biggs, M. L., Smith, A. H. Lung and kidney cancer mortality associated with arsenic in drinking water in Córdoba, Argentina. *Int. J. Epidemiol*. 1998; 27:561–9.

[210] Wu, M. M., Kuo, T. L., Hwang, Y. H., et al. Dose-response relation between arsenic concentration in well water and mortality from cancers and vascular diseases. *Am. J. Epidemiol*. 1989; 130:1123–32.

[211] Sohel, N., Persson, L. A., Rahman, M., et al. Arsenic in drinking water and adult mortality: a population-based cohort study in rural Bangladesh. *Epidemiology* 2009; 20: 824–30.

[212] Mostafa, M. G., Cherry, N. Arsenic in drinking water and renal cancers in rural Bangladesh. *Occup. Environ. Med*. 2013; 70:768-73.

[213] Mathew, A., Devesa, S. S., Fraumeni, J., et al. Global increases in kidney cancer incidence, 1973–1992. *Eur. J. Cancer Prev*. 2002; 11: 171–8.

[214] Chow, W. H., Lindblad, P., Gridley, G., Nyre´n, O., McLaughlin, J. K., Linet, M. S., et al. Risk of urinary tract cancers following kidney or ureter stones. *J. Natl. Cancer Inst*. 1997; 89:1453–7.

[215] Chung, S. D., Liu, S. P., Lin, H. C. A population-based study on the association between urinary calculi and kidney cancer. *Can. Urol. Assoc. J*. 2013; 7:E716–21.

[216] Yoshikawa, T. T., Nicolle, L. E., Norman, D. C. Management of complicated urinary tract infection in older patients. *J. Am. Geriatr. Soc*. 1996; 44:1235-41.
[217] Cheungpasitporn, W., Thongprayoon, C., O'Corragain, O. A., et al. The risk of kidney cancer in patients with kidney stones: a systematic review and meta-analysis. *QJM*. 2014 Sep. 9.
[218] Scales, C. D. Jr, Smith, A. C., Hanley, J. M., Saigal, C. S. Prevalence of kidney stones in the United States. *Eur. Urol*. 2012; 62:160–5.
[219] Siegel, R., Ward, E., Brawley, O., Jemal, A. Cancer statistics, 2011: the impact of eliminating socioeconomic and racial disparities on premature cancer deaths. *CA Cancer J. Clin*. 2011; 61:212–36.
[220] Roupret, M., Babjuk, M., Comperat, E., Zigeuner, R., Sylvester, R., Burger, M., et al. European guidelines on upper tract urothelial carcinomas: 2013 update. *Eur. Urol*. 2013; 63:1059–71.
[221] Daniel, C. R., Cross, A. J., Graubard, B. I., Park, Y., Ward, M. H., Rothman, N., et al. Large prospective investigation of meat intake, related mutagens, and risk of renal cell carcinoma. *Am. J. Clin. Nutr*. 2012; 95:155–62.
[222] Li, W. M., Chou, Y. H., Li, C. C., Liu, C. C., Huang, S. P., Wu, W. J., et al. Association of body mass index and urine pH in patients with urolithiasis. *Urol. Res*. 2009; 37:193–6.
[223] Rosenberg, L., Rao, R. S., Palmer, J. R., et al. Transitional cell cancer of the urinary tract and renal cell cancer in relation to acetaminophen use (United States). *Cancer Causes Control*. 1998; 9:83-8.
[224] McCredie, M., Pommer, W., McLaughlin, J. K., et al. International renal-cell cancer study. II. Analgesics. *Int. J. Cancer*. 1995; 60:345–9.
[225] Gago-Dominguez, M., Yuan, J. M., Castelao, J. E., et al. Regular use of analgesics is a risk factor for renal cell carcinoma. *Br. J. Cancer*. 1999; 81:542–8.
[226] Friis, S., Sørensen, H. T., McLaughlin, J. K., et al. A population-based cohort study of the risk of colorectal and other cancers among users of low-dose aspirin. *Br. J. Cancer*. 2003; 88:684–8.
[227] Tavani, A., Scotti, L., Bosetti, C., et al. Aspirin and risk of renal cell cancer in Italy. *Eur. J. Cancer Prev*. 2010; 19:272–4.
[228] Cho, E., Curhan, G., Hankinson, S. E., et al. Prospective evaluation of analgesic use and risk of renal cell cancer. *Arch. Intern. Med*. 2011; 171: 1487–93.
[229] Jacobs, E. J., Thun, M. J., Bain, E. B., et al. A large cohort study of long-term daily use of adult-strength aspirin and cancer incidence. *J. Natl. Cancer Inst*. 2007; 99:608–15.
[230] Rothwell, P. M., Fowkes, F. G., Belch, J. F., et al. Effect of daily aspirin on long-term risk of death due to cancer: analysis of individual patient data from randomised trials. *Lancet*. 2011; 377:31–41.
[231] Algra, A. M., Rothwell, P. M. Effects of regular aspirin on long-term cancer incidence and metastasis: a systematic comparison of evidence from observational studies versus randomized trials. *Lancet Oncol*. 2012; 13:518–27.
[232] Sørensen, H. T., Friis, S., Nørgard, B., et al. Risk of cancer in a large cohort of nonaspirin NSAID users: a population-based study. *Br. J. Cancer*. 2003; 88:1687–92.
[233] Lipworth, L., Friis, S., Blot, W. J., et al. A population-based cohort study of mortality among users of ibuprofen in Denmark. *Am. J. Ther*. 2004; 11:156–63.

[234] Liu, W., Park, Y., Purdue, M. P., Giovannucci, E., Cho, E. A large cohort study of nonsteroidal anti-inflammatory drugs and renal cell carcinoma incidence in the National Institutes of Health–AARP Diet and Health Study. *Cancer Causes Control.* 2013; 24: 1865–73.

[235] Cook, N. R., Lee, I. M., Gaziano, J. M., et al. Low-dose aspirin in the primary prevention of cancer: the Women's Health Study: a randomized controlled trial. *JAMA.* 2005; 294:47–55.

[236] van Dijk, B. A., Schouten, L. J., Kiemeney, L. A., Goldbohm, R. A., van den Brandt, P. A. Relation of height, body mass, energy intake, and physical activity to risk of renal cell carcinoma: results from the Netherlands Cohort Study. *Am. J. Epidemiol.* 2004; 60: 1159-67.

[237] Moore, S. C., Chow, W. H., Schatzkin, A., et al. Physical activity during adulthood and adolescence in relation to renal cell cancer. *Am. J. Epidemiol.* 2008; 68:149-57.

[238] Behrens, G., Leitzmann, M. F., et al. The association between physical activity and renal cancer: Systematic review and meta-analysis. *Br. J. Cancer.* 2013; 108:798–811.

[239] Richardson, C. R., Newton, T. L., Abraham, J. J., Sen, A., Jimbo, M., Swartz, A. M. A meta-analysis of pedometer-based walking interventions and weight loss. *Ann. Fam. Med.* 2008; 6:69-77.

[240] Pialoux, V., Brown, A. D., Leigh, R., Friedenreich, C. M., Poulin, M. J. Effect of cardiorespiratory fitness on vascular regulation and oxidative stress in postmenopausal women. *Hypertension.* 2009; 54:1014-20.

[241] Li, J. J., Weroha, S. J., Davis, M. F., Tawfik, O., Hou, X., Li, S. A. ER and PR in renomedullary interstitial cells during Syrian hamster estrogeninduced tumorigenesis: evidence for receptor-mediated oncogenesis. *Endocrinology* 2001; 142:4006–14.

[242] Cavalieri, E. L., Kumar, S., Todorovic, R., et al. Imbalance of estrogen homeostasis in kidney and liver of hamsters treated with estradiol: implications for estrogen-induced initiation of renal tumors. *Chem. Res. Toxicol.* 2001; 14:1041–50.

[243] Concolino, G., Marocchi, A., Conti, C., et al. Human renal cell carcinoma as a hormone-dependent tumor. *Cancer Res.* 1978; 38(11 Pt 2):4340–4.

[244] Ronchi, E., Pizzocaro, G., Miodini, P., et al. Steroid hormone receptors in normal and malignant human renal tissue: relationship with prog stin therapy. *J. Steroid Biochem.* 1984; 21:329–35.

[245] Zucchetto, A., Talamini, R., Dal Maso, L., et al. Reproductive, menstrual, and other hormone-related factors and risk of renal cell cancer. *Int. J. Cancer.* 2008; 123:2213–2216.

[246] Chow, W. H., McLaughlin, J. K., Mandel, J. S., et al. Reproductive factors and the risk of renal cell cancer among women. *Int. J. Cancer.* 1995; 60:321–324.

[247] Altman, D., Yin, L., Johansson, A., et al. Risk of renal cell carcinoma after hysterectomy. *Arch. Intern. Med.* 2010; 170:2011–6.

[248] Karami, S., Daugherty, S. E., Schonfeld, S. J., et al. Reproductive Factors and Kidney Cancer Risk in 2 US Cohort Studies, 1993–2010. *Am. J. Epidemiol.* 2013; 177:1368-77.

[249] Whiteman, M. K., Hillis, S. D., Jamieson, D. J., et al. Inpatient hysterectomy surveillance in the United States, 2000–2004. *Am. J. Obstet. Gynecol.* 2008; 198:34. e1–7.

[250] Lindblad, P., Mellemgaard, A., Schlehofer, B., et al. International renal-cell cancer study. V. Reproductive factors, gynecologic operations and exogenous hormones. *Int. J. Cancer.* 1995; 61:192–8.

[251] Melin, A., Sparén, P., Bergqvist, A. The risk of cancer and the role of parity among women with endometriosis. *Hum. Reprod.* 2007; 22(11): 3021–6.

[252] Mellemgaard, A., Engholm, G., McLaughlin, J. K., et al. Risk factors for renal-cell carcinoma in Denmark. III. Role of weight, physical activity and reproductive factors. *Int. J. Cancer.* 1994; 56(1):66–71.

[253] Lee, J. E., Hankinson, S. E., Cho, E. Reproductive factors and risk of renal cell cancer: the Nurses' Health Study. *Am. J. Epidemiol.* 2009; 169:1243–50.

[254] Setiawan, V. W., Kolonel, L. N., Henderson, B. E. Menstrual and reproductive factors and risk of renal cell cancer in the Multiethnic Cohort. *Cancer Epidemiol. Biomarkers Prev.* 2009; 18(1):337–40.

[255] Cavalieri, E. L., Kumar, S., Todorovic, R., et al. Imbalance of estrogen homeostasis in kidney and liver of hamsters treated with estradiol: implications for estrogen-induced initiation of renal tumors. *Chem. Res. Toxicol.* 2001; 14:1041–50.

[256] Pechere-Bertschi, A., Burnier, M. Gonadal steroids, saltsensitivity and renal function. *Curr. Opin. Nephrol. Hypertens.* 2007; 16:16–21.

[257] Guan, H. B., Wu, Q. J., Gong, T. T. Parity and Kidney Cancer Risk: Evidence from Epidemiologic Studies. *Cancer Epidemiol. Biomarkers Prev.* 2013; 22:2345-53.

[258] Chiu, H. F., Kuo, C. C., Kuo, H. W., Lee, I. M., Yang, C. Y. Parity, age at first birth and risk of death from kidney cancer: a population-based cohort study in Taiwan. *Eur. J. Public Health.* 2014 Apr; 24:249-52.

[259] Ramin, S. M., Vidaeff, A. C., Yeomans, E. R., et al. Chronic renal disease in pregnancy. *Obstet. Gynecol.* 2006; 108: 1531–9.

[260] Giubertoni, E., Bertelli, L., Bartolacelli, Y., Origliani, G., Modena, M. G. Parity as predictor of early hypertension during menopausal transition. *J. Hypertens.* 2013; 31: 501–7.

[261] Mansour, A. A., Ajeel, N. A. Parity is associated with increased waist circumference and other anthropometric indices of obesity. *Eat Weight Disord.* 2009; 14:e50–5.

[262] Gago-Dominguez, M., Yuan, J. M., Castelao, J. E., Ross, R. K., Yu, M. C. Family history and risk of renal cell carcinoma. *Cancer Epidemiol. Biomarkers Prev.* 2001; 10: 1001–4.

[263] Clague, J., Lin, J., Cassidy, A., Matin, S., Tannir, N. M., Tamboli, P., et al. Family history and risk of renal cell carcinoma: results from a case–control study and systematic meta-analysis. *Cancer Epidemiol. Biomarkers Prev.* 2009; 18:801–7.

[264] Latif, F., Tory, K., Gnarra, J. R., et al. Identification of the von Hippel-Lindau disease tumor suppressor gene. *Science.* 1993; 260:1317–20.

[265] Haas, N. B., Nathanson, K. L. Hereditary Kidney Cancer Syndromes. *Adv. Chronic Kidney Dis.* 2014; 21:81-90.

[266] Maher, E. R., Iselius, L., Yates, J. R., et al. Von Hippel-Lindau disease: a genetic study. *J. Med. Genet.* 1991; 28:443-7.

[267] Linehan, W. M., Walther, M. M., Zbar, B. The genetic basis of cancer of the kidney. *J. Urol.* 2003; 170:2163–72.

[268] Lonser, R. R., Glenn, G. M., Walther, M. M., et al. von Hippel-Lindau disease. *Lancet.* 2003; 361:2059–67.

[269] Cancer Genome Atlas Research Network. Comprehensive molecular characterization of clear cell renal cell carcinoma. *Nature*. 2013; 499: 43–9.

[270] Kim, W., Kaelin, W. G. Jr. The von Hippel-Lindau tumor suppressor protein: new insights into oxygen sensing and cancer. *Curr. Opin. Genet. Dev.* 2003; 13:55-60.

[271] Crossey, P. A., Foster, K., Richards, F. M., et al. Molecular genetic investigations of the mechanism of tumourigenesis in von Hippel-Lindau disease: analysis of allele loss in VHL tumours. *Hum. Genet.* 1994; 93: 53-8.

[272] Anglada Curado, F. J., Campos Hernández, P., Prieto Castro, R., Carazo Carazo, J. L., Regueiro López, J. C., Vela Jiménez, F., Requena Tapia, M. J. New epidemiologic patterns and risk factors in renal cáncer. *Actas Urol. Esp.* 2009; 33:459-67.

[273] Richards, F. M., Webster, A. R., McMahon, R., Woodward, E. R., Rose, S., Maher, E. R. Molecular genetic analysis of von Hippel-Lindau disease. *J. Intern. Med.* 1998; 243: 527-33.

[274] Banks, R. E., Tirukonda, P., Taylor, C., et al. Genetic and epigenetic analysis of von Hippel-Lindau (VHL) gene alterations and relationship with clinical variables in sporadic renal cancer. *Cancer Res.* 2006; 66: 2000-11.

[275] Goldfarb, D. A., Neumann, H. P., Penn, I., Novick, A. C. Results of renal transplantation in patients with renal cell carcinoma and von Hippel-Lindau disease. *Transplantation*. 1997; 64:1726-9.

[276] Walther, M. M., Choyke, P. L., Glenn, G., et al. Renal cancer in families with hereditary renal cancer: prospective analysis of a tumor size threshold for renal parenchymal sparing surgery. *J. Urol.* 1999; 161(5): 1475-9.

[277] Duffey, B. G., Choyke, P. L., Glenn, G., et al. The relationship between renal tumor size and metastases in patients with von Hippel-Lindau disease. *J. Urol.* 2004; 172(1): 63-5.

[278] Zbar, B., Glenn, G., Lubensky, I., et al. Hereditary papillary renal cell carcinoma: clinical studies in 10 families. *J. Urol.* 1995; 153(3 Pt 2): 907-12.

[279] Zbar, B., Tory, K., Merino, M., et al. Hereditary papillary renal cell carcinoma. *J. Urol.* 1994; 151(3):561-6.

[280] Linehan, W. M., Vasselli, J., Srinivasan, R., Walther, M. M., Merino, M., Choyke, P., et al. Genetic basis of cancer of the kidney: disease-specific approaches to therapy. *Clin. Cancer Res.* 2004; 10:6282S–9S.

[281] Dharmawardana, P. G., Giubellino, A., Bottaro, D. P. Hereditary papillary renal carcinoma type I. *Curr. Mol. Med.* 2004; 4:855-68.

[282] Smit, D. L., Mensenkamp, A. R., Badeloe, S., et al. Hereditary leiomyomatosis and renal cell cancer in families referred for fumarate hydratase germline mutation analysis. *Clin. Genet.* 2011; 79:49-59.

[283] Schmidt, L. S., Linehan, W. M. Hereditary leiomyomatosis and renal cell carcinoma. *Int. J. Nephrol. Renovasc. Dis.* 2014; 7:253-60.

[284] Stewart, L., Glenn, G. M., Stratton, P., et al. Association of germline mutations in the fumarate hydratase gene and uterine fibroids in women with hereditary leiomyomatosis and renal cell cancer. *Arch. Dermatol.* 2008; 144:1584-92.

[285] Wei, M. H., Toure, O., Glenn, G. M., et al. Novel mutations in FH and expansion of the spectrum of phenotypes expressed in families with hereditary leiomyomatosis and renal cell cancer. *J. Med. Genet.* 2006; 43:18–27.

[286] Merino, M. J., Torres-Cabala, C., Pinto, P., Linehan, W. M. The morphologic spectrum of kidney tumors in hereditary leiomyomatosis and renal cell carcinoma (HLRCC) syndrome. *Am. J. Surg. Pathol.* 2007; 31:1578-85.

[287] Grubb, R. L. III, Franks, M. E., Toro, J., et al. Hereditary leiomyomatosis and renal cell cancer: a syndrome associated with an aggressive form of inherited renal cancer. *J. Urol.* 2007; 177:2074–80.

[288] Shuch, B., Ricketts, C. J., Vocke, C. D., et al. Adrenal nodular hyperplasia in hereditary leiomyomatosis and renal cell cancer. *J. Urol.* 2013; 189: 430–5.

[289] Lamba, M., Verma, S., Prokopetz, R., Pierscianowski, T. A., Jabi, M., Moyana, T. Multiple cutaneous and uterine leiomyomas associated with gastric GIST. *J. Cutan. Med. Surg.* 2005; 9:332-5.

[290] Badeloe, S., van Spaendonck-Zwarts, K. Y., van Steensel, M. A., et al. Wilms tumour as a possible early manifestation of hereditary leiomyomatosis and renal cell cancer? *Br. J. Dermatol.* 2009; 160: 707-9.

[291] Schmidt, L. S., Warren, M. B., Nickerson, M. L., et al. Birt-Hogg-Dube syndrome, a genodermatosis associated with spontaneous pneumothorax and kidney neoplasia, maps to chromosome 17p11.2. *Am. J. Hum. Genet.* 2001; 69:876-882.

[292] Pavlovich, C. P., Walther, M. M., Eyler, R. A., et al. Renal tumors in the Birt-Hogg-Dubé syndrome. *Am. J. Surg. Pathol.* 2002; 26:1542–52.

[293] Pavlovich, C. P., Grubb, R. L. III, Hurley, K., et al. Evaluation and management of renal tumors in the Birt-Hogg-Dube syndrome. *J. Urol.* 2005; 173:1482-6.

[294] da Silva, N. F., Gentle, D., Hesson, L. B., Morton, D. G., Latif, F., Maher, E. R. Analysis of the Birt-Hogg-Dube (BHD) tumour suppressor gene in sporadic renal cell carcinoma and colorectal cancer. *J. Med. Genet.* 2003; 40:820-4.

[295] Linehan, W. M., Pinto, P. A., Bratslavsky, G., et al. Hereditary kidney cancer: unique opportunity for disease-based therapy. *Cancer.* 2009; 115 (suppl. 10):2252-2261.

[296] Dixon, B. P., Hulbert, J. C., Bissler, J. J. Tuberous sclerosis complex renal disease. *Nephron. Exp. Nephrol.* 2011; 118:e15-e20.

[297] Lynch, E. D., Ostermeyer, E. A., Lee, M. K., et al. Inherited mutations in PTEN that are associated with breast cancer, Cowden disease, and juvenile polyposis. *Am. J. Hum. Genet.* 1997; 61:1254-60.

[298] Amar, L., Baudin, E., Burnichon, N., et al. Succinate dehydrogenase B gene mutations predict survival in patients with malignant pheochromocytomas or paragangliomas. *J. Clin. Endocrinol. Metab.* 2007; 92:3822-8.

[299] Popova, T., Hebert, L., Jacquemin, V., et al. Germline BAP1 mutations predispose to renal cell carcinomas. *Am. J. Hum. Genet.*, http://dx.doi.org/10.1016/j.ajhg.2013.04.012.

[300] Bonne, A. C., Bodmer, D., Schoenmakers, E. F., van Ravenswaaij, C. M., Hoogerbrugge, N., van Kessel, A. G. Chromosome 3 translocations and familial renal cell cancer. *Curr. Mol. Med.* 2004; 4:849-54.

In: Renal Cell Carcinoma
Editors: J. M. Fernández-Gomez, J. García-Rodríguez ISBN: 978-1-63482-495-8

Chapter 2

Histology Types and Molecular Markers of Renal Carcinoma

V. Blanco, MD, V. Folgueras, PhD*, N. Fuentes, PhD, and B. Vivanco, PhD

Department of Pathology, Central de Asturias
University Hospital, Oviedo, Spain

Abstract

Renal cell carcinoma (RCC) is the most common malignancy in the kidney of adults with an incidence of 2-3% of cancers, corresponding mostly to tumors derived from the renal parenchyma. Advances in the understanding of molecular pathology in recent years, allowed the recognition of numerous genetic alterations associated with the known renal carcinomas, as well as the identification of new entities.

In this chapter, we will present a review of the most common tumors arising from the renal parenchyma, including both emerging and well-accepted tumors. Likewise, we will associate the tumor pathogenesis with new therapeutic avenues that could be of relevance for the future and helpful to change the prognosis of these tumors, but without forgetting the traditional prognostic factors that still remain in force.

Keywords: renal cell carcinoma, histology, molecular, immunohistochemistry, differential diagnosis

Introduction

Renal cell cancer is usually sporadic (no family history) and rarely is part of a hereditary syndrome (5% of cases). The exact causes of this disease remain to be elucidated. However,

* Corresponding author: Mª Victoria Folgueras, Avda Rubín s/n, 33011-Oviedo. E-mail: folgueras@hca.es.

several factors are associated with an increased incidence of this type of cancer. For instance, smoking (which doubles the risk of developing this disease), exposure to certain chemicals (cadmium, asbestos, oil), obesity (eating habits), hypertension, the acquired renal cystic disease (ARCD) in chronic dialysis patients (30% of these patients develop kidney cancer) and the indiscriminate use of analgesics (aspirin and phenacetin, which are more involved in the development of urinary tract cancer) are known to be associated with a higher incidence of renal cancer.

Origin of Each Tumor Type

The identification of the tumor origin of the most frequent variants present in different areas of the nephron, revealed a correlation with the prognosis and also with the genetic and molecular alterations established in recent years in this disease. In this sense, numerous molecular alterations were identified. As an example, from proximal tubule arise the clear cell renal cell carcinoma (CCRCC), which shows deletions and mutations in chromosome 3p, mainly associated with the VHL gene.

Also, from this region the papillary renal cell carcinoma (PRCC) is also derived, which is molecularly characterized by trisomies of chromosomes 7 and 17, loss of chromosome 3p and Y, and being associated Type I and Type II with mutations in MET and FH genes respectively. Cortical collecting ducts give rise to the chromophobe renal cell carcinoma (CHRCC), which presents multiple known mutations on chromosomes 1, 2, 3, 10 and 13 (generally associated to the loss of heterozygosity, LOH) and to the oncocytoma, with mutations in chromosomes Y and 1, and telomere alterations. Both, the CHRCC and the oncocytoma are linked to mutations in in the FLCN gene.

Finally, collecting duct carcinoma of Bellini (CDC) which arises from the renal medulla is characterized by mutations on chromosomes 1, 6, 14, 15 and 22.

Genetic Factors

Kidney cancer can occur, like most cancers, hereditary and non-hereditary or sporadic; with the latter being the most frequent (around 95% of all cases).

Several genes have been linked to the risk of sporadic renal cell cancer, as the gene encoding the protein glutathione-S-transferase, or several genes involved in cell cycle control, such as cyclin D1 and CHEK2.

Among hereditary factors, it has been described that patients with a first-degree relative diagnosed with renal cancer before the age of 40 years (patients with sporadic renal cancer have an average age of onset of the disease between 50-70 years) or with a bilateral or multifocal renal cancer in one kidney may have a hereditary component.

Additionally, there are 10 hereditary syndromes associated with different histological types of kidney cancer, however only four of them have a greater risk of developing renal carcinoma: von Hippel Lindau disease (VHL) -Multiple bilateral CCRCC, renal cysts-, hereditary leiomyomatosis -PRCC (non type 1)-, Birt-Hogg-Dubé syndrome -Multiple CHRCC, oncocytic adenoma, PRCC- and hereditary PRCC -Multiple, bilateral PRCC (type

1)-. The study of these hereditary syndromes has been a breakthrough in understanding the genetic basis of renal carcinoma [1, 2].

The identification of the genes involved in the process of renal carcinogenesis, as well as their expression pattern has allowed us to analyze its relationship with the different tumor types and their mechanisms of action.

The best known are the changes related to the inactivation of the VHL gene, which occur associated with both sporadic and hereditary carcinomas, mainly in CCRCC but also in papillary, playing an important role in the process of angiogenesis through the induction of the expression of vascular endothelial growth factor (VEGF) [3].

On the other hand, it is possible to find associations of kidney cancer with other neoplasms. Thus, studies in patient record series have shown an increased incidence of lymphomas in patients with RCC [4, 5].

Pathogenesis

The RCC is a highly vascularized tumor due to the genetic alterations that occur that promote angiogenesis. As examples are those mutations of VHL that cause overexpression of Hypoxia Inducible Factor (HIF) [6]. HIF is a factor which expression is usually restricted to hypoxic conditions. It regulates cell growth and angiogenesis by encoding the production of growth factors such as VEGF, PDGF and FGF.

MET mutations are also a pathological basis of hereditary papillary renal cancer, being HIF also a target gene of MET. The PI3K / AKT / mTOR signaling pathway is frequently deregulated in cancer. Approximately 70% of all cancers have alterations in a component of the mTOR pathway. mTOR also increases VEGF production and HIF. Currently, mTOR inhibitors are being investigated as new therapeutic opportunities in the treatment of several types of cancer including renal cell carcinoma [7].

Histological and Molecular Prognostic Factors

Surgical treatment remains as the first choice in the treatment of RCC. An accurate diagnosis of tumor type and the correct definition of other pathological features are accepted as significant prognostic factors. We discuss in this section the most important recommendations that The International Society of Urological Pathology (ISUP) has recently introduced by consensus in the meeting that took place in Vancouver 2013 [8]. Staging: It is one of the most important prognostic factors; therefore several recommendations have been made in relation to tumor sampling:

1. The tumor must be painted with ink in both total and partial nephrectomies.
2. The initial section should be longitudinal. Next, kidney sections should be performed perpendicularly to evaluate the affectation of perirenal fat (without detaching it from the tumor) and the perinephric sinus. Perform lymph node sampling in perihilar fat.

3. A compressive edge is not considered as infiltration of perinephric tissue. Infiltration is only considered if it extends into irregular protrusions with or without desmoplasia or if any focal location of tumoral cells is detected within the sinus fat.
4. Tumor sampling is related to tumor size (1 sample per cm, with a minimum of 3) and the uni or multifocality [9].
5. Remember those modifications of TNM 2010 regarding the adrenal gland.

Tumor Type: It is very important to make a detailed description of tumor type as these distinctions may represent prognostic features. See below some types that is important to remark:

- Identify the multilocular variant that is low grade in CCRCC.
- Distinguish between type I and II PRCC as they are recognized to have a different prognosis.
- Also identify as a different type the oncocytic variant.
- Hybrid oncocytomas and chromophobe tumors should be considered as chromophobe tumors although it is advisable to describe their characteristics [10, 11].

Fuhrman Grading: The ISUP meeting agreed to simplify the system of evaluation by focusing only in the description of the nucleolus. In this regard, the new grading system has been established as follows: a) ISUP Grade 1: invisible or small nucleolus at 400x magnification. b) ISUP Grade 2: visible nucleolus at 400 x but invisible or very small at 100x. c) ISUP Grade 3: visible nucleolus at 100 x. d) ISUP Grade 4: rhabdoid or sarcomatoid transformation or marked nuclear polymorphism. This grading should primarily be used for papillary and clear cell renal cell carcinoma, but it cannot be used in chromophobe renal cell carcinoma. Tumor necrosis (coagulative): Its presence should be noted in the report including its percentage. This is also considered as a prognosis factor. Necrosis secondary to vascular obstruction, areas of fibrosis, hemorrhage or hyalinization should be excluded.

In the papillary variant there is no correlation between tumor necrosis and prognosis.

Microscopic vascular infiltration: It is not considered as a prognostic factor although it is advisable to mention it. Molecular characteristics: A clear prognostic marker has not been validated yet, although recent research related to some classical markers such as the proliferation index Ki-67, or to others such as the loss of PBMR-1 or alterations in carbonic anhydrase IX (CA IX), suggest that some this molecular features will be possibly considered as prognostic markers in a near future [12, 13].

Another important molecular avenue that will affect the prognosis of patients are those therapies aimed to block specific signaling pathways such as the PI3K / Akt / mTOR and MET pathways, since both contribute to increase the expression of HIF [14]. These and other treatment options, such as new immunological therapies, will be discussed in depth in this chapter [15, 16].

New Classification

The classification of kidney tumors has evolved considerably in the latest decades. Since WHO classification in 1981 and Mainz classification in 1986 [17, 18] there have been many changes as a result of a better understanding of renal neoplasms related to their morphology, prognosis and genetic and molecular characteristics.

Recently, The ISUP introduced an amendment to the WHO classification of 2004, which we believe better classify the known tumor types, and incorporates new independent tumor types [19]. In our review, we will focus on renal cell parenchymal tumors in adults through the prism of this new classification.

CLEAR CELL RENAL CELL CARCINOMA

Definition

- Most common RCC, composed of cell with clear or eosinophilic cytoplasm and a prominent vascular network.

Epidemiology

- 2% of all malignant tumors.
- 60-70% of all RCC [18].
- All age groups, but primary adults (60-70 years).
- Male to female ratio 3:1 to 1.5: 1 [20, 21].
- Familiar settings [22].
    - VHL disease (1/36000 births). Autosomal dominant disease. 35-45% of affected patients develop bilateral multifocal RCC, always clear cell type. Patients are born with a germline defect in one of the two alleles located on chromosome 3p9.25-26 which functions as a tumor suppressor. Loss of the second allele results in clinical disease expression [23].
    - Families with constitutional chromosome 3 translocations [24].
    - Families with succinate dehydrogenase B (SDHB)-associated heritable paraganglioma [25].

Gross Findings

- Solitary. 4% of cases can be multiple. 3% bilateral. Normally multiple and bilateral forms are features of hereditary clear cell carcinoma [1].
- Variable size that ranges from few millimeters to several centimeters. They have an average size of 7 cm.
- Well circumscribed, with expansive and lobulated borders.
- Fibrous pseudocapsule of variable thickness.
- Normally are cortically located.
- Section surface shows golden yellow parenchyma (because of the abundance of cholesterol, phospholipids and lipids).
- Frequent necrosis (with secondary pseudocyst formation), hemorrhage and fibrosis [20, 22].

Histology

- Microscopically, clear cell carcinoma displays a variety of architectural patterns. Most frequent is tumor growth in sheets or compact nests of tumor cells separated by a vascular network.
- Vascular network is normally thin and delicate but often shows dilated vascular spaces.
- Cysts are frequently seen (with serosanguineous or sanguineous content).
- Other patterns of growth often seen are: trabecular, papillary (rare), tubular, microcystic, macrocystic and alveolar.
- Cells have clear cytoplasm due to lipid and glycogen content and distinct cell membranes.
- Sometimes cells may have eosinophilic or granular cytoplasm, more frequent in high grade tumors. And they may show also high nuclear grade.
- Nuclei shows considerable variation in size, is normally rounded and with prominent nucleoli. It has different characteristics depending on the nuclear grade of the tumor [22].
- Areas of sarcomatoid type may be seen in 5% of all cases [26].
- They may show rhabdoid differentiation with malignant spindle cells or heterologous elements like heterotopic bone formation [1].
- There is a unique subtype of RCC which consists of a classic CCRCC with prominent angioleiomyoma-like stromal proliferation composed of bundles of uniform spindle cells resembling mature smooth muscle merging with the walls of medium sized blood vessels [27].

Immunohistochemistry

- Positive for: CAM5.2 (cell adhesion molecule), Cytokeratin (Ck) AE1/AE3, EMA (epithelial membrane antigen), Vimentin, CD10 (cluster of differentiation), RCC-Ag (renal cell carcinoma), CA IX (carbonic anhydrase), PAX2 (paired box), and PAX8.
- Negative for: HMWCK (high molecular weight cytokeratin), K903, Ck7, Ck20, CD117, Mucin 1 cell surface associated (MUC1), Kidney-specific cadherin, parvalbumin, S100, and CEA (last two can be positive in isolated cases) [22, 28].

Differential Diagnosis

- Clear cell tubulopapillary RCC: Low nuclear grade. Positive for Ck7 but negative for CD10.
- CHRCC: Prominent cell borders, translucent and reticulated cytoplasm, raisinoid nuclear atypia, diffuse Ck7 positivity, positive Hale´s colloidal iron stain, CA IX negative.
- PRCC, solid variant: Papillary architecture with hemosiderin and histiocytes. Positive for Ck7 and AMACR and negative for CA IX.
- Xp11 translocation associated RCC/transcription factor E3 (TFE3) translocation: Children and young adults. Frequent psammomatous calcifications and hyaline fibrovascular cores. Negative epithelial markers and TFE3 positive.
- Adrenocortical carcinoma: Negative for epithelial markers (CkAE1/AE3 and EMA) and positive for calretinin and inhibin.

- Urothelial carcinoma: may be associated with pelvic urothelial carcinoma in situ or dysplasia. They are frequently positive for Ck7, Ck20, K903, and p63. Negative for PAX2 and PAX8.
- Pure epithelioid angiomyolipoma: Multinucleated giant cells and cells with ganglion like nuclei are often seen. Negative epithelial markers and melanocytic markers [20].

Molecular Genetic Studies

- Initiating events at 3p: [29-33]
  - 90% loss of 3p.
  - VHL gene alterations in 50-70% of sporadic CCRCC (3p25-26) [22]. Normally VHL is inactivated due to deletions, mutations or hypermethylation [34].
- Other genes located in 3p may act as tumor suppressors and may be involved in the development of clear cell carcinomas: Inactivation of FHIT gene (due to 3p14.2 deletion), and another tumor suppressor gene at 3p12 [35]. 96% patients may have a continuous deletion from 3p14.2-p25 including FHIT and VHL genes [36].
- Additional genetic alterations are associated with more aggressive behavior (higher histologic grade, higher pathologic stage): loss of 9p, 14q, loss of heterozygosity on 10q (PTEN/MAC locus) [37-40].

Prognosis

- 1/3 of the patients develop local or distant recurrence after surgery.
- 50% of the patients died of disease [20].

MULTILOCULAR CYSTIC RENAL CELL CARCINOMA OF LOW MALIGNANT POTENTIAL

Definition

- Multilocular cystic renal cell carcinoma (MCRCC) is a tumor of low malignant potential. This term should be restricted to encapsulated tumors composed entirely of multiple cysts the septa of which contain groups of clear cells indistinguishable from grade 1 CCRCC [41-43].

Epidemiology

- 4% of all CCRCCs [44].
- Affects middle age adults.
- Male to female ratio of 1.2-2.1:1 [22, 45, 46].

Gross Findings

- Unilateral and solitary.
- From 2.5 to 13 cm.
- Well-circumscribed, encapsulated mass.
- Composed entirely of small and large cysts containing serous, gelatinous or hemorrhagic fluid.

- No expansive nodules.
- Yellowish solid component limited to small areas.
- No necrosis [22, 42, 43, 46].
- Occasionally calcifications or osseous metaplasia.

Histology

- Neoplasm with fibrous pseudocapsule.
- Composed entirely of cysts lined by a single layer of epithelial cells or without epithelial lining.
- Less than 25% of solid clear cell tumor component.
- Tumor cells are flat or plump with clear or pale cytoplasm.
- Small, spherical nuclei with dense chromatin without nucleoli (nuclear grade 1 or 2).
- Septa with fibrous tissue, densely collagenous and with groups of epithelial cells similar to cyst-lining cells.
- 20% of tumors show calcifications within the septa and also metaplastic bone formation.
- Increased vascularity within the tumor cell clusters.
- No necrosis [22, 41, 42, 44].

Immunohistochemistry

- Positive for: CA IX, PAX2 [47], Ck (CAM 5.2, Ck7), CD10 and EMA [41, 48, 49].

Differential Diagnosis

- CCRCC: Absent or only focal staining for CK7 [49].
- PRCC with predominant cystic configuration: They share co-expression of CK7 and CA IX, but PRCC lack chromosomal alterations of 3p.
- RCC with cystic necrosis: Usually belongs to clear cell group. Gross solid tumor areas are frequent and aids the differential diagnosis [50].
- Tubulocystic renal cell carcinoma (TCRCC) of the kidney: In contrasts with MCRCC, cysts are uniform in size, lined by a single layer of carcinoma cells with eosinophilic cytoplasm and with prominent nucleoli, there is also necrosis and mitosis [51].
- Cystic nephroma: In contrast with MCRCC, clear cells lining the cyst are focal and there are no clusters of clear cells in the walls [52].
- Benign multilocular renal cortical cysts: Cysts are usually unilocular lined by a single layer of flattened or cuboid epithelium, without any mural clear cell clusters [53].

Molecular Genetic Studies

- Similar to low-grade CCRCC.
- 90% Diploid DNA content [54].
- VHL gene mutations (25%).
- Same 3p chromosome alterations (3p deletion) [22, 47, 55].

Prognosis

- Good prognosis.

- 5-year follow up series showed no recurrences, metastasis, or deaths because of the tumor after surgery [22, 56].

PAPILLARY RENAL CELL CARCINOMA

Definition

- Carcinoma of the kidney with a predominantly papillary growth pattern.

Epidemiology

- 10-15% of all RCC [57-59].
- 52-66 years of age.
- Male-Female: 2, 4:1.
- Most cases are sporadic. Hereditary PRCC are multiple and bilateral.

Gross Findings

- Well circumscribed.
- Thick fibrous pseudocapsule is present in up to two thirds of cases [60-62].
- Light grey tan to golden yellow to red brown.
- Haemorrhage and necrosis.

Histology

- Papillary and tubular structures. Cysts with papillary excrescences. Compact and tight packing in some tumors results in a solid or trabecular appearance [60].
- Solid areas composed of spindle cells with low-grade features [63, 64].
- Both types exhibit inflammation, extensive necrosis, recent haemorrhage, psammoma bodies, cholesterol clefts, foreign body-type giant cells and dystrophic calcification [65-67].
    - Type 1: 6 cm. Papillae are thin, delicate and short. Glomeruloid appearance. Single or double layer of small epithelial cells of low nuclear grade. Minimal pale or clear cytoplasm. Foamy macrophages within the papillae. Edema in fibrovascular cores. Type 1 tumor morphology is characteristic of HPRC [66].
    - Type 2: 9, 5 cm. High nuclear grade [65, 67]. Pseudostratification and complex papillary architecture. Abundant and eosinophilic cytoplasm. Dense and fibrous fibrovascular cores. Glomeruloid bodies and foamy macrophages are less prevalent.
- Some PRCC are composed of tumor cells with oncocytic cytoplasm and low-grade nuclei [68, 69].

Immunohistochemistry

- Positive for: CkAE1/AE3, AMACR (α-methyl-coenzyme A racemase), CD15, CD10, RCC-Ag, BerEP4 (epithelial specific antigen), PAX2.
- Negative for: CD117, HMWCK, CA IX.
- Type 1: Ck7 (80%), MUC1.

- Type 2: Ck7 (20%), E-cadherin, Ck20.

Differential Diagnosis

- Papillary adenoma: < 5 mm and low nuclear grade.
- CCRCC: positive for CD10 and CA IX; negative for AMACR and Ck7.
- t Xp11 associated RCC: positive for TFE3.
- Tubulopapillary renal cell carcinoma (TPRCC): negative for AMACR.
- Papillary urothelial carcinoma: negative for PAX2 and positive for p63.
- Metanephric adenoma: negative for Ck and positive for WT1.

Molecular Genetic Studies

- Hereditary PRCC is characterized by mutations in the MET oncogene at 7q31 [70-74].
- MET mutations in 13% of sporadic PRCC [66].
- Complex numeric chromosomal abnormalities: gains of chromosome 7, 8, 12q, 17 and 20q, and losses of chromosome 1p, 4q, 6q, 9p, 11p, 13q, 14q, 18, 21q, X and Y [75, 76].
- Trisomy or tetrasomy 7, trisomy 17 and loss of Y, in sporadic cases [77].
- Deletions of 9p in 20% of cases of PRCC; LOH in 9p13 has been linked to short patient survival [78].

Prognosis

- Five-year survival rate ranges from 49% to 91% [57, 58, 61].

CHROMOPHOBE RENAL CELL CARCINOMA

Definition

- A malignant epithelial neoplasm, which is believed to arise from the intercalated cells of the collecting duct system [79].

Variants

- Eosinophilic.

Epidemiology

- Represents a 4.9% of surgically excised renal epithelial neoplasms.
- Middle East patients have a higher incidence.
- Almost all cases are sporadic.
- Some have a hereditary etiology (as part of Birt-Hogg-Dubé syndrome).
- Accounts for 34% of the renal neoplasms that occur in patients with this syndrome [22].

Gross Findings

- Variable in size (1.5 - 25 cm diameter).
- Well circumscribed.

- At sections, solid, homogeneous and light brown parenchyma.
- Other colors: light pink or yellow-white [22, 80].
- Necrosis and hemorrhage are unusual.
- Just few cases have a central scar [81].

Histology

- Cells are arranged in solid sheets.
- Sporadically a tubulocystic pattern is present [82].
- Delicate fibrous septa and medium caliber blood vessels [83].
- Two types of cells: Chromophobe and eosinophilic.
- Chromophobe: large polygonal cells with abundant and transparent cytoplasm. Plant-like cell membranes.
- Eosinophilic: small cells with scant granular and eosinophilic cytoplasm. They have a perinuclear halo.
- Both types of cells have hyperchromatic and irregular nuclei.
- A sarcomatoid differentiation can occur (not common).
- This tumor should not be graded (there is no relation between nuclear grade and prognosis) [22].

EOSINOPHILIC VARIANT

- A variant of CHRCC which is practically entirely composed of intensely eosinophilic cells with prominent cell membranes [82].

Immunohistochemistry

- Positive for: CkAE1/AE3, EMA, Ck7, parvalbumin, PAX2 (sometimes negative), CD15, CD117 and E-cadherin.
- Negative for: Vimentin, AMACR, RCC-Ag, Ck20 and S100A1 [22, 84-87].
- Although it is a histochemical technique, a diffuse and granular cytoplasmic staining for Hale´s colloidal iron favors the diagnosis of CHRCC [22].
- A combination of these antibodies should be use to confirm the diagnosis, because any of them have demonstrated enough specificity to be used individually.

Differential Diagnosis

- CCRCC with eosinophilic areas.
- Oncocytoma.

Hematoxylin-Eosin (H and E) in some cases is not sufficient to differentiate between these neoplasms, hence a panel of antibodies is recommended to do the differential diagnosis. They are summarized in table 1 and 2.

- Fluorescent in situ hybridization (FISH) has permitted to differentiate between CHRCC and oncocytoma because the loss of chromosomes 2, 6, 10 or 17 support the diagnosis of the former and exclude the latter [22].

Table 1. Panel of usefull antibodies to differentiate CHCCR from oncocytoma

	Ck7	Parvalbumin	PAX2	Ck20	S100A1	CD15
Oncocytoma	- or +/-	+++ (47%)	+++	- or +(st)	+++	-
CHCCR	+++	+++	+++ or -(st)	-	-	+++

(+++: almost always positive staining) (+/-: weakly positive staining).
(st: sometimes) (-: negative staining).

Table 2. Panel of useful antibodies to differentiate CHCCR from CCRCC

	Ck7	RCC-Ag	CD10	Vimentin	CD117	Parvalbumin	E-Cadherin
CCRCC	-	+	+	+	-	-	-
CHRCC	+	-	-	-	+	+	+

(+: positive staining) (-: negative staining).

Molecular Genetic Studies

- Multiple losses of whole chromosomes Y, 1, 2, 6, 10, 13, 17 y 21 [22, 82, 88].
- Mutation of the tumor suppressor gene TP53 (minority of tumors). Does not seem to be a prognostic factor.
- The sarcomatoid variant has shown gains of multiple chromosomes (polysomy) 1, 2, 6, 10 and 17.
- Metastases have the same genetic abnormalities as its primary tumor [22].
- Those tumors associated with Birt-Hogg-Dubé syndrome have a point mutation in chromosome 17p11.2. This gene encodes folliculin protein, which is probably a tumor suppressor [89].

Prognosis

- Better prognosis than CCRCC because usually at diagnosis does not present metastases [22].
- Some authors point out as prognostic factors: tumor size, vascular invasion, sarcomatoid differentiation and macroscopic necrosis [90].
- Another study has demonstrated that only TNM stage and sarcomatoid differentiation provided significant prognostic information [91].
- Does not seem to exist differences between the classic variant of CHRCC and its eosinophilic variant [22].

HIBRID ONCOCYTIC CHROMOPHOBE TUMOR

Definition

- Renal neoplasia of mixed morphologies, with cells suggestive of oncocytoma and CHRCC in the same tumor [22].

Epidemiology

- This tumor occurs in three clinicopathologic situations:
  1. Renal oncocytosis (RO).

2. Birt-Hogg-Dubé syndrome.
3. Sporadic.

- ❖ In the three clinical settings adults are affected and do not have sex predilection.
- ❖ Renal oncocytosis occasionally occurs in long term hemodialysis patients.

Gross Findings

- ❖ Sporadic are solitary and unilateral tumors.
- ❖ Tumors in RO and Birt-Hogg-Dubé syndrome are often multiple and bilateral.
- ❖ Tumors are usually well circumscribed and non-encapsulated.
- ❖ Usually homogeneous tan to brown cut surface.
- ❖ Necrosis is not common.
- ❖ A central scar may be present [19, 22].

Histology

Sporadic

- ❖ Composed of cells arranged in solid-alveolar pattern.
- ❖ Nuclei showing mild nuclear pleomorphism.
- ❖ Abundant granular eosinophilic to oncocytic cytoplasm.
- ❖ Cells often have a perinuclear halo and are occasional binuclear.
- ❖ No raisinoid nuclei of the type seen in classic CHRCC are present.
- ❖ Usually cells resemble cells of RO with perinuclear cytoplasmic clearing.
- ❖ Small tubules may be present [19, 22].

Associated with RO

- ❖ Similar to sporadic tumors.
- ❖ Composed of sheets of cells separated by delicate blood vessels.
- ❖ Cells are round to polygonal with finely granular cytoplasm.
- ❖ Nuclei are pleomorphic and irregular with visible nucleoli.
- ❖ Raisinoid nuclei are not seen.
- ❖ Mitotic figures are infrequent [19, 22].

Associated with Birt-Hogg-Dubé Syndrome

- ❖ These types of tumors show three morphological patterns.
  - First: admixture of areas typical of RO and CHRCC.
  - Second: scattered chromophobe cells in the background of a typical RO.
  - Third: large eosinophilic cells with intracytoplasmic vacuoles.
- ❖ These tumors have pleomorphic cells and in contrast with the others, occasionally have raisinoid morphology [19, 92].

Immunohistochemistry

- ❖ Majority have a positive staining for: parvalbumin, antimitochondrial antigen and Ck7
- ❖ CD117 is always positive [19].

Differential Diagnosis

- Oncocytoma.
- CHRCC.
- Other tumors with oncocytic differentiation.

Molecular Genetic Studies

Sporadic

- These tumors have multiple monosomies and polysomies of chromosomes 1, 2, 6, 9, 10, 13, 17, 20, 21, and 22, with lack of mutations in the VHL, c-kit, PDGFRA (alpha-type platelet-derived growth factor receptor), and FLCN (folliculin) genes.
- Monosomy of chromosome 20 is the most frequent finding, and this is of importance as this is highly unusual for both RO and CHRCC [93].

Associated with RO

- These tumors have variable genetic profiles [19, 93, 94].
- The majority show no losses of chromosomes 1, 2, 6, 10, and 17; however, losses of chromosomes 1, 14, 21, and Y have been documented [95].

Associated with Birt-Hogg-Dubé Syndrome

- These tumors have a variable profile.
- Rarely, multiple abnormalities are seen in chromosomes 2, 3, 4, 5, 6, 13, and 18, although, to date, loss of chromosome 1 or translocation of 11q13 has not been reported.
- Loss of heterozygosity of 3p is rarely seen in this type of tumor.
- The most important molecular alteration seen in this group of tumors is an elevated expression of mitochondria and oxidative phosphorylation (OXPHOS)–associated genes and germline mutations in the FLCN gene [96, 97].

Prognosis

- Data indicates an indolent behavior.
- However, until new data become available, hybrid oncocytic chromophobe tumor should be treated as CHCCR [22].

CARCINOMA OF THE COLLECTING DUCTS OF BELLINI

Definition

- A renal cell carcinoma derived from collecting duct epithelium.

Epidemiology

- Less than 1% of all RCC.
- More than 200 cases have been reported.
- 6-87 years of age (mean age of 55 years) [20, 22].
- Male to female ratio 3:1 [98].

- Strong family history of various cancer types.
- Cases appear in horseshoe kidney, end-stage renal kidney (ESRD) and failed renal allografts [99].

Gross Findings

- 1-16 cm [98, 100].
- Indistinct borders.
- Gray white and firm.
- Necrosis.
- Satellite tumor nodules.
- Frequent involvement of the adrenal gland, perirenal fat, renal sinus fat, renal pelvis, Gerota fascia, renal vein, and/or regional lymph nodes.

Histology

- Complex tubulopapillary architecture.
- Cordlike areas.
- Microcystic with intracystic papillary proliferations of high-grade carcinoma.
- Stromal desmoplasia.
- Intratubular extension. Native ducts may show marked cytological atypia or carcinoma in situ.
- Always high nuclear grade with eosinophilic cytoplasm.
- Frequent mitosis.
- Hobnail appearance.
- Presence of extracellular or intracellular mucin deposition [101-103]
- 20% have involvement of renal vein [100].
- 16-36% have sarcomatoid differentiation [104-106].

Immunohistochemistry

- Positive for: Vimentin, PAX8 and Ulex Europaeus aglutinin-1 (UEA-1).
- < 50% positive for: Ck7, Ck20, Ck34βE12 and PAX2 [99].
- EMA and CD15 positivity is variable.
- Negative for: AMACR and CD10.

Differential Diagnosis

- Urothelial carcinoma: p63 positive/PAX8 negative [101].
- PRCC: Positive for CD10 and AMACR.
- Metastatic adenocarcinoma.

Molecular Genetic Studies

- Aneuploidy in a high percentage of tumors [107].
- LOH in 1q32, 6p, 8p, 13q, 21q and loss of Y, have been reported [53, 108-110].
- LOH in 3p was reported by some investigators [109, 111].
- 50% c-erbB-2 amplification [112].
- No distinctive molecular mechanism or pathway has been proposed [99].

Prognosis

- Normally diagnosed in advanced stage.
- 50% lymph node/distant metastases [98, 100].
- 2/3 died of cancer within 2 years [113].
- Mortality rates are as high as 83%.

RENAL MEDULLARY CARCINOMA

Definition

- An uncommon malignant epithelial neoplasm of highly aggressive behavior, which seems to have an origin in the terminal collecting ducts and their adjacent papillary epithelium [22].

Epidemiology

- Almost all cases are associated with sickle cell hemoglobinopathies (2% do not have this association).
- More than 100 patients have been described in the literature.
- Age range of presentation (5-58 years of age), mean age (20 years of age).
- Male to female ratio 2:1.
- Localized more frequently on the right kidney [22, 99].
- Almost exclusive of African descent. Less common in white patients (5%) [114].

Gross Findings

- Localized in the renal medulla.
- Variable in size. Mean diameter of 7 cm.
- Lobulated and poorly circumscribed.
- Firm to rubbery consistency.
- Tan to gray coloration.
- Often showed areas of hemorrhage and necrosis.
- Satellite nodules are usually present and also has perinephric and fat sinus infiltration [22, 115].

Histology

- Different type of patterns can be seen.
- The most characteristic is the reticular or microcystic pattern, giving the tumor an appearance similar to a yolk sac tumor [116].
- Other patterns: tubular growth, diffuse sheets and solid nodules.
- Pleomorphic cells with large nuclei and prominent nucleoli.
- Eosinophilic cytoplasm, in variable amounts.
- Cells sometimes adopt rhabdoid or squamous characteristics [117].
- Neutrophils are prominent in the transition zone between the tumor and the non-tumor renal parenchyma.
- The tumor induces an intense desmoplastic stromal reaction.
- Mucin production can be seen.

- In almost all histologic sections, the sickle erythrocytes are present [22].

Immunohistochemistry

- Positive staining for Vimentin, UEA-1, Ck7 and HMWCK, CEA, EMA, Ck20 and Ck8 [99, 118, 119].
- Generally positive for OCT 3/4 (this should be taken into account in the assessment of a poorly differentiated metastatic carcinoma because germinal tumors also have positive staining with OCT 3/4) [120].

Differential Diagnosis

- Carcinoma of the collecting ducts of Bellini (some authors point out this tumor as an aggressive variant of renal medullary carcinoma) [22].
- Papillary carcinoma of high grade.
- Urothelial carcinoma with renal parenchyma invasion.
- Metastases.

The clinical data, gross examination of the tumor, histology and immunohistochemistry should help in a definitive diagnosis of renal medullary carcinoma.

Molecular Genetic Studies

- Genetic abnormalities are different from those seen in CRCC and PRCC [22].
- Loss of expression of integrase interactor-1 (INI1), and hSNF5/SMARCB1/BAF47 (shared this profile with rhabdoid malignant tumor) [22, 121].
- The heterozygosity of SMARCG1 (tumor suppressor gene) has been described accompanied of lack of expression of SMARCB1 protein. This alteration may play an important role in the pathogenesis of renal medullary carcinoma [119, 121].

Prognosis

- Almost all patients debut with metastasis at diagnosis. This may explain the poor prognosis of this tumor.
- Long-term disease-free survival is rare. Mean survival of 19 weeks.
- Survival is quite longer in patients who underwent adjuvant therapy, but limited in duration.
- Even in those tumors with a complete response to adjuvant treatment, recurrence and death are very frequent [22, 122, 123].

MIT FAMILY TRANSLOCATION RENAL CELL CARCINOMA

Definition

- MiT family translocation renal cell carcinoma.
- Recognized as a new entity in 2004 [42].

Epidemiology

- 3% of all RCC [124].

- Most patients are younger than 50 years old.
- Male to female ratio 1:1.
- TFE3 rearrangements in 0.6% to 1.6% of adult renal cell carcinomas [125-127].

Gross Findings

- PRCC-TFE3: 3-4 cms. Fibrous pseudocapsule with calcification. Yellow or grey parenchyma.
- ASPL-TFE3: Well circumscribed but unencapsulated [128].

Histology

- PRCC-TFE3:
  - Papillary formations and nest surrounded by thin-walled capillary vessels. Alveolar appearance. Some nests have central lumina with fresh blood.
  - Foam cells are evident in a minority of papillae.
  - Psammoma bodies are isolated and often present.
  - Transitions between areas of nested and papillary architecture are sharply demarcated.
  - Tumor cells are polygonal, with sharply defined cell borders and with abundant clear, finely granular or eosinophilic cytoplasm. Fuhrman grade is 2 or 3.
  - Necrosis.
  - Mitotic activity is very limited.
- ASPL-TFE3:
  - Nested and pseudopapillary pattern.
  - Psammomatous calcifications.
  - Hyaline nodules.
  - Papillary structures lack foam cells and intracytoplasmic hemosiderin [129].
  - Epithelioid cells with well-defined cell borders and voluminous clear, granular or eosinophilic cytoplasm. Vesicular chromatin and single prominent nucleolus.
- Melanotic Xp11 translocation renal cell carcinoma:
  - Sheets and nests of polygonal epithelioid cells with clear or finely granular cytoplasm, containing melanin.

Immunohistochemistry

- Positive for: CD10, AMACR, RCC-Ag and TFE3.
- 50% focal positivity for EMA and Ck.
- Negative for: vimentin, CA IX and MiTF.
- 2/3 positivity for PAX2 and PAX8 [130].
- PRCC-TFE3: Positive for Cathepsin-K.
- ASPL-TFE3: Negative for Cathepsin-K [131].
- PSF-TFE3 and CLTC-TFE3: Positive for HMB45 and Melan A. Melanotic Xp11 translocation renal cancer [132-134].
- TFE3 is the most sensitive and specific. TFE3 immunostaining can show equivocal results; in such cases, a TFE3 break-apart FISH probe can be employed [135, 136].

Differential Diagnosis

- PRCC.
- CCRCC.

Molecular Genetic Studies

- Variety of chromosome translocations, all of which involve a breakpoint at Xp11.2 [134, 137, 138].
- PRCC-TFE3: t(X;1)(p11.2;q21).
- PSF-TFE3: t(X;1)(p11.2;p34).
- NonO-TFE3: inv(X)(p11; q12).
- CLTC-TFE3: t(X;17)(p11.2;q23).
- ASPL-TFE3: t(X;17)(p11.2;q25).
- Other fusions involving unknown genes have been reported [135].

Prognosis

- ASPL-TFE3 carcinoma is the most aggressive and has the worst prognosis [127].
- PRCC-TFE3 carcinoma has a uncertain prognosis, with late recurrences [137, 139].

T(6;11) ASSOCIATED RENAL CELL CARCINOMA

Definition

- MiT family translocation renal cell carcinoma.
- Distal nephron origin [140].

Epidemiology

- Fewer than 40 cases have been reported.
- 9-60 years (mean age of 17 years).

Gross Findings

- 2-12 cm.
- Pseudocapsule.
- Tan-yellow-brown color.
- Solid with focal cystic formations.
- Without necrosis.

Histology

- Solid and nested pattern.
- Predominant cell type is epithelioid with well-defined borders, abundant clear, finely granular or eosinophilic cytoplasm, and vesicular nuclei with prominent nucleoli.
- Second cell population (5% to 30% of the tumor), consisting of smaller cells with denser chromatin, clustered around nodules of hyaline basement membrane material (pseudorosettes).
- Mitotic figures are not apparent.

- Abortive papillae, brown pigmentations, psammomatous calcifications and well-formed tubules in the minority of cases.
- Areas of epithelioid angiomyolipoma-like [140].

Immunohistochemistry

- Positive for: Melan A, HMB45, Cathepsin-K, PAX8 and TFEB [141].
- CD10 positive focally [142].
- Negative for: EMA, Ck, RCC-Ag, s100 and TFE3 [142].
- TFEB break-apart FISH probe [140, 143].

Differential Diagnosis

- Epithelioid angiomyolipoma: Negative for PAX8.

Molecular Genetic Studies

- t(6,11)(p21;q12) translocation results in fusion of the 5´ portion of the alpha gene with the TFEB [140, 142-147].

Prognosis

- Less aggressive than tXp11 associated RCC [140, 143].

CARCINOMA ASSOCIATED WITH NEUROBLASTOMA

Definition

- A secondary renal carcinoma following treatment for neuroblastoma [22].

Epidemiology

- Affect patients with history of neuroblastoma treatment (chemotherapy, radiotherapy or both).
- The age range of presentation varied from 3 to 36 years old [22].

Gross Findings

- May be unilateral or bilateral and single or multiple.
- Size range from 1 to 8 cm.
- In multifocal neoplasm the tumors may be as small as 0.1 cm [22, 48].

Histology

- Cells are arranged in solid sheets or nests and in papillae.
- Occasional psammoma bodies are present.
- Tumor cells have sharply defined cell membranes and abundant eosinophilic granular cytoplasm.
- Small foci of cells with abundant reticular cytoplasm are present.
- Nuclei are medium sized and irregular, and have prominent nucleoli.
- Occasional mitotic figures are observed.

- Some cases have more prominent characteristics as high nuclear grade and diffuse parenchymal infiltration with desmoplastic reaction.
- Some cases have a "pseudosarcomatous" or "anaplastic" appearance [22].
- In recent years, tXp11 RCC and PRCC have been described in neuroblastoma survivors [48, 148].

Immunohistochemistry

- Positive staining for: EMA, CAM5.2 and patchy for vimentin.
- Inconsistent staining for: Ck8, Ck19 and Ck20.
- Negative staining for: S100, HMB45, Ck7 and Ck14 [22].

Molecular Genetic Studies

- Some researcher believed that these tumors have a genetic relationship or susceptibility.
- This hypothesis is supported by the finding that at least two patients with post-neuroblastoma renal cell carcinoma were never treated with chemotherapy or radiotherapy.
- Another finding that supported this hypothesis is the presence of similar genetic alterations in different tumors in patients with multiple neoplasms [22, 149].

Prognosis

- Due to the limited follow-up in this kind of tumors, it is difficult to make a conclusion concerning prognosis [22].
- Current data suggest that these neoplasms are minimally aggressive.
- Approximately one half of the patients were free of disease and even some patients with known metastases are reported to have stable disease after several years [150, 151].

MUCINOUS TUBULAR AND SPINDLE CELL CARCINOMA

Definition

- Mucinous tubular and spindle cell carcinoma (MTSCC) is a renal epithelial neoplasms with mucinous, tubular and spindle cell features.
- This tumor as first reported in 1997 under the name of "low-grade collecting duct carcinoma" and was included in the 2004 WHO classification [43, 152].

Epidemiology

- Mean age at the time of diagnosis was 53 years (range between 13 and 82 years) [22].
- The tumors occur predominantly in females with a male to female ratio of 1:4 [19].

Gross Findings

- From 2 to 12 cm.
- Well circumscribed tumors.

- Grey or light tan parenchyma.
- Sometimes with hemorrhage and/or necrosis.

Histology

- MTSCC is a very heterogeneous neoplasm.
- The histologic spectrum goes from: tubular appearance alone to spindle cell component alone. With intermediate tumors with different proportions of these two components.
- The tubular appearance shows: Small, elongated tubules separated by abundant mucinous stroma (Alcian blue positive). Cells are uniform, small, cuboidal or oval shaped and low-grade nuclear features (absent or inconspicuous nucleoli).
- The spindle cell appearance shows: Monotonous sheets of uniform cells with large eosinophilic cytoplasm (similar to spindle cell carcinomas o sarcomatoid carcinomas).
- MTSC can be spindle cell predominant or tubular predominant.
- Mitotic figures are rare.
- Occasionally you can see: areas of necrosis, foam cells, paucity of mucinous matrix (mucin poor MTSCC) [153], papillae (MSTCC with prominent papillary component) [154], clear cell change, oncocytic tubules, small vacuoles, psammomatous calcifications, heterotopic bone formation and chronic inflammation [1, 19, 22].

Immunohistochemistry

- Similar to PRCC
- Positive for: CAM 5.2, Ck7, Ck18, Ck19, and Ck34βE12.
- EMA, AMACR, vimentin, CD15, E-cadherin and weak for VHL (45%).
- Ki-67 <5%.
- Two cases with neuroendocrine differentiation: neuron-specific enolase (NSE), chromogranin and synaptophysin [155].
- Negative for: CD10, CD117, RCCAg, parvalbumin and Villin [1, 28].

Differential Diagnosis

- There is considerable overlap between the immunohistochemistry of MTSCC tumors and PRCC. Molecular alterations help making differential diagnosis. PRCC usually shows gains on chromosomes 7 and 17 and loss of Y, rarely seen in MTSCC. Some authors don't agree and conclude MTSC may be a subtype of PRCC [156].

Molecular Genetic Studies

- Different to PRCC.
- Losses involving chromosome 1, 4, 6, 8, 9, 11, 13, 14, 15, 18 and 22.
- Gains involving chromosome 2, 5, 7, 9, 10, 11, 12, 16, 17, 18, 19, 20, 21, 22 and X [157-159].

Prognosis

- MTSC is a low-grade entity [48].

- Usually are indolent with no tumor-related deaths and very rare metastasis, more frequent in patients with sarcomatoid change [160].

TUBULOCYSTIC RENAL CELL CARCINOMA

Definition

- Tumor subtype that was first considered a low-grade collecting duct carcinoma, but finally, clinical, pathological and molecular features pointed a different entity called tubulocystic carcinoma [152, 161-163].
- This entity is closely related to PRCC and sometimes may coexist with this neoplasm [164].
- Diagnosis must be restricted to tumors with macroscopic and microscopic features described below, if there are elements of PRCC or CDC admixed, this term should not be used.

Epidemiology

- More common in males (>7:1) [161].

Gross Findings

- Cortical (subcapsular) or cortico-medullary located.
- From 0.7-17 cm [22].
- Well circumscribed, encapsulated.
- Grossly cystic, white or gray parenchyma.
- No hemorrhage or necrosis [161].

Histology

- Tumor composed of small to medium size tubules, some of them cystically dilated ("bubble-wrap" appearance).
- Tubules are lined by a single layer of low cuboidal atypical cells with eosinophilic cytoplasm.
- Focally hobnail appearance.
- Nuclei enlarged and nucleoli (nuclear grade 1 or 2).
- Infrequent mitosis.
- No necrosis.
- Hypocellular stroma.
- Ultrastructural studies show features of proximal convoluted tubules and collecting ducts (short microvilli with a brush border configuration, complex cytoplasmic interdigitation) [22, 161, 162].

Immunohistochemistry

- Immunohistochemical studies show expression of proximal convoluted tubule-related markers: CD10 and AMACR.
- And collecting duct markers: Parvalbumin, Ck34βE12, and Ck19.

- Also positive for: Ck8, Ck18.
- Less frequent: Ck7, PAX2 and CA IX.

Differential Diagnosis

- Multilocular cystic renal cell carcinoma: Typically has lower Fuhrman grade nuclei and scattered cells will be seen within the intervening fibrous stroma [161].
- Cystic nephroma: Usually has larger cystic spaces and inconspicuous nucleoli.
- PRCC: Gene expression profiling data indicates tubulocystic renal cell carcinoma has different alterations [48].

Molecular Genetic Studies

- Gene expression profiling data indicates that tubulocystic carcinoma has unique molecular findings [161].
- Gains involving chromosomes: 7 and 17 [163].
- Loose of chromosome Y.

Prognosis

- They are indolent with less than 10% of metastasis and only one case with lymph node metastases, another with local recurrence, another with bone metastases and a fourth with bone and liver metastases who died of disease [51, 152, 161, 164, 165].

ACQUIRED CYSTIC DISEASE ASSOCIATED RENAL CELL CARCINOMA (ARCD-ASSOCIATED RCC)

Definition

- Most frequent epithelial tumor in ESRD kidneys, specifically in acquired renal cystic disease (ARCD) and with direct correlation on the duration of dialysis [48, 166].
- This tumor is only seen in patients with ESRD or ARCD.

Epidemiology

- Patients with ARCD have a risk 100 times higher than general population to develop carcinomas, with an incidence of 3-7% [166, 167].
- Young patients.
- Males [22].

Gross Findings

- Solitary or multifocal (50% of the cases).
- 20% bilateral.
- From 1 to 8 cm [22, 48].
- Well circumscribed masses with thick fibrous capsule.
- Some have calcified capsule.
- Often appear to arise within cysts.
- Tan to yellow parenchyma.
- Frequent hemorrhage and necrosis.

Histology

- ❖ RCCs associated to ESRD or ARCD may be the classic histologic types (CCRCC, PRCC, or CHRCC), but recently a unique subtype has been described: ARCD-associated RCC [166, 168-170].
- ❖ This subtype shows nodules arising in cyst walls or solid encapsulated masses separated from the cysts.
- ❖ It is composed of common growth patterns that can be combined: acinar, tubular, solid-alveolar, microcystic, macrocystic, papillary.
- ❖ Some tumors may have sarcomatoid or rhabdoid features [166, 171, 172].
- ❖ Tumor typically shows cribriform/sieve-like architecture because of the intra and/or intercellular microscopic cribriform lumina.
- ❖ 80% have intratumor calcium oxalate crystals [166, 169, 170, 173].
- ❖ Tumor cells have abundant eosinophilic granular cytoplasm. Round to oval nuclei, vesicular chromatin and prominent nucleoli.
- ❖ The background kidney shows numerous cysts, frequently unilocular, lined by large cells [22].

Immunohistochemistry

- ❖ Positive for: CkAE1/AE3, AMACR, CD10, RCC-Ag, CD57 and GST-α-glutathione S-Transferase.
- ❖ Negative or only focally positive for: Ck7 [19, 173-175].
- ❖ Non neoplastic renal parenchyma often contains cysts lined by large eosinophilic cells with similar immunophenotype to that of ARCD-associated RCC.

Molecular Genetic Studies

- ❖ Gains involving chromosomes 7 and/or 17 and 3. Sometimes Chr. 1, 2, 3, 6, 7, 16 and Y [175].
- ❖ Numeric abnormalities of chromosomes 3 and 16 (gains or loss) may be characteristic of ARCD-associated RCC [172, 176].
- ❖ Gains of chromosome 3 have been the more consistent findings [172, 175, 177, 178].

Prognosis

- ❖ Less aggressive than sporadic RCC.
- ❖ Indolent behavior as they are often diagnosed at a lower stage and have smaller size [179].
- ❖ Sarcomatoid morphology, metastases and death from cancer are infrequent but have been reported [166].

CLEAR CELL PAPILLARY (TUBULO-PAPILLARY) RENAL CELL CARCINOMA

Definition

- ❖ Origin in the distal convoluted tubule.
- ❖ Typically arising in end-stage kidneys. Tumors of this type are not restricted to a setting of ESRD [180].

Epidemiology

- 26-88 years of age (mean of age 60 years).
- Male to female ratio 1:1.

Gross Findings

- Small (mean diameter of 2 cm).
- Well circumscribed.
- Thin fibrous capsule.
- White tan to pale yellow.
- Cystic.
- Without haemorrhage or necrosis.

Histology

- Focal branching and small blunt papillae. Areas of a dense, compact arrangement of tubular structures.
- Nuclei aligned at the apical end of the cells. Clear cytoplasm and a low nuclear grade.
- Sarcomatoid change absent.
- Some cases show proliferation of smooth muscle bundles [20].

Immunohistochemistry

- Positive for: Ck7, K903, PAX8, CA IX, Ck34βE12 and BerEP4.
- Negative for: AMACR, CD10 and TFE3.

Differential Diagnosis

- Renal angiomyoadenomatous tumor (RAT): Studies suggest that RAT and TPRCC are two ends of a spectrum of a single nosologic entity [170, 181].
- CCRCC: Positive for CD10 and negative for CK7.
- PRCC: Positive for CD10 and AMACR.
- tXp11 associated RCC: Positive for TFE3.

Molecular Genetic Studies

- No alterations of chromosome 3p or the VHL gene.
- Rarely show low copy number gains of chromosome 7 or 17 and loss of Y [20].
- No specific characteristic genetic abnormality has been found.

Prognosis

- Stage T1.
- None have been reported to invade large vessels or perirenal fat.
- No patient has reportedly died or suffered recurrence of this neoplasm.

HEREDITARY LEIOMYOMATOSIS-ASSOCIATED RENAL CELL CARCINOMA

Definition

- An aggressive carcinoma which occur in the setting of hereditary leiomyomatosis and RCC syndrome [22].

Epidemiology

- Approximately 1/3 of patients with the syndrome will develop RCC.
- Patients who suffer of this syndrome will develop multiple cutaneous leimyomas, and female patients uterine leiomyomas and less frequently, uterine leiomyosarcoma [22].

Gross Findings

- Tumors are unilateral and solitary.
- Size range from 2.3 to 20 cm [19, 22].

Histology

- RCC arise in this syndrome have a papillary or tubulopapillary architecture.
- Some have a solid or cribriform pattern.
- Resemble sporadic type 2 papillary renal cell carcinoma, but actually is well known that it is a different entity.
- Large nucleus with prominent inclusion-like orangiophilic or eosinophilic nucleolus surrounded by a clear halo [19, 22].

Immunohistochemistry

- A recent study point out the 2-succino-cysteine (2SC) as a useful tool to differentiate the hereditary leiomyomatosis-associated renal cell carcinoma (HL-RCC) of others high grade neoplasm of the kidney [182].
- In this study 100% of HL-RCC stained with 2SC. In contrast 96% of unclassified high grade RCC and 78% of type 2 PRCC show no 2SC immunoreactivity [182].

Differential Diagnosis

- Sporadic type 2 PRCC.
- Others high grade RCC.

Molecular Genetic Studies

- These tumors occur in the setting of this autosomal dominant syndrome (HL-RCC) [19, 22].
- RCC and leiomyomas in the HL-RCC syndrome demonstrate biallelic inactivation of fumarate hydratase, with germline mutations in one allele and loss of the second allele, typical of a tumor-suppressor gene [19].
- The germline mutations occur in the fumarate hydratase gene at chromosome 1q42 [19, 22].
- Sporadic type 2 PRCC doesn´t have these mutations.

Prognosis

- Nowadays the prognosis is poor because these patients are diagnosed at an advanced stage of the disease, hence the importance of recognizing this entity.
- Patients with this syndrome (unlike patients with other hereditary RCC syndromes) may be followed closely for even small renal masses (<3 cm) and are taken to surgery early due to the highly aggressive nature of these neoplasms [19, 22].

RENAL CELL CARCINOMA UNCLASSIFIED (URCC)

Definition

- Aggressive form of RCCs that don´t fit in any of the accepted categories.

Epidemiology

- 0.7 to 5.7% of all RCC [42, 183, 184].

Gross Findings

- These tumors are generally large.

Histology

- Tumors in this category tend to be heterogeneous and high grade.
- They may be composed of:
  - Recognized types
  - Unrecognizable cell types
  - Entirely sarcomatoid morphology without recognizable epithelial elements
  - Rare mixtures of epithelial and stromal elements
- Mucin production.
- Usually exhibits high nuclear grade, necrosis and microvascular invasion [22, 184].

Immunohistochemistry

- There are no big series of Unclassified RCC, so immunohistochemical profile has not yet been defined, but we can make a few observations: Normally they have strong positive expression of p53, and partial expression of CD10 and Ck.
- They are negative for Ck7, chromogranin, AMACR, CD117, TFE3, EGFR (epidermal growth factor receptor), and MDM2 (mouse double minute 2 homolog).
- Vimentin expression is variable [22, 185, 186].

Molecular Genetic Studies

- Chromosomal losses were observed in chromosomes 1q22-23, 3p12-22, 5p30-ter, 6p, 11q, 16q18-22, 17p12-14, and 20p.
- Gains were observed in chromosomes 1p11-12, 1q12-13, 2q20-23, 3q22-23, 8p12, and 16q11-15.
- ABC (ATP-binding cassette) transporter pathway was associated with URCC [186].

Prognosis

- Heterogeneous category. Prognosis is influenced by the same clinical and histological features described in most of RCC [43, 183, 185, 187].

EMERGING PROVISIONAL ENTITIES

1) THYROID-LIKE FOLLICULAR RENAL CELL CARCINOMA

Definition

- Thyroid-like follicular renal cell carcinoma (TLF-RCC) is provisionally defined as a RCC resembling well-differentiated follicular carcinoma of the thyroid gland. Was first described in 2006 [188, 189].

Epidemiology

- Few cases reported.

Gross Findings

- From less than 4 cm to 12 cm.
- Well circumscribed.
- Encapsulated.
- Solid.
- Homogenous tan-brown.
- No necrosis or hemorrhage.

Histology

- Macro or micro-follicular pattern with dense colloid-like material (Tamm-Horsfall glycoprotein).
- No papillary architecture allowed for this diagnosis.
- Follicles lined by single layer of cuboidal to columnar cells with scant cytoplasm.
- Nuclei round and regular with enlarged nucleoli (nuclear grade 2 or 3).
- Intratumoral lymphocytic infiltration that may occasionally contain lymphoid follicles with reactive germinal centers.
- Absent mitotic activity [19, 22].

Immunohistochemistry

- Variable staining with Ck7, Ck19, vimentin, EMA, PAX2 and PAX8.
- Negative for thyroid transcription factor-1 (TTF1), thyroglobulin, HBME-1 and Galectin-3 (last two markers overexpressed in thyroid malignancies). And also negative for: WT-1, CD10, RCC-Ag, CEA and UEA-1 [188-190].

Differential Diagnosis

- Metastasis from follicular carcinoma of the thyroid which are positive for TTF1, thyroglobulin, HBME-1 and Galectin-3.

Molecular Genetic Studies

- Limited genetic studies have been performed in this neoplasm, so no distinctive pattern has been described.
- Using comparative genomic hybridization analysis, Jung et al. reported losses of chromosomes: 1, 3 and 9 and gains of chromosomes 7, 8, 12, 16, 17, 19, 20, 21, and X in their case [188].
- Using fluorescent in situ hybridization analysis, Sterlacci et al. found losses of chromosomes 1, 3, 7, 9, 12, 17, and X in this tumor [191].

Prognosis

- Generally good

2) ALK-TRANSLOCATION RENAL CELL CARCINOMA

Definition

- A malignant carcinoma characterized by translocations resulting in fusion of a variety of genes with the anaplastic lymphoma kinase (ALK) gene [22].

Epidemiology

- Few cases associated with the epidemiology have been described in literature [22].
- Two young patients with cytoskeletal protein vinculin (VCL)-ALK fusion (6-16 years old respectively), these cases were associated with sickle cell trait.
- Two older patients with (TPM3, EML4)-ALK fusion (36-53 years respectively), these cases were not associated with sickle cell trait [19].

Histology

- VCL-ALK (vinculin-anaplastic lymphoma kinase) fusion has shown polygonal to spindle cells with abundant eosinophilic cytoplasm and frequent intracytoplasmic lumina.
- In contrast, (TPM3, EML4)-ALK (tropomyosin alpha-3 chain echinoderm microtubule-associated protein-like *4*- Anaplastic Lymphoma Kinase Receptor) fusion have demonstrated papillary and unclassified histology.
- Two recent cases in adults were described by Mayo Clinic Group (fusion partner not determined). They have shown clear cells and papillary architecture [19].

Differential Diagnosis

- Renal Medullary Carcinoma

Molecular Genetic Studies

- Two cases harboring a t (2; 10) (p23; q22) translocation resulting in a fusion of the gene for the VCL with the ALK gene have been reported [19].
- A recent Japan study identifies two further renal cell carcinomas in adults associated with ALK fusions involving partner genes (TPM3, EML4) [19].

Prognosis

- The number of reported cases is too few to allow prognostication, although cases reported by Mayo Clinic Group were highly aggressive [19, 22].

3) SUCCINIC DEHYDROGENASE B DEFICIENCY-ASSOCIATED RENAL CELL CARCINOMA

Definition

- A recently described entity of RCC causes by a germline mutation in succinic dehydrogenase β (SDH-B) [22, 192].

Epidemiology

- 0.05-0.2% of all RCC [192].

Gross Findings

- Unencapsulated.
- Cystic.

Histopathology

- Compact nest or small tubules.
- Cuboidal cells with bubbly eosinophilic cytoplasm and indistinct cell borders.
- Within the cytoplasm it has vacuoles containing wispy eosinophilic material.
- The tumor is often surrounded by benign elements from the adjacent kidney.
- It has been reported two cases with atypical morphology [193].

Immunohistochemistry

- Positive for PAX8.
- Negative for SDH-B [193].

Genetic Features

- Different renal tumours may arise in patients with the pheocromocytoma-paraganglioma syndrome type [194, 195].

Prognosis

- Exceptionally good.

Conclusion

A correct diagnosis of renal cell carcinoma is the key to successful treatment. From the point of view of the pathologist, a correct report of these features provides the clinician key information about the prognosis and therapeutic alternatives in order to decide on the optimal management of kidney cancers.

In this chapter, the main pathological characteristics of the most frequent malignant epithelial neoplasms of the kidney have been presented, as well as those of provisional entities still not completely approved.

We have addressed some pathological features as the morphology, immunohistochemistry and special molecular characteristics of these tumors to provide a proper loco-regional stage and classification of the tumor. Therefore, the main characteristics of every tumor and their principal differential diagnosis has been described.

References

[1] Algaba, F., et al., Current pathology keys of renal cell carcinoma. *Eur. Urol.,* 2011. 60 (4): p. 634-43.

[2] Anglada Curado, F. J., et al., [New epidemiologic patterns and risk factors in renal cancer]. *Actas Urol. Esp.*, 2009. 33(5): p. 459-67.

[3] Zudaire Bergera, J. J., et al., [Renal cell carcinoma molecular biology. Prognostic and therapeutic usefulness]. *Arch. Esp. Urol.*, 2013. 66(1): p. 23-32.

[4] Lossos, C., et al., Association between non-Hodgkin lymphoma and renal cell carcinoma. *Leuk. Lymphoma*, 2011. 52(12): p. 2254-61.

[5] David, A. W., et al., Burkitt's lymphoma of the ileum with renal cell carcinoma. *Can. J. Surg.,* 2008. 51(4): p. E77-8.

[6] Baldewijns, M. M., et al., VHL and HIF signalling in renal cell carcinogenesis. *J. Pathol.*, 2010. 221(2): p. 125-38.

[7] Schultz, L., et al., Immunoexpression status and prognostic value of mTOR and hypoxia-induced pathway members in primary and metastatic clear cell renal cell carcinomas. *Am. J. Surg. Pathol.*, 2011. 35(10): p. 1549-56.

[8] Delahunt, B., et al., The International Society of Urological Pathology (ISUP) grading system for renal cell carcinoma and other prognostic parameters. *Am. J. Surg. Pathol.*, 2013. 37(10): p. 1490-504.

[9] Rioux-Leclercq, N., et al., [Renal tumors: The International Society of Urologic Pathology (ISUP) 2012 consensus conference recommendations]. *Ann. Pathol.*, 2014. 34(6): p. 448-61.

[10] Tan, P. H., et al., Renal tumors: diagnostic and prognostic biomarkers. *Am. J. Surg. Pathol.*, 2013. 37(10): p. 1518-31.

[11] Reuter, V. E., et al., Best practices recommendations in the application of immunohistochemistry in the kidney tumors: report from the International Society of Urologic Pathology consensus conference. *Am. J. Surg. Pathol.*, 2014. 38(8): p. e35-49.

[12] Rubio-Briones, J., et al., [Immunohistochemical expression of microvascular density and carbonic anhidrase IX in renal carcinoma. Relation to histological type and tumoral progression]. *Actas Urol. Esp.*, 2011. 35(2): p. 80-6.

[13] Pawlowski, R., et al., Loss of PBRM1 expression is associated with renal cell carcinoma progression. *Int. J. Cancer*, 2013. 132(2): p. E11-7.

[14] Iliopoulos, O., Molecular biology of renal cell cancer and the identification of therapeutic targets. *J. Clin. Oncol.*, 2006. 24(35): p. 5593-600.

[15] Kaelin, W. G., Jr., Treatment of kidney cancer: insights provided by the VHL tumor-suppressor protein. *Cancer*, 2009. 115(10 Suppl.): p. 2262-72.
[16] Rini, B. I. and M. B. Atkins, Resistance to targeted therapy in renal-cell carcinoma. *Lancet Oncol.*, 2009. 10(10): p. 992-1000.
[17] Mostofi, F. K., C. J. Davis and Springer Link (Online service), Histological Typing of Kidney Tumours In Collaboration with L. H. Sobin and Pathologists in 6 Countries, In: *WHO World Health Organization International Histological Classification of Tumours* 1998, Springer Berlin Heidelberg,: Berlin, Heidelberg. p. 1 online resource.
[18] Thoenes, W., S. Storkel and H. J. Rumpelt, Histopathology and classification of renal cell tumors (adenomas, oncocytomas and carcinomas). The basic cytological and histopathological elements and their use for diagnostics. *Pathol. Res. Pract.*, 1986. 181 (2): p. 125-43.
[19] Srigley, J. R., et al., The International Society of Urological Pathology (ISUP) Vancouver Classification of Renal Neoplasia. *Am. J. Surg. Pathol.*, 2013. 37(10): p. 1469-89.
[20] Zhou, M., G. J. Netto and J. I. Epstein, *Uropathology high-yield pathology*, 2012, Elsevier/Saunders,: Philadelphia. p. 1 online resource (xiv, 539 p.).
[21] Jemal, A., et al., Cancer statistics, 2007. *CA Cancer J. Clin.*, 2007. 57(1): p. 43-66.
[22] Bostwick, D. G. and L. Cheng, *Urologic surgical pathology*. Third ed. Copyright©2014, 2006, 1998 by Saunders, an imprint of Elsevier Inc, Chapter 2 pp. 74-156.
[23] Linehan, W. M., M. M. Walther and B. Zbar, The genetic basis of cancer of the kidney. *J. Urol.*, 2003. 170(6 Pt 1): p. 2163-72.
[24] Van Erp, F., et al., Chromosome 3 translocations and the risk to develop renal cell cancer: a Dutch intergroup study. *Genet. Couns.*, 2003. 14(2): p. 149-54.
[25] Vanharanta, S., et al., Early-onset renal cell carcinoma as a novel extraparaganglial component of SDHB-associated heritable paraganglioma. *Am. J. Hum. Genet.*, 2004. 74 (1): p. 153-9.
[26] Cheville, J. C., et al., Sarcomatoid renal cell carcinoma: an examination of underlying histologic subtype and an analysis of associations with patient outcome. *Am. J. Surg. Pathol.*, 2004. 28(4): p. 435-41.
[27] Kuhn, E., et al., Renal cell carcinoma associated with prominent angioleiomyoma-like proliferation: Report of 5 cases and review of the literature. *Am. J. Surg. Pathol.*, 2006. 30(11): p. 1372-81.
[28] Shen, S. S., et al., Role of immunohistochemistry in diagnosing renal neoplasms: when is it really useful? *Arch. Pathol. Lab. Med.*, 2012. 136(4): p. 410-7.
[29] Kovacs, G., et al., Specific chromosome aberration in human renal cell carcinoma. *Int. J. Cancer*, 1987. 40(2): p. 171-8.
[30] Yoshida, M. A., et al., Cytogenetic studies of tumor tissue from patients with nonfamilial renal cell carcinoma. *Cancer Res.*, 1986. 46(4 Pt 2): p. 2139-47.
[31] Anglard, P., et al., Molecular analysis of genetic changes in the origin and development of renal cell carcinoma. *Cancer Res.*, 1991. 51(4): p. 1071-7.
[32] Teyssier, J. R. and D. Ferre, Chromosomal changes in renal cell carcinoma. No evidence for correlation with clinical stage. *Cancer Genet. Cytogenet.*, 1990. 45(2): p. 197-205.

[33] Whaley, J. M., et al., Germ-line mutations in the von Hippel-Lindau tumor-suppressor gene are similar to somatic von Hippel-Lindau aberrations in sporadic renal cell carcinoma. *Am. J. Hum. Genet.*, 1994. 55(6): p. 1092-102.

[34] Gnarra, J. R., et al., Mutations of the VHL tumour suppressor gene in renal carcinoma. *Nat. Genet.*, 1994. 7(1): p. 85-90.

[35] Velickovic, M., et al., VHL and FHIT locus loss of heterozygosity is common in all renal cancer morphotypes but differs in pattern and prognostic significance. *Cancer Res.*, 2001. 61(12): p. 4815-9.

[36] Sukosd, F., et al., Deletion of chromosome 3p14.2-p25 involving the VHL and FHIT genes in conventional renal cell carcinoma. *Cancer Res.*, 2003. 63(2): p. 455-7.

[37] Schraml, P., et al., CDKNA2A mutation analysis, protein expression, and deletion mapping of chromosome 9p in conventional clear-cell renal carcinomas: evidence for a second tumor suppressor gene proximal to CDKN2A. *Am. J. Pathol.*, 2001. 158(2): p. 593-601.

[38] Beroud, C., et al., Correlations of allelic imbalance of chromosome 14 with adverse prognostic parameters in 148 renal cell carcinomas. *Genes Chromosomes Cancer*, 1996. 17(4): p. 215-24.

[39] Herbers, J., et al., Significance of chromosome arm 14q loss in nonpapillary renal cell carcinomas. *Genes Chromosomes Cancer*, 1997. 19(1): p. 29-35.

[40] Velickovic, M., et al., Intragenic PTEN/MMAC1 loss of heterozygosity in conventional (clear-cell) renal cell carcinoma is associated with poor patient prognosis. *Mod. Pathol.*, 2002. 15(5): p. 479-85.

[41] Eble, J. N. and S. M. Bonsib, Extensively cystic renal neoplasms: cystic nephroma, cystic partially differentiated nephroblastoma, multilocular cystic renal cell carcinoma, and cystic hamartoma of renal pelvis. *Semin. Diagn. Pathol.*, 1998. 15(1): p. 2-20.

[42] Eble, J. N., *Pathology and genetics of tumours of the urinary system and male genital organs*. 2004, Lyon: IARC Press; Oxford: Oxford University Press [distributor].

[43] Lopez-Beltran, A., et al., 2004 WHO classification of the renal tumors of the adults. *Eur. Urol.*, 2006. 49(5): p. 798-805.

[44] Montironi, R., et al., Update on selected renal cell tumors with clear cell features. With emphasis on multilocular cystic clear cell renal cell carcinoma. *Histol. Histopathol.*, 2013. 28(12): p. 1555-66.

[45] You, D., et al., Multilocular cystic renal cell carcinoma: clinicopathological features and preoperative prediction using multiphase computed tomography. *BJU Int.*, 2011. 108(9): p. 1444-9.

[46] Suzigan, S., et al., Multilocular cystic renal cell carcinoma : a report of 45 cases of a kidney tumor of low malignant potential. *Am. J. Clin. Pathol.*, 2006. 125(2): p. 217-22.

[47] Halat, S., et al., Multilocular cystic renal cell carcinoma is a subtype of clear cell renal cell carcinoma. *Mod. Pathol.*, 2010. 23(7): p. 931-6.

[48] Crumley, S. M., et al., Renal cell carcinoma: Evolving and emerging subtypes. *World J. Clin. Cases,* 2013. 1(9): p. 262-75.

[49] Williamson, S. R., et al., Multilocular cystic renal cell carcinoma: similarities and differences in immunoprofile compared with clear cell renal cell carcinoma. *Am. J. Surg. Pathol.*, 2012. 36(10): p. 1425-33.

[50] Williamson, S. R., et al., Cystic partially regressed clear cell renal cell carcinoma: a potential mimic of multilocular cystic renal cell carcinoma. *Histopathology*, 2013. 63 (6): p. 767-79.
[51] MacLennan, G. T. and L. Cheng, Tubulocystic carcinoma of the kidney. *J. Urol.*, 2011. 185(6): p. 2348-9.
[52] Stamatiou, K. N. and F. Sofras, Multilocular cystic nephroma and multicystic clear cell carcinoma: two faces of the Roman god Janus? *Int. J. Surg. Pathol.*, 2009. 17(2): p. 170-1.
[53] Chen, Y. B. and S. K. Tickoo, Spectrum of preneoplastic and neoplastic cystic lesions of the kidney. *Arch. Pathol. Lab. Med.*, 2012. 136(4): p. 400-9.
[54] Corica, F. A., et al., Cystic renal cell carcinoma is cured by resection: a study of 24 cases with long-term followup. *J. Urol.*, 1999. 161(2): p. 408-11.
[55] von Teichman, A., et al., VHL mutations and dysregulation of pVHL- and PTEN-controlled pathways in multilocular cystic renal cell carcinoma. *Mod. Pathol.*, 2011. 24 (4): p. 571-8.
[56] Verine, J., Re: Rodolfo Montironi, Antonio Lopez-Beltran, Liang Cheng, Marina Scarpelli. Re: Multilocular cystic renal cell carcinoma with focus on clinical and pathobiological aspects. *Eur. Urol.* 2013;63: 400-1. *Eur. Urol.*, 2013. 63(6): p. e72-3.
[57] Lohse, C. M., et al., Comparison of standardized and nonstandardized nuclear grade of renal cell carcinoma to predict outcome among 2,042 patients. *Am. J. Clin. Pathol.*, 2002. 118(6): p. 877-86.
[58] del Vecchio, M. T., et al., DNA ploidy pattern in papillary renal cell carcinoma. Correlation with clinicopathological parameters and survival. *Pathol. Res. Pract.*, 1998. 194(5): p. 325-33.
[59] Mydlo, J. H. and R. H. Bard, Analysis of papillary renal adenocarcinoma. *Urology*, 1987. 30(6): p. 529-34.
[60] Amin, M. B., et al., Papillary (chromophil) renal cell carcinoma: histomorphologic characteristics and evaluation of conventional pathologic prognostic parameters in 62 cases. *Am. J. Surg. Pathol.*, 1997. 21(6): p. 621-35.
[61] Mancilla-Jimenez, R., R. J. Stanley and R. A. Blath, Papillary renal cell carcinoma: a clinical, radiologic, and pathologic study of 34 cases. *Cancer*, 1976. 38(6): p. 2469-80.
[62] el-Naggar, A. K., J. Y. Ro and L. G. Ensign, Papillary renal cell carcinoma: clinical implication of DNA content analysis. *Hum. Pathol.*, 1993. 24(3): p. 316-21.
[63] Argani, P., G. J. Netto and A. V. Parwani, Papillary renal cell carcinoma with low-grade spindle cell foci: a mimic of mucinous tubular and spindle cell carcinoma. *Am. J. Surg. Pathol.*, 2008. 32(9): p. 1353-9.
[64] Cantley, R., P. Gattuso and D. Cimbaluk, Solid variant of papillary renal cell carcinoma with spindle cell and tubular components. *Arch. Pathol. Lab. Med.*, 2010. 134(8): p. 1210-4.
[65] Delahunt, B., et al., Morphologic typing of papillary renal cell carcinoma: comparison of growth kinetics and patient survival in 66 cases. *Hum. Pathol.*, 2001. 32(6): p. 590-5.
[66] Lubensky, I. A., et al., Hereditary and sporadic papillary renal carcinomas with c-met mutations share a distinct morphological phenotype. *Am. J. Pathol.*, 1999. 155(2): p. 517-26.
[67] Delahunt, B. and J. N. Eble, Papillary renal cell carcinoma: a clinicopathologic and immunohistochemical study of 105 tumors. *Mod. Pathol.*, 1997. 10(6): p. 537-44.

[68] Kunju, L. P., et al., Papillary renal cell carcinoma with oncocytic cells and nonoverlapping low grade nuclei: expanding the morphologic spectrum with emphasis on clinicopathologic, immunohistochemical and molecular features. *Hum. Pathol.*, 2008. 39(1): p. 96-101.
[69] Park, B. H., et al., Oncocytic papillary renal cell carcinoma with inverted nuclear pattern: distinct subtype with an indolent clinical course. *Pathol. Int.*, 2009. 59(3): p. 137-46.
[70] Zbar, B., et al., Hereditary papillary renal cell carcinoma. *J. Urol.*, 1994. 151(3): p. 561-6.
[71] Ornstein, D. K., et al., Prevalence of microscopic tumors in normal appearing renal parenchyma of patients with hereditary papillary renal cancer. *J. Urol.*, 2000. 163(2): p. 431-3.
[72] Fischer, J., et al., Duplication and overexpression of the mutant allele of the MET proto-oncogene in multiple hereditary papillary renal cell tumours. *Oncogene*, 1998. 17 (6): p. 733-9.
[73] Zhuang, Z., et al., Trisomy 7-harbouring non-random duplication of the mutant MET allele in hereditary papillary renal carcinomas. *Nat. Genet.*, 1998. 20(1): p. 66-9.
[74] Schmidt, L., et al., Two North American families with hereditary papillary renal carcinoma and identical novel mutations in the MET proto-oncogene. *Cancer Res.*, 1998. 58(8): p. 1719-22.
[75] Ramphal, R., et al., Pediatric renal cell carcinoma: clinical, pathologic, and molecular abnormalities associated with the members of the mit transcription factor family. *Am. J. Clin. Pathol.*, 2006. 126(3): p. 349-64.
[76] Kattar, M. M., et al., Clinicopathologic and interphase cytogenetic analysis of papillary (chromophilic) renal cell carcinoma. *Mod. Pathol.*, 1997. 10(11): p. 1143-50.
[77] Kovacs, G., et al., Cytogenetics of papillary renal cell tumors. *Genes Chromosomes Cancer*, 1991. 3(4): p. 249-55.
[78] Ishikawa, I. and G. Kovacs, High incidence of papillary renal cell tumours in patients on chronic haemodialysis. *Histopathology*, 1993. 22(2): p. 135-9.
[79] Storkel, S., et al., The human chromophobe cell renal carcinoma: its probable relation to intercalated cells of the collecting duct. *Virchows Arch. B Cell Pathol. Incl. Mol. Pathol.*, 1989. 56(4): p. 237-45.
[80] Moch, H., et al., Prognostic utility of the recently recommended histologic classification and revised TNM staging system of renal cell carcinoma: a Swiss experience with 588 tumors. *Cancer*, 2000. 89(3): p. 604-14.
[81] Akhtar, M., et al., Chromophobe cell carcinoma of the kidney. A clinicopathologic study of 21 cases. *Am. J. Surg. Pathol.*, 1995. 19(11): p. 1245-56.
[82] Thoenes, W., et al., Chromophobe cell renal carcinoma and its variants--a report on 32 cases. *J. Pathol.*, 1988. 155(4): p. 277-87.
[83] Abrahams, N. A., et al., Chromophobe renal cell carcinoma: a comparative study of histological, immunohistochemical and ultrastructural features using high throughput tissue microarray. *Histopathology*, 2004. 45(6): p. 593-602.
[84] Rocca, P. C., et al., Diagnostic utility of S100A1 expression in renal cell neoplasms: an immunohistochemical and quantitative RT-PCR study. *Mod. Pathol.*, 2007. 20(7): p. 722-8.

[85] Carvalho, J. C., et al., Cluster analysis of immunohistochemical profiles delineates CK7, vimentin, S100A1 and C-kit (CD117) as an optimal panel in the differential diagnosis of renal oncocytoma from its mimics. *Histopathology*, 2011. 58(2): p. 169-79.

[86] Memeo, L., et al., Immunohistochemical analysis for cytokeratin 7, KIT, and PAX2: value in the differential diagnosis of chromophobe cell carcinoma. *Am. J. Clin. Pathol.*, 2007. 127(2): p. 225-9.

[87] Adley, B. P., et al., Diagnostic value of cytokeratin 7 and parvalbumin in differentiating chromophobe renal cell carcinoma from renal oncocytoma. *Anal. Quant. Cytol. Histol.*, 2006. 28(4): p. 228-36.

[88] Brunelli, M., et al., Eosinophilic and classic chromophobe renal cell carcinomas have similar frequent losses of multiple chromosomes from among chromosomes 1, 2, 6, 10, and 17, and this pattern of genetic abnormality is not present in renal oncocytoma. *Mod. Pathol.*, 2005. 18(2): p. 161-9.

[89] Nickerson, M. L., et al., Mutations in a novel gene lead to kidney tumors, lung wall defects, and benign tumors of the hair follicle in patients with the Birt-Hogg-Dube syndrome. *Cancer Cell*, 2002. 2(2): p. 157-64.

[90] Przybycin, C. G., et al., Chromophobe renal cell carcinoma: a clinicopathologic study of 203 tumors in 200 patients with primary resection at a single institution. *Am. J. Surg. Pathol.*, 2011. 35(7): p. 962-70.

[91] Cheville, J. C., et al., Chromophobe renal cell carcinoma: the impact of tumor grade on outcome. *Am. J. Surg. Pathol.*, 2012. 36(6): p. 851-6.

[92] Murakami, T., et al., Identification and characterization of Birt-Hogg-Dube associated renal carcinoma. *J. Pathol.*, 2007. 211(5): p. 524-31.

[93] Petersson, F., et al., Sporadic hybrid oncocytic/chromophobe tumor of the kidney: a clinicopathologic, histomorphologic, immunohistochemical, ultrastructural, and molecular cytogenetic study of 14 cases. *Virchows Arch.*, 2010. 456(4): p. 355-65.

[94] Al-Saleem, T., et al., The genetics of renal oncocytosis: a possible model for neoplastic progression. *Cancer Genet. Cytogenet.*, 2004. 152(1): p. 23-8.

[95] Cossu-Rocca, P., et al., Interphase cytogenetic analysis with centromeric probes for chromosomes 1, 2, 6, 10, and 17 in 11 tumors from a patient with bilateral renal oncocytosis. *Mod. Pathol.*, 2008. 21(4): p. 498-504.

[96] Adley, B. P., et al., Birt-Hogg-Dube syndrome: clinicopathologic findings and genetic alterations. *Arch. Pathol. Lab. Med.*, 2006. 130(12): p. 1865-70.

[97] Pavlovich, C. P., et al., Renal tumors in the Birt-Hogg-Dube syndrome. *Am. J. Surg. Pathol.*, 2002. 26(12): p. 1542-52.

[98] Tokuda, N., et al., Collecting duct (Bellini duct) renal cell carcinoma: a nationwide survey in Japan. *J. Urol.*, 2006. 176(1): p. 40-3; discussion 43.

[99] Gupta, R., et al., Carcinoma of the collecting ducts of Bellini and renal medullary carcinoma: clinicopathologic analysis of 52 cases of rare aggressive subtypes of renal cell carcinoma with a focus on their interrelationship. *Am. J. Surg. Pathol.*, 2012. 36(9): p. 1265-78.

[100] Chao, D., et al., Collecting duct renal cell carcinoma: clinical study of a rare tumor. *J. Urol.*, 2002. 167(1): p. 71-4.

[101] Albadine, R., et al., PAX8 (+)/p63 (-) immunostaining pattern in renal collecting duct carcinoma (CDC): a useful immunoprofile in the differential diagnosis of CDC versus urothelial carcinoma of upper urinary tract. *Am. J. Surg. Pathol.*, 2010. 34(7): p. 965-9.

[102] Kennedy, S. M., et al., Collecting duct carcinoma of the kidney. *Hum. Pathol.*, 1990. 21 (4): p. 449-56.

[103] Halenda, G., et al., Atypical renal adenocarcinoma with features suggesting collecting duct origin and mimicking a mucinous adenocarcinoma. *Urology*, 1993. 41(2): p. 165-8.

[104] Baer, S. C., et al., Sarcomatoid collecting duct carcinoma: a clinicopathologic and immunohistochemical study of five cases. *Hum. Pathol.*, 1993. 24(9): p. 1017-22.

[105] de Peralta-Venturina, M., et al., Sarcomatoid differentiation in renal cell carcinoma: a study of 101 cases. *Am. J. Surg. Pathol.*, 2001. 25(3): p. 275-84.

[106] Carter, M. D., et al., Collecting duct carcinoma of the kidney: a case report and review of the literature. *J. Urol.*, 1992. 147(4): p. 1096-8.

[107] Dimopoulos, M. A., et al., Collecting duct carcinoma of the kidney. *Br. J. Urol.*, 1993. 71(4): p. 388-91.

[108] Schoenberg, M., et al., Frequent loss of chromosome arms 8p and 13q in collecting duct carcinoma (CDC) of the kidney. *Genes Chromosomes Cancer*, 1995. 12(1): p. 76-80.

[109] Hadaczek, P., et al., Losses at 3p common deletion sites in subtypes of kidney tumours: histopathological correlations. *Virchows Arch.*, 1996. 429(1): p. 37-42.

[110] Steiner, G. and D. Sidransky, Molecular differential diagnosis of renal carcinoma: from microscopes to microsatellites. *Am. J. Pathol.*, 1996. 149(6): p. 1791-5.

[111] Fogt, F., et al., Collecting duct carcinomas of the kidney: a comparative loss of heterozygosity study with clear cell renal cell carcinoma. *Oncol. Rep.*, 1998. 5(4): p. 923-6.

[112] Selli, C., et al., Retrospective evaluation of c-erbB-2 oncogene amplification using competitive PCR in collecting duct carcinoma of the kidney. *J. Urol.*, 1997. 158(1): p. 245-7.

[113] Srigley, J. R. and J. N. Eble, Collecting duct carcinoma of kidney. *Semin. Diagn. Pathol.*, 1998. 15(1): p. 54-67.

[114] Kalyanpur, A., et al., Renal medulla carcinoma in a white adolescent. *AJR Am. J. Roentgenol.*, 1997. 169(4): p. 1037-8.

[115] Simpson, L., et al., Renal medullary carcinoma and ABL gene amplification. *J. Urol.*, 2005. 173(6): p. 1883-8.

[116] Khan, A., et al., Renal medullary carcinoma: sonographic, computed tomography, magnetic resonance and angiographic findings. *Eur. J. Radiol.*, 2000. 35(1): p. 1-7.

[117] Selby, D. M., et al., Renal medullary carcinoma: can early diagnosis lead to long-term survival? *J. Urol.*, 2000. 163(4): p. 1238.

[118] Mathur, S. C. and A. M. Schwartz, Pathologic quiz case: a 33-year-old man with an abdominal mass. *Arch. Pathol. Lab. Med.*, 2000. 124(10): p. 1561-3.

[119] Liu, Q., et al., Renal medullary carcinoma: molecular, immunohistochemistry, and morphologic correlation. *Am. J. Surg. Pathol.*, 2013. 37(3): p. 368-74.

[120] Rao, P., N. M. Tannir and P. Tamboli, Expression of OCT3/4 in renal medullary carcinoma represents a potential diagnostic pitfall. *Am. J. Surg. Pathol.*, 2012. 36(4): p. 583-8.

[121] Cheng, J. X., et al., Renal medullary carcinoma: rhabdoid features and the absence of INI1 expression as markers of aggressive behavior. *Mod. Pathol.*, 2008. 21(6): p. 647-52.

[122] Pirich, L. M., P. Chou and D. O. Walterhouse, Prolonged survival of a patient with sickle cell trait and metastatic renal medullary carcinoma. *J. Pediatr. Hematol. Oncol.*, 1999. 21(1): p. 67-9.
[123] Stahlschmidt, J., et al., Renal medullary carcinoma: prolonged remission with chemotherapy, immunohistochemical characterisation and evidence of bcr/abl rearrangement. *Med. Pediatr. Oncol.*, 1999. 33(6): p. 551-7.
[124] Cao, Y., et al., Renal neoplasms in younger adults: analysis of 112 tumors from a single institution according to the new 2004 World Health Organization classification and 2002 American Joint Committee on Cancer Staging System. *Arch. Pathol. Lab. Med.*, 2005. 129(4): p. 487-91.
[125] Sukov, W. R., et al., TFE3 rearrangements in adult renal cell carcinoma: clinical and pathologic features with outcome in a large series of consecutively treated patients. *Am. J. Surg. Pathol.*, 2012. 36(5): p. 663-70.
[126] Macher-Goeppinger, S., et al., Molecular heterogeneity of TFE3 activation in renal cell carcinomas. *Mod. Pathol.*, 2012. 25(2): p. 308-15.
[127] Komai, Y., et al., Adult Xp11 translocation renal cell carcinoma diagnosed by cytogenetics and immunohistochemistry. *Clin. Cancer Res.*, 2009. 15(4): p. 1170-6.
[128] Argani, P., et al., Primary renal neoplasms with the ASPL-TFE3 gene fusion of alveolar soft part sarcoma: a distinctive tumor entity previously included among renal cell carcinomas of children and adolescents. *Am. J. Pathol.*, 2001. 159(1): p. 179-92.
[129] Renshaw, A. A., et al., Renal cell carcinomas in children and young adults: increased incidence of papillary architecture and unique subtypes. *Am. J. Surg. Pathol.*, 1999. 23 (7): p. 795-802.
[130] Argani, P., et al., Xp11 translocation renal cell carcinoma (RCC): extended immunohistochemical profile emphasizing novel RCC markers. *Am. J. Surg. Pathol.*, 2010. 34(9): p. 1295-303.
[131] Martignoni, G., et al., Differential expression of cathepsin K in neoplasms harboring TFE3 gene fusions. *Mod. Pathol.*, 2011. 24(10): p. 1313-9.
[132] Kovacs, G., et al., Cytogenetics of renal cell carcinomas associated with von Hippel-Lindau disease. *Genes Chromosomes Cancer*, 1991. 3(4): p. 256-62.
[133] Argani, P., et al., Melanotic Xp11 translocation renal cancers: a distinctive neoplasm with overlapping features of PEComa, carcinoma, and melanoma. *Am. J. Surg. Pathol.*, 2009. 33(4): p. 609-19.
[134] Chang, I. W., H. Y. Huang and M. T. Sung, Melanotic Xp11 translocation renal cancer: a case with PSF-TFE3 gene fusion and up-regulation of melanogenetic transcripts. *Am. J. Surg. Pathol.*, 2009. 33(12): p. 1894-901.
[135] Rao, Q., et al., TFE3 break-apart FISH has a higher sensitivity for Xp11.2 translocation-associated renal cell carcinoma compared with TFE3 or cathepsin K immunohistochemical staining alone: expanding the morphologic spectrum. *Am. J. Surg. Pathol.*, 2013. 37(6): p. 804-15.
[136] Zhong, M., et al., Dual-color, break-apart FISH assay on paraffin-embedded tissues as an adjunct to diagnosis of Xp11 translocation renal cell carcinoma and alveolar soft part sarcoma. *Am. J. Surg. Pathol.*, 2010. 34(6): p. 757-66.
[137] Argani, P. and M. Ladanyi, Translocation carcinomas of the kidney. *Clin. Lab. Med.*, 2005. 25(2): p. 363-78.

[138] Argani, P. and M. Ladanyi, The evolving story of renal translocation carcinomas. *Am. J. Clin. Pathol.*, 2006. 126(3): p. 332-4.

[139] Argani, P., et al., PRCC-TFE3 renal carcinomas: morphologic, immunohistochemical, ultrastructural, and molecular analysis of an entity associated with the t(X;1) (p11.2; q21). *Am. J. Surg. Pathol.*, 2002. 26(12): p. 1553-66.

[140] Rao, Q., et al., Renal cell carcinomas with t(6;11)(p21;q12): A clinicopathologic study emphasizing unusual morphology, novel alpha-TFEB gene fusion point, immunobiomarkers, and ultrastructural features, as well as detection of the gene fusion by fluorescence in situ hybridization. *Am. J. Surg. Pathol.*, 2012. 36(9): p. 1327-38.

[141] Smith, N. E., et al., t(6;11) renal cell carcinoma (RCC): expanded immunohistochemical profile emphasizing novel RCC markers and report of 10 new genetically confirmed cases. *Am. J. Surg. Pathol.*, 2014. 38(5): p. 604-14.

[142] Argani, P., et al., Renal carcinomas with the t(6;11)(p21;q12): clinicopathologic features and demonstration of the specific alpha-TFEB gene fusion by immunohistochemistry, RT-PCR, and DNA PCR. *Am. J. Surg. Pathol.,* 2005. 29(2): p. 230-40.

[143] Argani, P., et al., Molecular confirmation of t(6;11)(p21;q12) renal cell carcinoma in archival paraffin-embedded material using a break-apart TFEB FISH assay expands its clinicopathologic spectrum. *Am. J. Surg. Pathol.,* 2012. 36(10): p. 1516-26.

[144] Argani, P., et al., A distinctive pediatric renal neoplasm characterized by epithelioid morphology, basement membrane production, focal HMB45 immunoreactivity, and t(6;11)(p21.1;q12) chromosome translocation. *Am. J. Pathol.*, 2001. 158(6): p. 2089-96.

[145] Kuiper, R. P., et al., Upregulation of the transcription factor TFEB in t(6;11)(p21;q13)-positive renal cell carcinomas due to promoter substitution. *Hum. Mol. Genet.*, 2003. 12 (14): p. 1661-9.

[146] Petersson, F., et al., A distinctive translocation carcinoma of the kidney; "rosette forming," t(6;11), HMB45-positive renal tumor: a histomorphologic, immunohistochemical, ultrastructural, and molecular genetic study of 4 cases. *Hum. Pathol.*, 2012. 43(5): p. 726-36.

[147] Davis, I. J., et al., Cloning of an Alpha-TFEB fusion in renal tumors harboring the t(6;11)(p21;q13) chromosome translocation. *Proc. Natl. Acad. Sci. US*, 2003. 100(10): p. 6051-6.

[148] Hedgepeth, R. C., M. Zhou and J. Ross, Rapid development of metastatic Xp11 translocation renal cell carcinoma in a girl treated for neuroblastoma. *J. Pediatr. Hematol. Oncol.*, 2009. 31(8): p. 602-4.

[149] Medeiros, L. J., et al., Oncocytoid renal cell carcinoma after neuroblastoma: a report of four cases of a distinct clinicopathologic entity. *Am. J. Surg. Pathol.*, 1999. 23(7): p. 772-80.

[150] Koyle, M. A., et al., Long-term urological complications in survivors younger than 15 months of advanced stage abdominal neuroblastoma. *J. Urol.*, 2001. 166(4): p. 1455-8.

[151] Fleitz, J. M., et al., Renal cell carcinoma in long-term survivors of advanced stage neuroblastoma in early childhood. *Pediatr. Radiol.*, 2003. 33(8): p. 540-5.

[152] MacLennan, G. T., G. M. Farrow and D. G. Bostwick, Low-grade collecting duct carcinoma of the kidney: report of 13 cases of low-grade mucinous tubulocystic renal carcinoma of possible collecting duct origin. *Urology*, 1997. 50(5): p. 679-84.

[153] Fine, S. W., et al., Expanding the histologic spectrum of mucinous tubular and spindle cell carcinoma of the kidney. *Am. J. Surg. Pathol.*, 2006. 30(12): p. 1554-60.

[154] Alexiev, B. A., et al., Mucinous tubular and spindle cell carcinoma of the kidney with prominent papillary component, a non-classic morphologic variant. A histologic, immunohistochemical, electron microscopic and fluorescence in situ hybridization study. *Pathol. Res. Pract.*, 2014. 210(7): p. 454-8.

[155] Jung, S. J., et al., Mucinous tubular and spindle cell carcinoma of the kidney with neuroendocrine differentiation: report of two cases. *Am. J. Clin. Pathol.*, 2006. 125(1): p. 99-104.

[156] Shen, S. S., et al., Mucinous tubular and spindle cell carcinoma of kidney is probably a variant of papillary renal cell carcinoma with spindle cell features. *Ann. Diagn. Pathol.*, 2007. 11(1): p. 13-21.

[157] Rakozy, C., et al., Low-grade tubular-mucinous renal neoplasms: morphologic, immunohistochemical, and genetic features. *Mod. Pathol.*, 2002. 15(11): p. 1162-71.

[158] Ferlicot, S., et al., Mucinous tubular and spindle cell carcinoma: a report of 15 cases and a review of the literature. *Virchows Arch.*, 2005. 447(6): p. 978-83.

[159] Brandal, P., et al., Genomic aberrations in mucinous tubular and spindle cell renal cell carcinomas. *Mod. Pathol.*, 2006. 19(2): p. 186-94.

[160] Dhillon, J., et al., Mucinous tubular and spindle cell carcinoma of the kidney with sarcomatoid change. *Am. J. Surg. Pathol.*, 2009. 33(1): p. 44-9.

[161] Amin, M. B., et al., Tubulocystic carcinoma of the kidney: clinicopathologic analysis of 31 cases of a distinctive rare subtype of renal cell carcinoma. *Am. J. Surg. Pathol.*, 2009. 33(3): p. 384-92.

[162] Osunkoya, A. O., et al., Comparison of gene expression profiles in tubulocystic carcinoma and collecting duct carcinoma of the kidney. *Am. J. Surg. Pathol.*, 2009. 33 (7): p. 1103-6.

[163] Zhou, M., et al., Renal tubulocystic carcinoma is closely related to papillary renal cell carcinoma: implications for pathologic classification. *Am. J. Surg. Pathol.*, 2009. 33 (12): p. 1840-9.

[164] Yang, X. J., et al., Tubulocystic carcinoma of the kidney: clinicopathologic and molecular characterization. *Am. J. Surg. Pathol.*, 2008. 32(2): p. 177-87.

[165] Azoulay, S., et al., Tubulocystic carcinoma of the kidney: a new entity among renal tumors. *Virchows Arch.*, 2007. 451(5): p. 905-9.

[166] Tickoo, S. K., et al., Spectrum of epithelial neoplasms in end-stage renal disease: an experience from 66 tumor-bearing kidneys with emphasis on histologic patterns distinct from those in sporadic adult renal neoplasia. *Am. J. Surg. Pathol.*, 2006. 30(2): p. 141-53.

[167] Truong, L. D., et al., Renal neoplasm in acquired cystic kidney disease. *Am. J. Kidney Dis.*, 1995. 26(1): p. 1-12.

[168] Matson, M. A. and E. P. Cohen, Acquired cystic kidney disease: occurrence, prevalence, and renal cancers. *Medicine* (Baltimore), 1990. 69(4): p. 217-26.

[169] Rohan, S. M., et al., Clear-cell papillary renal cell carcinoma: molecular and immunohistochemical analysis with emphasis on the von Hippel-Lindau gene and hypoxia-inducible factor pathway-related proteins. *Mod. Pathol.*, 2011. 24(9): p. 1207-20.

[170] Aydin, H., et al., Clear cell tubulopapillary renal cell carcinoma: a study of 36 distinctive low-grade epithelial tumors of the kidney. *Am. J. Surg. Pathol.,* 2010. 34 (11): p. 1608-21.

[171] Srigley, J. R. and B. Delahunt, Uncommon and recently described renal carcinomas. *Mod. Pathol.*, 2009. 22 Suppl. 2: p. S2-S23.

[172] Kuroda, N., et al., Acquired cystic disease-associated renal cell carcinoma: an immunohistochemical and fluorescence in situ hybridization study. *Med. Mol. Morphol.*, 2011. 44(4): p. 228-32.

[173] Sule, N., et al., Calcium oxalate deposition in renal cell carcinoma associated with acquired cystic kidney disease: a comprehensive study. *Am. J. Surg. Pathol.*, 2005. 29 (4): p. 443-51.

[174] Cossu-Rocca, P., et al., Acquired cystic disease-associated renal tumors: an immunohistochemical and fluorescence in situ hybridization study. *Mod. Pathol.*, 2006. 19(6): p. 780-7.

[175] Pan, C. C., et al., Immunohistochemical and molecular genetic profiling of acquired cystic disease-associated renal cell carcinoma. *Histopathology*, 2009. 55(2): p. 145-53.

[176] Tajima, S., et al., Acquired cystic disease-associated renal cell carcinoma with a focal sarcomatoid component: Report of a case showing more pronounced polysomy of chromosomes 3 and 16 in the sarcomatoid component. *Pathol. Int.*, 2014.

[177] Kuntz, E., et al., Oligoarray comparative genomic hybridization of renal cell tumors that developed in patients with acquired cystic renal disease. *Hum. Pathol.*, 2010. 41(9): p. 1345-9.

[178] Kuroda, N., et al., Acquired cystic disease-associated renal cell carcinoma with sarcomatoid change and rhabdoid features. *Ann. Diagn. Pathol.,* 2011. 15(6): p. 462-6.

[179] Ishikawa, I., et al., Twenty-year follow-up of acquired renal cystic disease. *Clin. Nephrol.*, 2003. 59(3): p. 153-9.

[180] Alexiev, B. A. and C. B. Drachenberg, Clear cell papillary renal cell carcinoma: Incidence, morphological features, immunohistochemical profile, and biologic behavior: A single institution study. *Pathol. Res. Pract.*, 2014. 210(4): p. 234-41.

[181] Petersson, F., et al., Renal cell carcinoma with areas mimicking renal angiomyoadenomatous tumor/clear cell papillary renal cell carcinoma. *Hum. Pathol.*, 2013. 44(7): p. 1412-20.

[182] Chen, Y. B., et al., Hereditary leiomyomatosis and renal cell carcinoma syndrome-associated renal cancer: recognition of the syndrome by pathologic features and the utility of detecting aberrant succination by immunohistochemistry. *Am. J. Surg. Pathol.*, 2014. 38(5): p. 627-37.

[183] Karakiewicz, P. I., et al., Unclassified renal cell carcinoma: an analysis of 85 cases. *BJU Int.*, 2007. 100(4): p. 802-8.

[184] Lopez-Beltran, A., et al., Unclassified renal cell carcinoma: a report of 56 cases. *BJU Int.*, 2012. 110(6): p. 786-93.

[185] Zisman, A., et al., Unclassified renal cell carcinoma: clinical features and prognostic impact of a new histological subtype. *J. Urol.*, 2002. 168 (3): p. 950-5.

[186] Hu, Z. Y., et al., Unclassified renal cell carcinoma: a clinicopathological, comparative genomic hybridization, and whole-genome exon sequencing study. *Int. J. Clin. Exp. Pathol.*, 2014. 7(7): p. 3865-75.

[187] Skolarus, T. A., et al., The distribution of histological subtypes of renal tumors by decade of life using the 2004 WHO classification. *J. Urol.*, 2008. 179(2): p. 439-43; discussion 443-4.
[188] Jung, S. J., et al., Thyroid follicular carcinoma-like tumor of kidney: a case report with morphologic, immunohistochemical, and genetic analysis. *Am. J. Surg. Pathol.*, 2006. 30(3): p. 411-5.
[189] Amin, M. B., et al., Primary thyroid-like follicular carcinoma of the kidney: report of 6 cases of a histologically distinctive adult renal epithelial neoplasm. *Am. J. Surg. Pathol.*, 2009. 33(3): p. 393-400.
[190] Alessandrini, L., et al., Thyroid-like follicular carcinoma of the kidney: report of two cases with detailed immunohistochemical profile and literature review. *Virchows Arch.*, 2012. 461(3): p. 345-50.
[191] Sterlacci, W., et al., Thyroid follicular carcinoma-like renal tumor: a case report with morphologic, immunophenotypic, cytogenetic, and scintigraphic studies. *Virchows Arch.*, 2008. 452(1): p. 91-5.
[192] Gill, A. J., et al., Succinate Dehydrogenase (SDH)-deficient Renal Carcinoma: A Morphologically Distinct Entity: A Clinicopathologic Series of 36 Tumors From 27 Patients. *Am. J. Surg. Pathol.*, 2014. 38(12): p. 1588-602.
[193] Miettinen, M., et al., Mapping of succinate dehydrogenase losses in 2258 epithelial neoplasms. *Appl. Immunohistochem. Mol. Morphol.*, 2014. 22(1): p. 31-6.
[194] Gill, A. J., et al., Renal tumors associated with germline SDHB mutation show distinctive morphology. *Am. J. Surg. Pathol.*, 2011. 35(10): p. 1578-85.
[195] Ricketts, C. J., et al., Succinate dehydrogenase kidney cancer: an aggressive example of the Warburg effect in cancer. *J. Urol.*, 2012. 188 (6): p. 2063-71.

In: Renal Cell Carcinoma ISBN: 978-1-63482-495-8
Editors: J. M. Fernández-Gomez, J. García-Rodríguez

Chapter 3

Prognostic Factors and Predictive Tools in Localized and Advanced Renal Cancer

O. Rodriguez Faba, PhD, A. Breda, MD and J. Palou, PhD
Department of Urology, Fundació Puigvert, Barcelona, Spain

Abstract

The search for predictive and prognostic markers rises from the unpredictable biological behaviour of Renal Cell Carcinoma (RCC) in the localized, locally advanced and metastatic stages. The advances in the treatment of RCC over the last years have stimulated urologists to evaluate new predictive markers in order to clarify the selection of patients for optimal treatment. Classical prognostic factors in RCC include anatomical (TNM classification, tumor size), histological (Fuhrman grade, histologic subtype, sarcomatoid features, necrosis), clinical (symptoms and performance status), and molecular (CAIX, VEGF, B7-H1, Matrix Metalloproteinases). All these markers are not perfectly accurate when used alone. Therefore an increasing number of prognostic models or nomograms that include several combined prognostic factors have been designed in order to improve predictive accuracy. UCLA Integrated Staging System (UISS) and the Mayo Clinic's SSIGN score are the two most used prognostic models for localized RCC. In the setting of metastatic RCC, the drugs from the group of tyrosine kinase inhibitors have played a decisive role. The classical anatomical and histological tumor markers have little predictive value. However, accurate prognostic models have been designed to predict response to therapy, and progression-free and overall survival. So far, the Motzer and Heng models, grouping the prognostic factors, are the most commonly used in clinical practice.

1. Introduction

Renal cell carcinoma (RCC) represents one of the most important therapeutic challenges in oncology. It is predominantly refractory to treatment with traditional cytotoxic chemotherapies, and until recently, management options were limited to immunotherapy or palliative care. However, in the past few years we have experienced an important change in the treatment of advanced RCC with the introduction of targeted therapies that derive their efficacy at least in part through alterations in tumor angiogenesis. The tyrosine kinase inhibitors sunitinib, pazopanib, and sorafenib, the monoclonal antibody bevacizumab (in combination with interferon-α), and the rapamycin analogs, temsirolimus and everolimus, are now approved agents for the treatment of metastatic RCC [1].

Efforts to expand upon these successes include developing novel antiangiogenic agents, optimizing concomitant and sequential regimens, identifying predictors of response to specific treatments, and further dissecting the underlying molecular pathogenesis of RCC to reveal novel therapeutic targets. RCC remains one of the most lethal urologic tumours, with up to 40% of patients eventually dying of cancer progression [2].

Despite the advances in diagnosis staging and treatment a third of patients who undergo surgery with curative intent, will present recurrence [3]. Timely identification of recurrence is mandatory. Numerous studies have demonstrated that certain clinical, pathological and molecular factors, can improve the prediction of tumour recurrence [4]. The incorporation of these prognostic factors into stage-based stratification models should be better than stage alone in attempting to provide a rational approach to identify treatable recurrences and minimize unnecessary exams. Lastly molecular markers should in the near future improve surveillance protocols for RCC by tailoring follow-up to specific molecular classifications.

2. Anatomical Factors

The 5-year cancer specific survival for stage T3 locally advanced disease ranges from 37% to 67% [5]. In T3 stage tumour extends into major veins or directly invades adrenal gland or perinephric tissues but not into the ipsilateral adrenal gland and not beyond Gerota's fascia [6]. Perinephric and renal sinus fat invasion are classified as T3a RCC.

Nevertheless accumulating data suggest that renal sinus fat invasion carries a worse prognosis than perinephric fat invasion. Thompson et al. [7] reported that patients with sinus fat involvement were 1.6 times more likely to die compared with patients with perinephric invasion. In patients with stage T3b with renal vein involvement those with concomitant perirenal fat invasion presented worse prognosis than those without [8].

It has been shown that patients with adrenal involvement from direct extension appear to have similar outcomes to those of patients with T4 disease, being adrenal invasion an independent predictor for survival in non-metastatic RCC [9].

Lam et al., also reported that subclassify T3a according to size may have significant implications (patients with T3a tumors > 7 cm with fat involvement had significantly poorer survival compared with patients with T3a tumors ≤7 cm with fat involvement) [10]. Up to 10% of patients with RCC develop tumor thrombus involving the renal vein or vena cava [11].

Even with extensive surgery, the survival of patients with RCC and inferior vena cava thrombus is poor, with survival rates of 40–65% at 5 years, dropping to 0–17% in patients with metastases [12]. Wagner et al. did not find tumor thrombus level to be a predictive indicator of worse outcomes. Nevertheless, tumor size, fat invasion, lymph node invasion, and presence of metastasis were independent prognostic factors [13]. Papillary subtype has also recently been reported to present a worse prognosis in this subgroup of patients [14].

The overall risk of lymph node involvement is approximately 20%, and life expectancy decreases considerably when lymph node metastases are present with overall 5-year survival rates of 11% to 35% [15]. Patients with metastatic RCC face a poor prognosis, with a median survival of 6–10 months and a 2-year survival of 10–20% [16]. Distant metastases can present anywhere throughout the body, but most frequently involve the lungs and bone [16]. Patients with bone metastases have been shown to have a significantly shorter median survival compared to those without [17]. More recent data demonstrates that the number of metastatic sites of RCC rather than actual location dictates the overall prognosis [16].

3. Histopathological Factors

Fuhrman et al. [18] developed a four tier grading system based on nuclear and nucleolar size, shape, and content. Nuclear grade has been correlated with tumor stage, size, metastases, lymph node, vascular, and perirenal fat involvement. Despite criticisms to the reproducibility, it is the most widely used internationally assessing CSS survival rates of 89%, 65% and 46% for grades 1,2 and 3-4 respectively [19]. Subdividing the four grades into low grade (1-2) and high grade (3-4), interobserver and intraobserver variability is improved [20]. Among papillary RCC, two subgroups with different outcomes have been identified: Type 1 are low-grade tumours with a chromophilic cytoplasm and a favourable prognosis, type 2 are mostly high-grade tumours with an eosinophilic cytoplasm and a great propensity for developing metastases [21]. In chromophobe subtype, Fuhrman grade is often reported worse due to the presence of irregular nuclei and prominent nucleoli. In fact, some authors have adapted the classification for this subtype with the redefinition of three grades accepting that the more pleomorphic nuclear aspects in low grade correlates better with pT category [22, 23]. The question of whether different histological subtypes of RCC confer different survival outcomes remains controversial. According to the WHO classification [6], three major histological subtypes of RCC exist: Conventional (clear cell) (80-90%); Papillary (10-15%); and Chromophobe (4-5%). In univariate analysis, there is a trend towards a better prognosis for patients with chromophobe versus papillary versus conventional [24]. However, the prognostic information provided by the RCC subtype is lost when stratified to tumour stage [25]. A retrospective review of 2385 RCC patients treated by radical nephrectomy, demonstrated worse CSS for clear cell RCC compared to papillary or chromophobe, with 5-year CSS rates of 69%, 87%, and 87%, respectively [25]. Another international, multicenter study of 4063 RCC patients treated by surgical resection reported chromophobe subtype prognosis to be better than clear cell or papillary. Collecting duct carcinoma is an aggressive and rare variant accounting for less than 1% of tumors [24]. The sarcomatoid variant is not considered a distinct histological subtype [26].

It represents a relatively rare and high grade variant typified by a spindle cell growth pattern evident in less than 5% of RCC cases associated with a poor outcome [27]. Recently, Kim et al. [28] have reported that percentage of sarcomatoid component at 25% level is a predictive factor for recurrence and death in localized RCC. Tumor necrosis has been associated with markers of advanced disease. Lam et al. [29] reported in 310 patients with localized or metastatic disease that both, the presence and extent of histologic necrosis in tumor specimens were independent predictors of survival only in patients with localized disease. Furthermore, tumor necrosis was associated with markers of poor outcome including lymph node involvement, presence of distant metastases, greater tumor size, and higher grade [30]. Overall incidence of collecting system involvement is 14%. Tumors with collecting system involvement are associated with clear cell histology, higher grade, higher TNM stage, and larger size. Collecting system invasion in high stage tumors (≥T3) did not affect prognosis, whereas in low stage tumors (T1 and T2) was associated with poor prognosis with a median survival of only 46 months [31]. Incidence of MVI (microvascular invasion) in RCC has been reported to be 12–28% [32]. It was previously believed that MVI did not play a prognostic role in RCC. However, Van Poppel et al. [33] assessed in 180 patients with 4 years follow-up that 39.2% of patients with MVI presented disease progression compared to 6.2% of patients without MVI. Yildiz et al. [34] in a retrospective analysis of 54 specimens of RCC pT1-pT3 assessed that low MVD (microvascular density) and the presence of MVI appears to be a marker for identifying patients with an adverse prognosis (Table I).

4. Clinical Predictive Factors

It has been reported that approximately 20% of all patients diagnosed with RCC present with paraneoplastic symptoms.

Table 1. Clinical and pathological prognostic factors

Marker	Prognostic value
Nuclear grade	Independent predictor of poor prognosis
Histologic subtype	Type 2 papillary RCC associated with poorer prognosis compared type 1 papillary RCC. Chromophobe subtype associated with favorable prognosis
Sarcomatoid component	Associated with poor prognosis
Tumor necrosis	Presence and extent of histologic tumor necrosis associated with poorer prognosis
Collecting system invasion	Associated with poorer prognosis in low stage tumors (T1-2)
Microvascular invasion (MVI)	Associated with higher disease progression, recurrence, and death.
Paraneoplastic symptoms	Presence of cachexia-related findings portends poorer prognosis
Thrombocytosis	Independent predictor of poor prognosis
Elevated serum C-reactive protein (CPR) and erythrocyte sedimentation rate (ESR)	Associated with poorer prognosis

Another 10–40% of patients will develop paraneoplastic symptoms during the course of their disease [35]. Kim et al. [36] examined a cohort of 1046 patients with localized and metastatic RCC undergoing nephrectomy. Of the paraneoplastic symptoms examined, hypoalbuminemia, weight loss, anorexia and malaise were identified as predictors of poor prognosis that were independent of stage, grade and PS. Several studies have compared the prognostic significance of symptomatic presentation. When symptoms are grouped together, conclusions reveal no difference in prognosis for patients presenting with or without symptoms [37, 38]. Nevertheless, other authors have reported that symptomatic presentation predicts a worse prognosis [39]. These conflicting results suggest that specific signs and symptoms (cachexia related symptoms), and not simply the presence or absence, have a most accurate prognostic significance. ECOG-PS has demonstrated to be an independent prognostic factor of survival in patients with metastatic RCC at presentation with higher scores ($\geq$ 2) correlating with poorer survival [40]. Thrombocytosis (platelet count >400,000mm3) and Serum C-reactive protein (CRP) have been shown to be independent predictors of poor outcome in metastatic RCC treated with nephrectomy plus adjuvant therapy [41]. Patients with an elevated pre-treatment serum CRP ($\geq$1.0 ng/mL) who underwent surgery had a better prognosis compared to those who did not [42]. Furthermore, anaemia and Erythrocyte Sedimentation Rate (ESR) values >70mm at 2 h are also associated with a significantly poorer prognosis [43, 44] (Table I).

5. Molecular Factors

Molecular biomarkers may prove more effective for predicting survival than traditional clinical parameters such as tumor stage and grade [45]. Methods based on gene arrays, which screen for differential expression of thousands of genes, have identified large numbers of potential prognostic biomarkers [46].

These biomarkers require validation on larger patient populations, and validated biomarkers can be integrated into a multimarker prognostic system. The evaluation of protein expression in a high-throughput TMA is a natural extension to the efforts for molecular staging. Sections of the TMA provide targets for parallel in situ detection of DNA, RNA and protein in the same set of specimens, which can be correlated to clinical data with respect to disease progression, treatment response, and survival.

By better understanding the genetic alterations at the molecular level, clinicians will be able to tailor treatment. These tumor specific treatment plans will be more effective at targeting the genotypic alterations unique to each cancer with less systemic side effects.

Currently, there are a variety of molecular targets that have been identified to be important in RCC prognosis and specific therapies have been created to combat these alterations (Table II).

Carbonic Anhydrase IX

Carbonic anhydrase IX (CA IX) plays a role in the regulation of intracellular and extracellular pH during periods of hypoxia in tumor cells [47].

CA IX expression varies among different RCC subtypes and positive immunohistochemical staining has been shown in clear cell, granular, spindle, and papillary RCC, but is absent in chromophobe RCC and oncocytoma [48]. Bui et al. [49] reported the high specificity of CA IX. High CA IX expression is associated with a better prognosis in localised and metastatic RCC and low CA IX staining was found to be an independent prognostic indicator of survival in patients with metastatic RCC [50].

CA IX expression has also been combined with Ki67 (marker of cellular proliferation), to further stratify patients into low (high CA IX/low Ki67), intermediate (high Ki67 or low CA IX) and high-risk (high Ki67/low CA IX) groups to predict survival in RCC [51].

The association was a significant independent predictor of survival. CA IX expression in the peripheral blood has also been shown to be associated with decreased CSS [52].

Hypoxia-Inducible Factor (HIF)

HIF accumulates either in hypoxic cell conditions or when the pVHL gene is deficient [53]. Investigators showed a high percentage of HIF-expression regardless of VHL mutation status, and an equal or higher percentage of HIF-expression when analysis was restricted to the VHL-mutated subset [54].

Table 2. Molecular prognostic factors

Marker	Biological function	Prognostic value
CA IX.	Regulation of intra- and extra-cellular pH during hipoxia.	Low expression independent predictor of poor survival in clear cell RCC.
HIF	Up-regulates several genes to promote survival in low oxygen conditions.	High expression of HIF-1 is a favorable independent predictor of survival in clear cell RCC.
B7-H1	T-cell costimulatory molecule implicated as a potent negative regulator of antitumor immunity	High expression associated with adverse prognostic factors and poor survival.
B7-H4	Coregulatory ligand implicated as an inhibitor of T-cell-mediated immunity	Expression associated with adverse clinical and pathologic features, as well as poor survival.
p53	Tumor suppressor gene that regulates cell cycle and induces apoptosis when DNA damage occur.	Overexpression associated with poor survival. High expression independent predictor of recurrence.
bcl-2	Inhibits apoptosis.	Remains controversial
Survivin	Inhibits apoptosis.	High expression associated with poor survival.
Matrix metalloproteinases (MMP)	Zinc-dependent proteolytic enzymes capable to cleaving extracellular matrix components.	MMP-2 and MMP-9 affect malignant aggressiveness of RCC. Elevated MMP-7 independent predictor of poor survival.

HIF-expression was not detected in normal renal tissue, and non-clear cell RCC tumors were not found to have VHL mutations [55]. For clear cell RCC, increased HIF-1 expression was a favourable independent predictor of survival [56].

Von Hippel-Lindau Gene (VHL)

The Von Hippel-Lindau (VHL) gene was originally identified as a tumour suppressor gene on chromosome 3p isolated in deficient protein isoforms pVHL19 and pVHL30 [45]. Its absence, in the VHL familial tumour syndrome predisposes to retinal angiomas, central nervous system hemangioblastomas, pancreatic tumours, pheochromocytomas, and multiple bilateral clear cell RCC lesions [35]. VHL is inactivated in almost all patients with VHL syndrome and approximately 70% of sporadic clear cell RCC [53]. The presence of VHL alterations (mutation or hypermethylation) predicts longer progression-free survival and lower mortality for stage I–III clear cell RCC [57]. However, the survival rate of patients with VHL mutations was not different from patients without VHL mutations in other analyses [58].

Vascular Endothelial Growth Factor (VEGF)

Is a dimeric glycoprotein and a member of the platelet-derived growth factor [59]. VEGF affects tumour angiogenesis in both normal and pathologic conditions [35, 53]. In tumours, angiogenesis is induced by VEGF [59]. In clear cell RCC, the upregulation of VEGF mRNA is expected due to the dysregulation of HIF-1a as a result of the loss of VHL protein in addition to the hypoxic environment [59]. VEGF expression correlates with tumour size, Fuhrman grade, tumour necrosis, tumour stage, microvessel invasion, progression rate, and CSS [60].

p27

Regulates proliferation in the G1/S transition by modulating the action of cyclin-dependent kinases [53]. Migita et al. [61] examined the role of p27 in a cohort of 67 patients with clear cell RCC. Decreased p27 expression was associated with larger tumor size. Moreover, low p27 expression was found to be an independent predictor of poor disease specific survival (DSS) [62].

Phosphatase and Tensin Homologue Deleted on Chromosome 10 (PTEN)

PTEN is a tumor suppressor gene important in cell cycle regulation and apoptosis and is absent in many different types of tumors [53].

PTEN plays an important role in the phosphatidylinositol 3-kinase-protein kinase B-mammalian target of Rapamycin (PI3K-AKT-mTOR) signalling pathway [45].

Decreased PTEN expression has been reported to be an independent predictor of poor survival in patients with metastatic clear cell RCC [63].

B7-H1

B7-H1 is a cell surface glycoprotein that acts as a T-cell stimulatory molecule that has been implicated as a potent negative regulator of antitumor immunity by inducing T cell apoptosis, inhibiting cytokine production, and decreasing the cytotoxic effect of activated T-cells [35]. A high percentage of RCC metastases were shown to carry B7-H1 [64].

In an analysis of 306 patients who underwent nephrectomy for clear cell RCC, B7-H1 was associated with disease-specific death even after adjusting for TNM stage, grade, and PS [64].

B7-H4

Aberrant B7-H4 expression has also been reported in several tumours. Krambeck et al. [65] examined B7-H4 expression in 259 RCC specimens from patients treated with nephrectomy. B7-H4 expression was associated with adverse clinical and pathologic features, including constitutional symptoms, tumor necrosis, and advanced tumor size, stage, and grade. Patients with tumors expressing B7-H4 were also three times more likely to die from RCC compared with patients lacking B7-H4 [53].

p53

The tumor suppressor gene p53 plays a vital role in regulating the cell cycle and inducing apoptosis when DNA damage occurs [66]. Expression of p53 in RCC has been reported to be 16–57% [67].

Overexpression of p53 varies with histological subtype as is more frequently seen in papillary compared to chromophobe or clear cell RCC [68]. Zingeuner et al. [69] analyzed 184 primary and 56 metastatic RCC specimens and reported that overexpression of p53 was more frequently seen in metastatic specimens and was found to be an independent prognostic marker for disease progression for clear cell RCC.

Bcl-2

The bcl-2 gene encodes a survival protein that is known to inhibit of apoptosis [35]. Lee et al. [70] published a cohort of patients with stage T3 clear cell RCC that underwent nephrectomy and resection of metastases when needed. The immunohistochemical pattern of bcl-2 expression was observed to be either expressed at low levels or absent and expression of bcl-2 did not predict DFS or DSS. Nevertheless, metastases displayed much greater expression of bcl-2 and could serve as a future target of therapy.

Survivin

Survivin is an inhibitor of apoptosis that is expressed in a cell cycle dependent manner and is abundantly expressed in tumors of unfavorable histology [71].

Parker et al. [72] analyzed the association of survivin expression with disease progression and CSS. Patients who had high survivin expression levels were at significantly increased risk of death from RCC. In multivariate analysis, survivin expression remained associated with death from RCC even after adjusting for the ECOG-PS, TNM stage, grade, and the Mayo Clinic SSIGN score.

Matrix Metalloproteinases (MMPs)

The matrix metalloproteinase (MMP) family of enzymes is composed of critically important extracellular matrix remodelling proteases whose activity has been implicated in a number of key normal and pathologic processes. These functions include tumour growth, progression, and metastasis as well as the dysregulated angiogenesis associated with these events. As a result, these proteases have come to represent important therapeutic and diagnostic targets for the treatment and detection of human cancers [73]. In RCC, MMP-2 and MMP-9 were found to be overexpressed in 67–76% and 43% of tumours, respectively [74]. In addition, overexpression of MMP-2 and MMP-9 was more common in non–clear cell RCC tumours. MMP-2 and MMP-9 overexpression was associated with aggressive behaviour, tumour grade, and survival [75]. These associations are important because there are several synthetic (i.e., batimastat, marimastat) and natural (ie, bryostatins) MMP inhibitors that could help prevent and/or treat MMP-overexpressing cancers [76].

5. Predictive Nomograms

Many studies have aimed to integrate these independent prognostic indicators into comprehensive outcome models for both localized and metastatic RCC to assist urologist in facilitating patient counselling and identifying those patients who might benefit from adjuvant treatment [77]. The first report addressing this issue appeared in 1986 in which the factors predicting outcome for patients with metastatic RCC included PS, presence of pulmonary metastases, and metastatic-free interval [78]. Later, several groups have created similar models designed to include patients with localized and metastatic disease. Elson, et al. [79] presented an analysis of 610 patients with recurrent or metastatic RCC who were treated with chemotherapy. A scoring system was developed to stratify patients into 5 categories based on PS (0 to 1 vs. 2 to 3), time from initial diagnosis (>1 year vs. 1 year), number of metastatic sites, prior cytotoxic chemotherapy, and recent weight loss. Using this system, median survival times ranging from 2.1 to 12.8 months were observed across the five separate categories. Motzer, et al. [80] developed a model based on 670 patients with advanced RCC treated in 24 separate clinical trials at the Memorial Sloan-Kettering Cancer Center (MSKCC) including 394 patients treated with IFN-α or IL-2.

This model was created to define the relationship of pre-treatment clinical features and survival, which included the following risk factors: Low Karnofsky PS status, high serum LDH levels, low haemoglobin levels, hypercalcemia, and prior nephrectomy. The median survival rate was 10 months and significantly shorter survival occurred in patients with poor PS (Karnofsky scale <80%), high lactate dehydrogenase (>1.5 times the upper limit of normal), low haemoglobin, high-corrected calcium (>10 mg/dL), and absence of prior nephrectomy. Patients were stratified into favourable, intermediate, and poor risk groups according to the number of risk factors present. Patients at poor risk with 3 or more risk factors had a median survival of 4 months, whereas median survival improved to 20 months in those with no risk factors. Moreover, Motzer, et al. [81] reviewed 137 patients with metastatic RCC enrolled in clinical trials at MSKCC from 1990 onwards. The median overall survival rate for this group was 12.7 months. Independent predictors of worse survival rates were poor PS (Karnofsky scale <80%), low haemoglobin levels (less than or equal to 13 g/dL in males and 11.5 g/dL. in females), and elevated corrected serum calcium (≥10 mg/dL). The number of poor prognostic variables stratified patients into favourable risk (no risk factors), intermediate risk (one risk factor), and poor risk (two or three risk factors) groups. The favourable, intermediate, and poor risk groups demonstrated overall 1 and 3 years survival rates of 76% and 25%, 49% and 11%, and 11% and 0%, respectively. A study of 353 patients with previously untreated advanced RCC at the Cleveland Clinic was conducted to assess and validate the model proposed from MSKCC [82]. Four of five prognostic factors (time from diagnosis to entry into the study, serum lactate dehydrogenase, corrected serum calcium, and haemoglobin) identified by the MSKCC group were independent predictors of survival. In addition, prior radiotherapy and the presence of hepatic, lung, and retroperitoneal nodal metastases were found to be independent prognostic factors. Using the number of metastatic sites as surrogates for individual sites (none or one vs. two or three sites), the MSKCC definitions of risk groups were expanded to accommodate these two additional prognostic factors. Using this expanded criteria, favourable risk was defined as zero or one poor prognostic factor, intermediate-risk was defined as two poor prognostic factors, and poor-risk was defined as more than two poor prognostic factors.

The Kattan postoperative prognostic nomogram [39] was created to predict the probability of tumor recurrence within 5 years in patients undergoing a radical nephrectomy for RCC. The nomogram assigns numerical scores to various prognostic indicators that include presence of symptoms, histology, tumor size, and TNM staging criteria. In a study of 601 patients with RCC who were treated with a nephrectomy, the nomogram appeared accurate and discriminating with an area under the curve of 0.74. This nomogram was later modified to exclude histologic subtype and the analysis was limited to clear cell RCC [83].

The 5-year probability of freedom from recurrence for the patient cohort was 80.9%. This nomogram has a concordance index of 0.82 and external validation revealed it to be accurate and discriminating. The UCLA integrated staging system (UISS) is an extensive prognostic system that has been created for both localized and metastatic RCC [84].

The initial UISS contained 5 groups based on TNM stage, Fuhrman grade, and ECOG-PS all found to be independent predictors of survival. The two years survival rates and 5 years survival rates for patients in UISS Groups I through V were 96% and 94%, 89% and 67%, 66% and 39%, 42% and 23%, and 9% and 0%, respectively. The UISS was internally validated using a bootstrapping technique and an expanded database of patients treated at UCLA between 1989 and 2000 [85], external data from patients treated at MD Anderson

Cancer Center, patients treated in Nijmegen, Netherlands [86], and later with 4,202 patients from 8 international centers [5]. The Mayo Clinic created an extensive outcome prediction model for patients with clear cell RCC who are undergoing a radical nephrectomy [87]. According to an analysis of data from 1,801 patients, TNM stage, tumor size smaller than 5 cm, nuclear grade, and the presence of histological tumor necrosis were all found to be independent predictors of survival. Histologic necrosis is defined as any degree of microscopic tumor necrosis exclusive of degenerative changes such as hyalinization, hemorrhage, or fibrosis.

In the metastatic setting, it is well accepted that PS is a strong predictor for survival. Similarly, several studies have shown that cancer-related symptoms were independent prognostic parameters in localized RCC [88]. Based on symptoms at diagnosis, renal tumors were stratified into three groups: asymptomatic tumors (S1), tumors with isolated local symptoms (S2), and tumors with systemic symptoms (S3). The S classification appeared to predict cancer-specific survival independent of tumor stage and grade [89]. Karakiewicz, et al. [90] proposed a highly accurate (86.3%) prognostic nomogram that consisted of TNM stage, Fuhrman grade, tumor size, and symptom classification. External validation of the nomogram at 1, 2, 5, and 10 years after a nephrectomy revealed predictive accuracy of 87.8%, 89.2%, 86.7%, and 88.8%, respectively [91].

Furthermore, the Karakiewicz model provides accurate predictions that span a 10-year period after a nephrectomy, which exceeds the prognostic range of other models. Recently, Cindolo et al. [92] analyzed the accuracy and generalizability of the pre and postoperative Karakiewicz nomograms for predicting CSS. The study included 3231 patients between 1992 and 2010, and results suggested that the postoperative Karakiewicz nomogram discriminates substantially better than the preoperative one. Another recent validation by Zastrow et al. [93] has considered that the Karakiewicz model may overestimate CSS in high-risk patients, which should be kept in mind when counseling patients. A positive net benefit of nomogram predictions was proven. The presence of distant metastases at diagnosis substantially changes the prognosis of patients with RCC. Leibovich, et al. [94] reported that in patients with non-metastatic clear cell RCC who were treated with a radical nephrectomy, the median time to distant metastases was 1.3 years and of those who progressed to distant metastases, 77% died from RCC. Hutterer, et al. [95] developed a nomogram based on symptom classification and tumor size derived from a multi-institutional database. This nomogram was 85.2% accurate in predicting the individual probability of distant metastases in an external validation cohort and may assist in identifying patients at high risk of having metastatic RCC. The outcome of patients with RCC nodal metastases is substantially worse than that of patients with localized disease. Hutterer, et al. [96] also developed and externally validated a nomogram based on age, symptom classification, and tumor size that is accurate (78.4%) in predicting RCC nodal metastases in patients without radiographic evidence of distant metastases. This tool can help to risk adjust the need and the extent of nodal staging in patients without known distant metastases.

Heng et al. [97] developed a predictive model for overall survival (OS) in patients with metastatic renal cell carcinoma (RCC) treated with VEGF-targeted therapy. Four of the five adverse prognostic factors according to the Memorial Sloan-Kettering Cancer Center (MSKCC) were independent predictors of short survival: hemoglobin less than the lower limit of normal, corrected calcium greater than the upper limit of normal, Karnofsky performance status less than 80%, and time from diagnosis to treatment of less than 1 year.

In addition, neutrophils greater than the upper limit and platelets greater than the upper limit were independent adverse prognostic factors. Patients were segregated into three risk categories. Kwon et al. [98] studied 106 patients with metastatic renal cell carcinoma who were treated with sunitinib, to validate the MSKCC and Heng models.

Results revelaled that the MSKCC and Heng models were both valid models for predicting OS. The no nephrectomy, no hypertension at baseline, and high C-reactive protein levels were independently associated with poorer OS.

Conclusion

Over the last years, there has been a gradual transition from the use of solitary clinical factors as prognostic markers for patients with RCC to the introduction of systems that integrate multiple factors to the introduction of molecular and genetic markers with the goal of improving patient prognostication. The field of RCC is rapidly undergoing a revolution led by molecular biomarkers. The understanding of tumor biology gleaned from molecular biomarker research will be critical to the future treatment of patients with RCC.

References

[1] Heng, D. Y., Kollmannsberger, C., Chi, K. N.: Targeted therapy for metastatic renal cell carcinoma: current treatment and future directions. *Therapeutic advances in medical oncology* 2010, 2(1):39-49.

[2] Jemal, A., Siegel, R., Ward, E., Murray, T., Xu, J., Thun, M. J.: Cancer statistics, 2007. *CA Cancer J. Clin.* 2007, 57(1):43-66.

[3] Rabinovitch, R. A., Zelefsky, M. J., Gaynor, J. J., Fuks, Z.: Patterns of failure following surgical resection of renal cell carcinoma: implications for adjuvant local and systemic therapy. *Journal of clinical oncology: official journal of the American Society of Clinical Oncology* 1994, 12(1):206-212.

[4] Breda, A., Konijeti, R., Lam, J. S.: Patterns of recurrence and surveillance strategies for renal cell carcinoma following surgical resection. *Expert Rev. Anticancer Ther.* 2007, 7 (6):847-862.

[5] Patard, J. J., Kim, H. L., Lam, J. S., Dorey, F. J., Pantuck, A. J., Zisman, A., Ficarra, V., Han, K. R., Cindolo, L., De La Taille, A., et al.: Use of the University of California Los Angeles integrated staging system to predict survival in renal cell carcinoma: an international multicenter study. *Journal of clinical oncology: official journal of the American Society of Clinical Oncology* 2004, 22(16):3316-3322.

[6] Ljungberg, B., Cowan, N. C., Hanbury, D. C., Hora, M., Kuczyk, M. A., Merseburger, A. S., Patard, J. J., Mulders, P. F., Sinescu, I. C., European Association of Urology Guideline G: EAU guidelines on renal cell carcinoma: the 2010 update. *European urology* 2010, 58(3):398-406.

[7] Thompson, R. H., Leibovich, B. C., Cheville, J. C., Webster, W. S., Lohse, C. M., Kwon, E. D., Frank, I., Zincke, H., Blute, M. L.: Is renal sinus fat invasion the same as

perinephric fat invasion for pT3a renal cell carcinoma? *The Journal of urology* 2005, 174(4 Pt 1):1218-1221.

[8] Leibovich, B. C., Cheville, J. C., Lohse, C. M., Zincke, H., Kwon, E. D., Frank, I., Thompson, R. H., Blute, M. L.: Cancer specific survival for patients with pT3 renal cell carcinoma-can the 2002 primary tumor classification be improved? *The Journal of urology* 2005, 173(3):716-719.

[9] Thompson, R. H., Leibovich, B. C., Cheville, J. C., Lohse, C. M., Frank, I., Kwon, E. D., Zincke, H., Blute, M. L.: Should direct ipsilateral adrenal invasion from renal cell carcinoma be classified as pT3a? *The Journal of urology* 2005, 173(3):918-921.

[10] Lam, J. S., Klatte, T., Patard, J. J., Goel, R. H., Guille, F., Lobel, B., Abbou, C. C., De La Taille, A., Tostain, J., Cindolo, L., et al.: Prognostic relevance of tumour size in T3a renal cell carcinoma: a multicentre experience. *European urology* 2007, 52(1):155-162.

[11] Blute, M. L., Leibovich, B. C., Lohse, C. M., Cheville, J. C., Zincke, H.: The Mayo Clinic experience with surgical management, complications and outcome for patients with renal cell carcinoma and venous tumour thrombus. *BJU international* 2004, 94 (1):33-41.

[12] Lambert, E. H., Pierorazio, P. M., Shabsigh, A., Olsson, C. A., Benson, M. C., McKiernan, J. M.: Prognostic risk stratification and clinical outcomes in patients undergoing surgical treatment for renal cell carcinoma with vascular tumor thrombus. *Urology* 2007, 69(6):1054-1058.

[13] Wagner, B., Patard, J. J., Mejean, A., Bensalah, K., Verhoest, G., Zigeuner, R., Ficarra, V., Tostain, J., Mulders, P., Chautard, D., et al.: Prognostic value of renal vein and inferior vena cava involvement in renal cell carcinoma. *European urology* 2009, 55 (2):452-459.

[14] Tilki, D., Nguyen, H. G., Dall'Era, M. A., Bertini, R., Carballido, J. A., Chromecki, T., Ciancio, G., Daneshmand, S., Gontero, P., Gonzalez, J., et al.: Impact of histologic subtype on cancer-specific survival in patients with renal cell carcinoma and tumor thrombus. *European urology* 2014, 66(3):577-583.

[15] Pantuck, A. J., Zisman, A., Dorey, F., Chao, D. H., Han, K. R., Said, J., Gitlitz, B. J., Figlin, R. A., Belldegrun, A. S.: Renal cell carcinoma with retroperitoneal lymph nodes: role of lymph node dissection. *The Journal of urology* 2003, 169(6):2076-2083.

[16] Han, K. R., Pantuck, A. J., Bui, M. H., Shvarts, O., Freitas, D. G., Zisman, A., Leibovich, B. C., Dorey, F. J., Gitlitz, B. J., Figlin, R. A., et al.: Number of metastatic sites rather than location dictates overall survival of patients with node-negative metastatic renal cell carcinoma. *Urology* 2003, 61(2):314-319.

[17] Seaman, E., Goluboff, E. T., Ross, S., Sawczuk, I. S.: Association of radionuclide bone scan and serum alkaline phosphatase in patients with metastatic renal cell carcinoma. *Urology* 1996, 48(5):692-695.

[18] Fuhrman, S. A., Lasky, L. C., Limas, C.: Prognostic significance of morphologic parameters in renal cell carcinoma. *The American journal of surgical pathology* 1982, 6 (7):655-663.

[19] Scanga, L. R., Maygarden, S. J.: Utility of fine-needle aspiration and core biopsy with touch preparation in the diagnosis of renal lesions. *Cancer cytopathology* 2014, 122(3): 182-190.

[20] Bretheau, D., Lechevallier, E., de Fromont, M., Sault, M. C., Rampal, M., Coulange, C.: Prognostic value of nuclear grade of renal cell carcinoma. *Cancer* 1995, 76(12): 2543-2549.

[21] Delahunt, B., Eble, J. N., McCredie, M. R., Bethwaite, P. B., Stewart, J. H., Bilous, A. M.: Morphologic typing of papillary renal cell carcinoma: comparison of growth kinetics and patient survival in 66 cases. *Human pathology* 2001, 32(6):590-595.

[22] Steffens, S., Janssen, M., Roos, F. C., Becker, F., Steinestel, J., Abbas, M., Steinestel, K., Wegener, G., Siemer, S., Thuroff, J. W., et al.: The Fuhrman grading system has no prognostic value in patients with nonsarcomatoid chromophobe renal cell carcinoma. *Human pathology* 2014, 45(12):2411-2416.

[23] Pardo, P., Rodriguez-Faba, O., Palou, J., Algaba, F., Breda, A., Esquena, S., Villavicencio, H.: [Relevance of the clinical-pathological predictive factors in force in chromophobe renal cell cancer]. *Actas urologicas espanolas* 2012, 36(9):527-531.

[24] Patard, J. J., Leray, E., Rioux-Leclercq, N., Cindolo, L., Ficarra, V., Zisman, A., De La Taille, A., Tostain, J., Artibani, W., Abbou, C. C., et al.: Prognostic value of histologic subtypes in renal cell carcinoma: a multicenter experience. *Journal of clinical oncology: official journal of the American Society of Clinical Oncology* 2005, 23(12): 2763-2771.

[25] Cheville, J. C., Lohse, C. M., Zincke, H., Weaver, A. L., Blute, M. L.: Comparisons of outcome and prognostic features among histologic subtypes of renal cell carcinoma. *The American journal of surgical pathology* 2003, 27(5):612-624.

[26] Farrow, G. M., Harrison, E. G., Jr., Utz, D. C.: Sarcomas and sarcomatoid and mixed malignant tumors of the kidney in adults. 3. *Cancer* 1968, 22(3):556-563.

[27] Cangiano, T., Liao, J., Naitoh, J., Dorey, F., Figlin, R., Belldegrun, A.: Sarcomatoid renal cell carcinoma: biologic behavior, prognosis, and response to combined surgical resection and immunotherapy. *Journal of clinical oncology: official journal of the American Society of Clinical Oncology* 1999, 17(2):523-528.

[28] Kim, T., Zargar-Shoshtari, K., Dhillon, J., Lin, H. Y., Yue, B., Fishman, M., Sverrisson, E. F., Spiess, P. E., Gupta, S., Poch, M. A., et al.: Using Percentage of Sarcomatoid Differentiation as a Prognostic Factor in Renal Cell Carcinoma. *Clinical genitourinary cancer* 2014.

[29] Lam, J. S., Shvarts, O., Said, J. W., Pantuck, A. J., Seligson, D. B., Aldridge, M. E., Bui, M. H., Liu, X., Horvath, S., Figlin, R. A., et al.: Clinicopathologic and molecular correlations of necrosis in the primary tumor of patients with renal cell carcinoma. *Cancer* 2005, 103(12):2517-2525.

[30] Ito, K., Seguchi, K., Shimazaki, H., Takahashi, E., Tasaki, S., Kuroda, K., Sato, A., Asakuma, J., Horiguchi, A., Asano, T.: Tumor necrosis is a strong predictor for recurrence in patients with pathological T1a renal cell carcinoma. *Oncology letters* 2015, 9(1):125-130.

[31] Uzzo, R. G., Cherullo, E., Myles, J., Novick, A. C.: Renal cell carcinoma invading the urinary collecting system: implications for staging. *The Journal of urology* 2002, 167 (6):2392-2396.

[32] Goncalves, P. D., Srougi, M., Dall'lio, M. F., Leite, K. R., Ortiz, V., Hering, F.: Low clinical stage renal cell carcinoma: relevance of microvascular tumor invasion as a prognostic parameter. *The Journal of urology* 2004, 172(2):470-474.

[33] Van Poppel, H., Vandendriessche, H., Boel, K., Mertens, V., Goethuys, H., Haustermans, K., Van Damme, B., Baert, L.: Microscopic vascular invasion is the most relevant prognosticator after radical nephrectomy for clinically nonmetastatic renal cell carcinoma. *The Journal of urology* 1997, 158(1):45-49.

[34] Yildiz, E., Ayan, S., Goze, F., Gokce, G., Gultekin, E. Y.: Relation of microvessel density with microvascular invasion, metastasis and prognosis in renal cell carcinoma. *BJU international* 2008, 101(6):758-764.

[35] Lam, J. S., Klatte, T., Kim, H. L., Patard, J. J., Breda, A., Zisman, A., Pantuck, A. J., Figlin, R. A.: Prognostic factors and selection for clinical studies of patients with kidney cancer. *Crit. Rev. Oncol. Hematol.* 2008, 65(3):235-262.

[36] Kim, H. L., Belldegrun, A. S., Freitas, D. G., Bui, M. H., Han, K. R., Dorey, F. J., Figlin, R. A.: Paraneoplastic signs and symptoms of renal cell carcinoma: implications for prognosis. *The Journal of urology* 2003, 170(5):1742-1746.

[37] Jayson, M., Sanders, H.: Increased incidence of serendipitously discovered renal cell carcinoma. *Urology* 1998, 51(2):203-205.

[38] Schlomer, B., Figenshau, R. S., Yan, Y., Venkatesh, R., Bhayani, S. B.: Pathological features of renal neoplasms classified by size and symptomatology. *The Journal of urology* 2006, 176(4 Pt 1):1317-1320; discussion 1320.

[39] Kattan, M. W., Reuter, V., Motzer, R. J., Katz, J., Russo, P.: A postoperative prognostic nomogram for renal cell carcinoma. *The Journal of urology* 2001, 166(1):63-67.

[40] Hamada, S., Ito, K., Kuroda, K., Sato, A., Asakuma, J., Horiguchi, A., Seguchi, K., Asano, T.: Clinical characteristics and prognosis of patients with renal cell carcinoma and liver metastasis. *Molecular and clinical oncology* 2015, 3(1):63-68.

[41] Symbas, N. P., Townsend, M. F., El-Galley, R., Keane, T. E., Graham, S. D., Petros, J. A.: Poor prognosis associated with thrombocytosis in patients with renal cell carcinoma. *BJU international* 2000, 86(3):203-207.

[42] Dai, J., Tang, K., Xiao, W., Yu, G., Zeng, J., Li, W., Zhang, Y. Q., Xu, H., Chen, Z. Q., Ye, Z. Q.: Prognostic significance of C-reactive protein in urological cancers: a systematic review and meta-analysis. *Asian Pacific journal of cancer prevention: APJCP* 2014, 15(8):3369-3375.

[43] Choi, Y., Park, B., Kim, K., Jeong, B. C., Seo, S. I., Jeon, S. S., Choi, H. Y., Lee, J. E., Lee, H. M.: Erythrocyte sedimentation rate and anaemia are independent predictors of survival in patients with clear cell renal cell carcinoma. *British journal of cancer* 2013, 108(2):387-394.

[44] Lehmann, J., Retz, M., Nurnberg, N., Schnockel, U., Raffenberg, U., Krams, M., Kellner, U., Siemer, S., Weichert-Jacobsen, K., Stockle, M.: The superior prognostic value of humoral factors compared with molecular proliferation markers in renal cell carcinoma. *Cancer* 2004, 101(7):1552-1562.

[45] Lam, J. S., Leppert, J. T., Figlin, R. A., Belldegrun, A. S.: Role of molecular markers in the diagnosis and therapy of renal cell carcinoma. *Urology* 2005, 66(5 Suppl.):1-9.

[46] Kononen, J., Bubendorf, L., Kallioniemi, A., Barlund, M., Schraml, P., Leighton, S., Torhorst, J., Mihatsch, M. J., Sauter, G., Kallioniemi, O. P.: Tissue microarrays for high-throughput molecular profiling of tumor specimens. *Nature medicine* 1998, 4(7): 844-847.

[47] Takacova, M., Bartosova, M., Skvarkova, L., Zatovicova, M., Vidlickova, I., Csaderova, L., Barathova, M., Breza, J., Jr., Bujdak, P., Pastorek, J., et al.: Carbonic

anhydrase IX is a clinically significant tissue and serum biomarker associated with renal cell carcinoma. *Oncology letters* 2013, 5(1):191-197.

[48] Liao, S. Y., Aurelio, O. N., Jan, K., Zavada, J., Stanbridge, E. J.: Identification of the MN/CA9 protein as a reliable diagnostic biomarker of clear cell carcinoma of the kidney. *Cancer research* 1997, 57(14): 2827-2831.

[49] Bui, M. H., Seligson, D., Han, K. R., Pantuck, A. J., Dorey, F. J., Huang, Y., Horvath, S., Leibovich, B. C., Chopra, S., Liao, S. Y., et al.: Carbonic anhydrase IX is an independent predictor of survival in advanced renal clear cell carcinoma: implications for prognosis and therapy. *Clinical cancer research: an official journal of the American Association for Cancer Research* 2003, 9(2):802-811.

[50] Atkins, M., Regan, M., McDermott, D., Mier, J., Stanbridge, E., Youmans, A., Febbo, P., Upton, M., Lechpammer, M., Signoretti, S.: Carbonic anhydrase IX expression predicts outcome of interleukin 2 therapy for renal cancer. *Clinical cancer research: an official journal of the American Association for Cancer Research* 2005, 11(10):3714-3721.

[51] Bui, M. H., Visapaa, H., Seligson, D., Kim, H., Han, K. R., Huang, Y., Horvath, S., Stanbridge, E. J., Palotie, A., Figlin, R. A., et al.: Prognostic value of carbonic anhydrase IX and KI67 as predictors of survival for renal clear cell carcinoma. *The Journal of urology* 2004, 171(6 Pt 1): 2461-2466.

[52] Gilbert, S. M., Whitson, J. M., Mansukhani, M., Buttyan, R., Benson, M. C., Olsson, C. A., Sawczuk, I. S., McKiernan, J. M.: Detection of carbonic anhydrase-9 gene expression in peripheral blood cells predicts risk of disease recurrence in patients with renal cortical tumors. *Urology* 2006, 67(5):942-945.

[53] Sun, M., Shariat, S. F., Cheng, C., Ficarra, V., Murai, M., Oudard, S., Pantuck, A. J., Zigeuner, R., Karakiewicz, P. I.: Prognostic factors and predictive models in renal cell carcinoma: a contemporary review. *European urology* 2011, 60(4):644-661.

[54] Turner, K. J., Moore, J. W., Jones, A., Taylor, C. F., Cuthbert-Heavens, D., Han, C., Leek, R. D., Gatter, K. C., Maxwell, P. H., Ratcliffe, P. J., et al.: Expression of hypoxia-inducible factors in human renal cancer: relationship to angiogenesis and to the von Hippel-Lindau gene mutation. *Cancer research* 2002, 62(10):2957-2961.

[55] Wiesener, M. S., Munchenhagen, P. M., Berger, I., Morgan, N. V., Roigas, J., Schwiertz, A., Jurgensen, J. S., Gruber, G., Maxwell, P. H., Loning, S. A., et al.: Constitutive activation of hypoxia-inducible genes related to overexpression of hypoxia-inducible factor-1alpha in clear cell renal carcinomas. *Cancer research* 2001, 61(13):5215-5222.

[56] Lidgren, A., Hedberg, Y., Grankvist, K., Rasmuson, T., Bergh, A., Ljungberg, B.: Hypoxia-inducible factor 1alpha expression in renal cell carcinoma analyzed by tissue microarray. *European urology* 2006, 50(6):1272-1277.

[57] Yao, M., Yoshida, M., Kishida, T., Nakaigawa, N., Baba, M., Kobayashi, K., Miura, T., Moriyama, M., Nagashima, Y., Nakatani, Y., et al.: VHL tumor suppressor gene alterations associated with good prognosis in sporadic clear-cell renal carcinoma. *Journal of the National Cancer Institute* 2002, 94(20):1569-1575.

[58] Schraml, P., Struckmann, K., Hatz, F., Sonnet, S., Kully, C., Gasser, T., Sauter, G., Mihatsch, M. J., Moch, H.: VHL mutations and their correlation with tumour cell proliferation, microvessel density, and patient prognosis in clear cell renal cell carcinoma. *The Journal of pathology* 2002, 196(2):186-193.

[59] Song, S. H., Jeong, I. G., You, D., Hong, J. H., Hong, B., Song, C., Jung, W. Y., Cho, Y. M., Ahn, H., Kim, C. S.: VEGF/VEGFR2 and PDGF-B/PDGFR-beta expression in non-metastatic renal cell carcinoma: a retrospective study in 1,091 consecutive patients. *International journal of clinical and experimental pathology* 2014, 7(11):7681-7689.

[60] Rioux-Leclercq, N., Fergelot, P., Zerrouki, S., Leray, E., Jouan, F., Bellaud, P., Epstein, J. I., Patard, J. J.: Plasma level and tissue expression of vascular endothelial growth factor in renal cell carcinoma: a prospective study of 50 cases. *Human pathology* 2007, 38(10):1489-1495.

[61] Migita, T., Oda, Y., Naito, S., Tsuneyoshi, M.: Low expression of p27 (Kip1) is associated with tumor size and poor prognosis in patients with renal cell carcinoma. *Cancer* 2002, 94(4):973-979.

[62] Sgambato, A., Camerini, A., Genovese, G., De Luca, F., Viacava, P., Migaldi, M., Boninsegna, A., Cecchi, M., Sepich, C. A., Rossi, G., et al.: Loss of nuclear p27(kip1) and alpha-dystroglycan is a frequent event and is a strong predictor of poor outcome in renal cell carcinoma. *Cancer science* 2010, 101(9):2080-2086.

[63] Kim, H. L., Seligson, D., Liu, X., Janzen, N., Bui, M. H., Yu, H., Shi, T., Belldegrun, A. S., Horvath, S., Figlin, R. A.: Using tumor markers to predict the survival of patients with metastatic renal cell carcinoma. *The Journal of urology* 2005, 173(5):1496-1501.

[64] Thompson, R. H., Gillett, M. D., Cheville, J. C., Lohse, C. M., Dong, H., Webster, W. S., Chen, L., Zincke, H., Blute, M. L., Leibovich, B. C., et al.: Costimulatory molecule B7-H1 in primary and metastatic clear cell renal cell carcinoma. *Cancer* 2005, 104 (10): 2084-2091.

[65] Krambeck, A. E., Thompson, R. H., Dong, H., Lohse, C. M., Park, E. S., Kuntz, S. M., Leibovich, B. C., Blute, M. L., Cheville, J. C., Kwon, E. D.: B7-H4 expression in renal cell carcinoma and tumor vasculature: associations with cancer progression and survival. *Proceedings of the National Academy of Sciences of the United States of America* 2006, 103(27):10391-10396.

[66] Lane, D. P.: Cancer. p53, guardian of the genome. *Nature* 1992, 358(6381):15-16.

[67] Shvarts, O., Seligson, D., Lam, J., Shi, T., Horvath, S., Figlin, R., Belldegrun, A., Pantuck, A. J.: p53 is an independent predictor of tumor recurrence and progression after nephrectomy in patients with localized renal cell carcinoma. *The Journal of urology* 2005, 173(3):725-728.

[68] Vasavada, S. P., Novick, A. C., Williams, B. R.: P53, bcl-2, and Bax expression in renal cell carcinoma. *Urology* 1998, 51(6):1057-1061.

[69] Zigeuner, R., Ratschek, M., Rehak, P., Schips, L., Langner, C.: Value of p53 as a prognostic marker in histologic subtypes of renal cell carcinoma: a systematic analysis of primary and metastatic tumor tissue. *Urology* 2004, 63(4):651-655.

[70] Lee, C. T., Genega, E. M., Hutchinson, B., Fearn, P. A., Kattan, M. W., Russo, P., Reuter, V. E.: Conventional (clear cell) renal carcinoma metastases have greater bcl-2 expression than high-risk primary tumors. *Urologic oncology* 2003, 21(3):179-184.

[71] Takamizawa, S., Scott, D., Wen, J., Grundy, P., Bishop, W., Kimura, K., Sandler, A.: The survivin:fas ratio in pediatric renal tumors. *Journal of pediatric surgery* 2001, 36 (1):37-42.

[72] Parker, A. S., Kosari, F., Lohse, C. M., Houston Thompson, R., Kwon, E. D., Murphy, L., Riehle, D. L., Blute, M. L., Leibovich, B. C., Vasmatzis, G., et al.: High expression

levels of survivin protein independently predict a poor outcome for patients who undergo surgery for clear cell renal cell carcinoma. *Cancer* 2006, 107(1):37-45.

[73] Bonnans, C., Chou, J., Werb, Z.: Remodelling the extracellular matrix in development and disease. *Nature reviews Molecular cell biology* 2014, 15(12):786-801.

[74] Girgin, C., Tarhan, H., Hekimgil, M., Sezer, A., Gurel, G.: P53 mutations and other prognostic factors of renal cell carcinoma. *Urologia internationalis* 2001, 66(2):78-83.

[75] Kugler, A., Hemmerlein, B., Thelen, P., Kallerhoff, M., Radzun, H. J., Ringert, R. H.: Expression of metalloproteinase 2 and 9 and their inhibitors in renal cell carcinoma. *The Journal of urology* 1998, 160(5): 1914-1918.

[76] Curran, S., Murray, G. I.: Matrix metalloproteinases: molecular aspects of their roles in tumour invasion and metastasis. *European journal of cancer* 2000, 36(13 Spec. No): 1621-1630.

[77] Lam, J. S., Klatte, T., Breda, A.: Staging of renal cell carcinoma: Current concepts. *Indian journal of urology: IJU: journal of the Urological Society of India* 2009, 25(4): 446-454.

[78] Maldazys, J. D., deKernion, J. B.: Prognostic factors in metastatic renal carcinoma. *The Journal of urology* 1986, 136(2):376-379.

[79] Elson, P. J., Witte, R. S., Trump, D. L.: Prognostic factors for survival in patients with recurrent or metastatic renal cell carcinoma. *Cancer research* 1988, 48(24 Pt 1):7310-7313.

[80] Motzer, R. J., Mazumdar, M., Bacik, J., Berg, W., Amsterdam, A., Ferrara, J.: Survival and prognostic stratification of 670 patients with advanced renal cell carcinoma. *Journal of clinical oncology: official journal of the American Society of Clinical Oncology* 1999, 17(8):2530-2540.

[81] Motzer, R. J., Bacik, J., Schwartz, L. H., Reuter, V., Russo, P., Marion, S., Mazumdar, M.: Prognostic factors for survival in previously treated patients with metastatic renal cell carcinoma. *Journal of clinical oncology: official journal of the American Society of Clinical Oncology* 2004, 22(3):454-463.

[82] Mekhail, T. M., Abou-Jawde, R. M., Boumerhi, G., Malhi, S., Wood, L., Elson, P., Bukowski, R.: Validation and extension of the Memorial Sloan-Kettering prognostic factors model for survival in patients with previously untreated metastatic renal cell carcinoma. *Journal of clinical oncology: official journal of the American Society of Clinical Oncology* 2005, 23(4):832-841.

[83] Sorbellini, M., Kattan, M. W., Snyder, M. E., Reuter, V., Motzer, R., Goetzl, M., McKiernan, J., Russo, P.: A postoperative prognostic nomogram predicting recurrence for patients with conventional clear cell renal cell carcinoma. *The Journal of urology* 2005, 173(1):48-51.

[84] Zisman, A., Pantuck, A. J., Dorey, F., Said, J. W., Shvarts, O., Quintana, D., Gitlitz, B. J., deKernion, J. B., Figlin, R. A., Belldegrun, A. S.: Improved prognostication of renal cell carcinoma using an integrated staging system. *Journal of clinical oncology: official journal of the American Society of Clinical Oncology* 2001, 19(6):1649-1657.

[85] Zisman, A., Pantuck, A. J., Figlin, R. A., Belldegrun, A. S.: Validation of the ucla integrated staging system for patients with renal cell carcinoma. *Journal of clinical oncology: official journal of the American Society of Clinical Oncology* 2001, 19(17): 3792-3793.

[86] Han, K. R., Bleumer, I., Pantuck, A. J., Kim, H. L., Dorey, F. J., Janzen, N. K., Zisman, A., Dinney, C. P., Wood, C. G., Swanson, D. A., et al.: Validation of an integrated staging system toward improved prognostication of patients with localized renal cell carcinoma in an international population. *The Journal of urology* 2003, 170(6 Pt 1): 2221-2224.

[87] Frank, I., Blute, M. L., Cheville, J. C., Lohse, C. M., Weaver, A. L., Zincke, H.: An outcome prediction model for patients with clear cell renal cell carcinoma treated with radical nephrectomy based on tumor stage, size, grade and necrosis: the SSIGN score. *The Journal of urology* 2002, 168(6):2395-2400.

[88] Sengupta, S., Lohse, C. M., Leibovich, B. C., Frank, I., Thompson, R. H., Webster, W. S., Zincke, H., Blute, M. L., Cheville, J. C., Kwon, E. D.: Histologic coagulative tumor necrosis as a prognostic indicator of renal cell carcinoma aggressiveness. *Cancer* 2005, 104(3):511-520.

[89] Patard, J. J., Dorey, F. J., Cindolo, L., Ficarra, V., De La Taille, A., Tostain, J., Artibani, W., Abbou, C. C., Lobel, B., Chopin, D. K., et al.: Symptoms as well as tumor size provide prognostic information on patients with localized renal tumors. *The Journal of urology* 2004, 172(6 Pt 1):2167-2171.

[90] Karakiewicz, P. I., Briganti, A., Chun, F. K., Trinh, Q. D., Perrotte, P., Ficarra, V., Cindolo, L., De la Taille, A., Tostain, J., Mulders, P. F., et al.: Multi-institutional validation of a new renal cancer-specific survival nomogram. *Journal of clinical oncology: official journal of the American Society of Clinical Oncology* 2007, 25(11): 1316-1322.

[91] Gontero, P., Sun, M., Antonelli, A., Bertini, R., Carini, M., Carmignani, G., Longo, N., Martorana, G., Minervini, A., Mirone, V., et al.: External validation of the preoperative Karakiewicz nomogram in a large multicentre series of patients with renal cell carcinoma. *World journal of urology* 2013, 31(5):1285-1290.

[92] Cindolo, L., Chiodini, P., Brookman-May, S., De Cobelli, O., May, M., Squillacciotti, S., De Nunzio, C., Tubaro, A., Coman, I., Feciche, B., et al.: Assessing the accuracy and generalizability of the preoperative and postoperative Karakiewicz nomograms for renal cell carcinoma: results from a multicentre European and US study. *BJU international* 2013, 112(5):578-584.

[93] Zastrow, S., Brookman-May, S., Cong, T. A., Jurk, S., von Bar, I., Novotny, V., Wirth, M.: Decision curve analysis and external validation of the postoperative Karakiewicz nomogram for renal cell carcinoma based on a large single-center study cohort. *World journal of urology* 2014.

[94] Leibovich, B. C., Blute, M. L., Cheville, J. C., Lohse, C. M., Frank, I., Kwon, E. D., Weaver, A. L., Parker, A. S., Zincke, H.: Prediction of progression after radical nephrectomy for patients with clear cell renal cell carcinoma: a stratification tool for prospective clinical trials. *Cancer* 2003, 97(7):1663-1671.

[95] Hutterer, G. C., Patard, J. J., Jeldres, C., Perrotte, P., de La Taille, A., Salomon, L., Verhoest, G., Tostain, J., Cindolo, L., Ficarra, V., et al.: Patients with distant metastases from renal cell carcinoma can be accurately identified: external validation of a new nomogram. *BJU international* 2008, 101(1):39-43.

[96] Hutterer, G. C., Patard, J. J., Perrotte, P., Ionescu, C., de La Taille, A., Salomon, L., Verhoest, G., Tostain, J., Cindolo, L., Ficarra, V., et al.: Patients with renal cell carcinoma nodal metastases can be accurately identified: external validation of a new

nomogram. *International journal of cancer Journal international du cancer* 2007, 121 (11):2556-2561.

[97] Heng, D. Y., Xie, W., Regan, M. M., Warren, M. A., Golshayan, A. R., Sahi, C., Eigl, B. J., Ruether, J. D., Cheng, T., North, S., et al.: Prognostic factors for overall survival in patients with metastatic renal cell carcinoma treated with vascular endothelial growth factor-targeted agents: results from a large, multicenter study. *Journal of clinical oncology: official journal of the American Society of Clinical Oncology* 2009, 27(34): 5794-5799.

[98] Kwon, W. A., Cho, I. C., Yu, A., Nam, B. H., Joung, J. Y., Seo, H. K., Lee, K. H., Chung, J.: Validation of the MSKCC and Heng risk criteria models for predicting survival in patients with metastatic renal cell carcinoma treated with sunitinib. *Annals of surgical oncology* 2013, 20(13):4397-4404.

In: Renal Cell Carcinoma
Editors: J. M. Fernández-Gomez, J. García-Rodríguez
ISBN: 978-1-63482-495-8

Chapter 4

Advances in Imaging Studies for Diagnosis of Renal Carcinoma

A. Mesa, MD, R. Menendez-Llano, MD, A. Prieto, MD, and E. Nava, PhD*

Department of Radiology, University Hospital of Asturias, Oviedo, Spain

Abstract

Renal cell carcinoma (RCC) is the most common primary renal malignant neoplasm in adults, which constitutes 80 to 85 percent of primary renal neoplasms.

The past two decades have witnessed significant changes in the manifestations, diagnosis and management of renal cell carcinoma. With the widespread use of abdominal imaging modalities such as ultrasound (US), computed tomography (CT) and magnetic resonance imaging (MRI) performed for unrelated indications, as many as one-half of such carcinomas are discovered incidentally with a median tumor size of less than 5cm and in early-stage lesion. The diagnosis of renal masses, especially the incidentally detected ones, remains problematic.

Optimal images to assess a renal lesion (diagnosis, staging, treatment evaluation and follow up) involve a protocol-specified dedicated renal CT or MRI. CT is considered the modality of choice for detection and diagnosis of renal carcinoma. The advent of Multidetector CT (MDCT) has helped refine the diagnostic work-up of renal masses by allowing image acquisition in various phases of renal enhancement after intravenous administration of contrast material.

Currently, the Dual-energy CT is a promising new development in computed tomography that could improve lesion detection and characterization.

Other modalities, including ultrasound and PET, can also be utilized complimentarily.

Although ultrasonography is less sensitive than CT in detecting a renal mass, it is useful to distinguish a simple benign cyst from a more complex cyst or a solid tumor.

* Corresponding author: E. Nava PhD. Department of Radiology, University Hospital of Asturias, Avda. de Roma sn. 33011, Oviedo, Spain. E-mail: roengen97@gmail.com.

Ultrasound and cross-sectional imaging modalities complement each other in the characterization of renal lesion. In patients whose renal lesion is "indeterminate" on US a dedicated protocol CT or MRI may help characterize the lesion further. Conversely, US may prove useful for lesion that is considered "indeterminate" on CT.

The treatment of renal carcinoma depends on whether the disease is clinically localized or advanced at initial presentation. The TNM staging system correlates with prognosis and provides information for patient management. Surgery is curative in patients without metastatic renal carcinoma and is therefore the preferred treatment for them. For patients who are not surgical candidates, thermal ablation (radiofrequency ablation and cryotherapy) is an appropriate alternative to resection.

Additionally, tissue diagnosis provides information about the histopathological type of RCC, which may have important implications for prognosis and treatment. Although percutaneous needle biopsy of renal tumors has been reserved traditionally to selected cases, in recent years has increasing indications and can significantly contribute to manage these lesions.

The aim of this chapter is to provide an updated review of the role of imaging in the management of renal cell carcinoma.

Keywords: Rrenal cell carcinoma (RCC), kidney neoplasm, diagnosis, kidney neoplasm, CT, MR, renal carcinoma, radiofrequency ablation (RF)

1. Introduction

Renal cell carcinoma (RCC) is the most common cancer of the kidney. It constitutes up to 85-90% of all malignant renal tumors in adults and 1-3% of adult malignancies [1], with 65000 new cases in the United States in 2013 [2]. There is a 1.5:1 gender predominance of new cases diagnosed in men over women [3]. The median age of onset is in the mid-60s [4], and generally above the fifth decade of life. The management of the disease has improved in the last years due to recent advances in different medical fields such as imaging, pathology, urology and oncology which facilitate early diagnosis.

Accordingly, RCC incidence is gradually increasing [5] and it is noted that up to 70% of solid renal cortical masses are detected incidentally on imaging studies [6]. RCC is now considered a clinical and pathologically heterogeneous disease.

Its classification distinguishes: Clear Cell (70%), Papillary (10-15%), Chromophobe (4-6%), and minor subtypes as renal hereditary [7].

Lifestyle factors such as smoking, hypertension and obesity have been found to be etiologically related to this cancer. Nevertheless, RCC can be found associated to different hereditary conditions: Von Hippel-Lindau disease, syndrome of hereditary papillary RCC, Birt Hogg Dube syndrome, hereditary leiomyomatosis, tuberous sclerosis, and constitutional chromosome 3 translocation [8].

In order to develop an appropriate management of the disease an accurate staging is mandatory. TNM classification is utilized for formal staging and was updated in 2010. Furthermore, staging imaging has gained prominence in assessment of therapy response and postoperative outcome [9].

Due to recent advances, the therapeutical approach includes different options such as open or laparoscopic radical or partial nephrectomy, percutaneous image-guided ablative procedures (radiofrequency ablation and cryoablation) and biopsy of the mass for further evaluation or imaging surveillance [10, 11].

Multiple detectors computed tomography (MDCT) is the best technique for characterizing and staging renal lesion, although it lacks of accurate discrimination between benign and malignant solid renal lesions. MRI is a valuable diagnostic tool in further characterization of renal lesions masses [9].

Dual Energy MDCT offers an improvement of the diagnosis of renal tumors, by representing a potential shift from a merely attenuation-based to a material-specific spectral imaging investigation [12].

Nevertheless, great advances have been developed in recent years, including intraoperative and ultrasonography-guided biopsy [13].

2. Diagnosis

An annual increase of 2% in the incidence of RCC has been observed throughout the past two decades both in Europe and North America [3]. As mentioned previously, this fact results from the increased incidental detection of renal lesions in asymptomatic patients who undergo abdominal imaging due to several conditions unrelated with the disease [14].

Most of these incidentally detected tumors are small lesion (<4 cm) and are first detected by abdominal ultrasound, albeit in presence of solid or complex cystic lesions an accurate assessment of the mass by CT or MRI is needed.

Percutaneous renal tumors biopsies are increasingly being used in order to establish the diagnosis of indeterminate renal masses by CT or MRI, to obtain histology in patients who are not candidates for surgical treatment, and to set the most suitable targeted therapy for metastatic renal tumor.

2.1. Ultrasound

Ultrasound (US) represents a first-line imaging technique in the assessment of the kidney. Its advantages over the other imaging techniques are well known and comprise low cost, portability, availability, lack of restrictions in performing frequent serial examinations at short intervals, and absence of exposure to radiation or nuclear tracers.

Operator dependence and technical limitations, depending on patient body habit and bowel gas, may hamper US utility for focusing small renal lesions. Moreover, limitations of the assessment of retroperitoneum and renal vasculature may difficult the accurate staging [15, 16].

Ultrasound can differentiate a renal mass as cystic or solid showing particular utility in the characterization of minimally complicated cysts to rule out a cystic tumor.

The renal cyst is the most common renal lesion incidentally found at US. They frequently present a simple cystic pattern at US being any further imaging investigations or surgical procedures unnecessary. However, a complex cyst pattern can occasionally be observed and the malignant potential should be established according to the number and thickness of intracystic septations, presence of mural nodules and thick nodular calcifications [13-19]. In detail, a thickened cystic wall (>2 mm), numerous septations, thickened (>2 mm) or nodular septations, irregular or central calcifications, and the presence of flow in the septations or cystic wall on Doppler imaging are US features suggestive of malignancy.

A malignant tumor can present as a complex cystic mass up to 10% of RCC so cystic renal carcinomas and benign complicated cyst can be indistinguishable at gross inspection. In these cases, extended imaging examinations such as contrast-enhanced CT and MRI are recommended to evaluate the presence of contrast enhancement, a crucial criterion in the choice of management option [17, 20].

Solid renal tumors may present all the possible degrees of echogenicity, albeit the most typical pattern is the homogeneous hyperechogenicity of renal angiomyolipoma. Echogenicity and tumor vascularity do not correlate to cell differentiation and cell architecture. These lesions may appear hypo, iso or hyperechoic in comparison with the renal parenchyma (Figure 1). Nonetheless, the hypoechoic appearance is frequently observed in renal cell carcinoma, sometimes with evidence of an anechoic rim or small intratumoral cysts (Figure 2). Intratumoral necrosis, calcifications and hemorrhage, often present in Clear Cell RCC larger than 3 cm, lead to a heterogeneous US appearance.

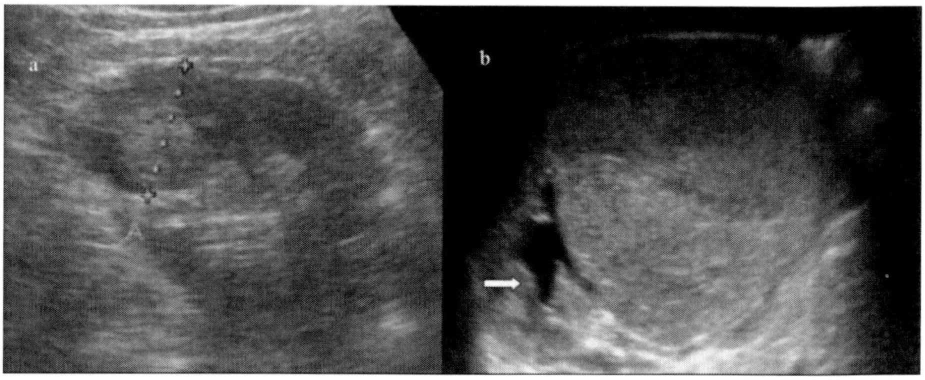

Figure 1. US image. (a) US image demonstrates a well-defined, echogenic, solid mass at the middle of the kidney. (b) US image shows a large, echogenic, solid mass with associated dilatation of adjacent collecting system (arrow).

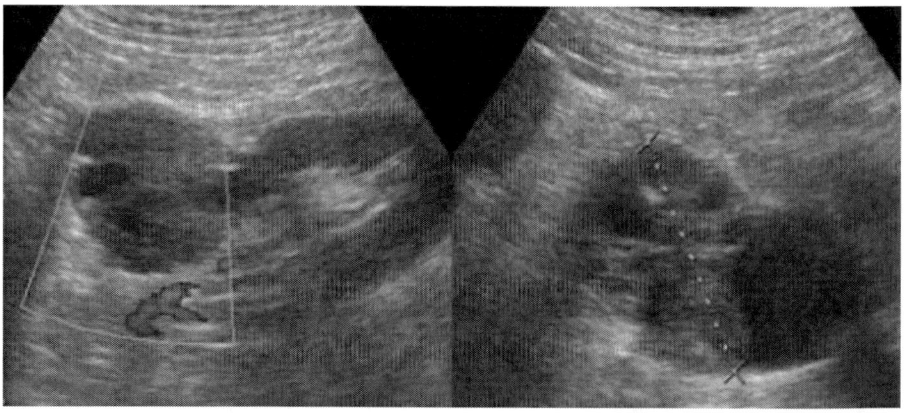

Figure 2. US images demonstrate a well-defined, heterogeneous renal mass with small intratumoral cysts.

A recently introduced diagnostic tool is the contrast enhanced ultrasound (CEUS) consisting in the intravenous injection of microbubble contrast agents which can pass through the pulmonary capillar bed due to their small diameter (3-10 mm) below that of red blood cells. The main advantage is the real time assessment of normal and abnormal renal perfusions. This US contrast media are not nephrotoxic and can be employed safely even in situations of impaired renal function.

CEUS can play an important role in certain clinical scenarios since it represents a low-cost and scarcely invasive tool. These situations include renal atypical masses, follow-up of cystic lesions managed conservative, and pseudo-tumors sometimes misdiagnosed as a renal mass (e.g., prominent Bertin column, a persistent fetal lobulation…).

Contrast-enhanced US had been useful in classifying renal cystic lesions into the Bosniak classification [13]. Recent studies have demonstrated it can differentiate between benign complex cysts and other lesions which will require further investigations [18]. Moreover, CEUS has demonstrated its utility in the diagnosis of renal cortical tumors and in the detection of tumor blood flow especially in hypovascular renal mass [19].

CEUS may provide a valuable help making additional examinations unnecessary [13, 21]. In spite of its already mentioned advantages, CEUS should not be used for evaluating large solid renal masses since it doesn't avoid CT and MRI evaluation, which will still be necessary. Pre-surgical CT study must be performed in order to evaluate extension into renal vein, contralateral kidney status and TNM staging [21].

In recent years, intraoperative sonography has appeared as a useful tool. It helps to characterize the primary tumor and to assess in real time the extent of renal involvement, especially in central tumors that are not visible during surgical resection, even avoiding partial nephrectomy [22].

Furthermore, clinical management of renal tumors has been increasingly influenced by the contribution of percutaneous biopsies, often guided by imaging techniques such as CT and ultrasound, which can be useful in selected patients to handle treatment approaching and guide surveillance strategies [23].

2.2. Multidetector Computer Tomography

Advances in CT and MRI technology have significantly improved the diagnostic accuracy in the diagnosis and staging of RCC [9].

MRI has demonstrated to be a useful technique for characterizing renal masses and staging RCC. However, CT offers several advantages such as its widespread availability, lower costs and faster scanning times and it is, therefore, more commonly used in many centers. CT is considered the modality of choice for detection and diagnosis of renal cortical tumors [24], and defined by the American College of Radiology as "the most important technique for evaluating the indeterminate renal mass" [25].

The achievement of high resolution multiplanar reformations and three-dimensional volume-rendered reformations from isotropic voxels with multidetector Computer tomography (MDCT) has clearly improved its value, especially regarding the preoperative planning for RCC [26].

The challenges of renal tumor imaging include not only reliable differentiation between benign and malignant lesions but also accurate delineation of the extent of the disease.

2.2.1. CT Techniques

Protocol-specified dedicated CT exam is required for further assessment of these lesions. Protocol optimization implicates attention to several data acquisition, reconstruction, and display parameters. Specifically, multiple acquisitions with varying coverage, careful timing of each contrast-enhanced phase and use of 2D and 3D multiplanar displays are required [27].

The increased ionizing radiation which the patient may undergo through the multiphasic protocol is a certain concern, considering the recent evidence supporting risks of radiation-induced cancers after imaging-related exposures [28, 29].

In order to minimize radiation exposure, a relatively thin slice thickness of 2.5 mm may be obtained through the kidneys, while for the rest of the study a standard slice thickness of 5 mm is obtained in case of simultaneous performing [30].

The renal mass CT protocol varies by centers, but standard imaging comprises an unenhanced acquisition combined with two or more contrast-enhanced phases (corticomedullary, nephrographic or excretory phases) (Figure 3) [24, 26, 27]. In general, 100–150 mL of iodinated IV contrast medium is used at a flow rate of 3-4 mL/s [27].

- Precontrast phase is essential to provide a base-line density measurement for evaluating the degree and pattern of enhancement in renal lesion. Despite it does not directly improve staging, it helps to distinguish between RCC from hiperdense cyst (Figure 4) and angiomyolipoma (i.e., presence of macroscopic fat with attenuation of -10HU or less) (Figure 5) [31].

Most renal cell carcinomas are solid lesions with attenuation values of 20 HU or greater at unenhanced CT [32].

- The cortico-medullary images, which take place between 25 and 70 seconds after the start of injection, are the most informative images for vascularity lesion and can depict with accuracy the renal vascular anatomy (Figure 6), being therefore useful for the staging and the subsequent preoperative planning [33].

However, not all renal tumors are well delineated during the corticomedullary phase. For instance, small hypervascular cortical RCC may enhance to the same degree as the normal cortex (Figure 7), whereas hypovascular tumor of the renal medulla may not enhance during this phase as the renal medulla, consequently may be difficult to detect [30, 33-35].

- The nephrographic phase is best imaged after a scanning delay of at least 80 seconds and lasts up to 180 seconds after the start of injection.

During this phase the renal parenchyma enhances homogenously being the most valuable phase tool for discrimination between the normal renal medulla and masses (Figure 8), and characterizing indeterminate lesions [35-37].

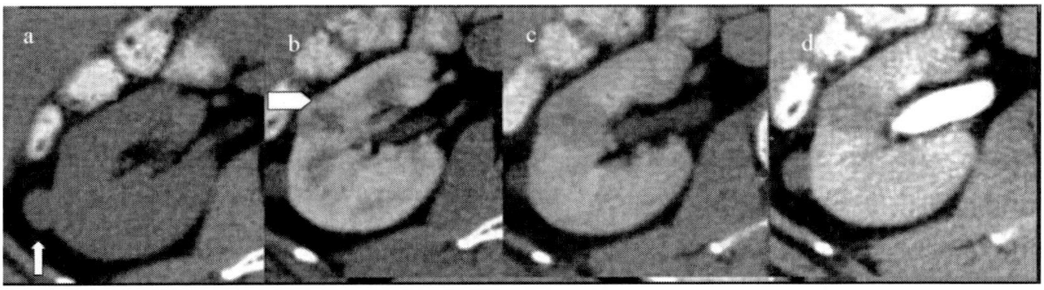

Figure 3. Unenhanced (a), corticomedullary phase (b), nephrographic phase (c), and excretory phase (d) CT scan show an exophytic simple cyst (thin arrow) and a clear cell RCC (arrow).

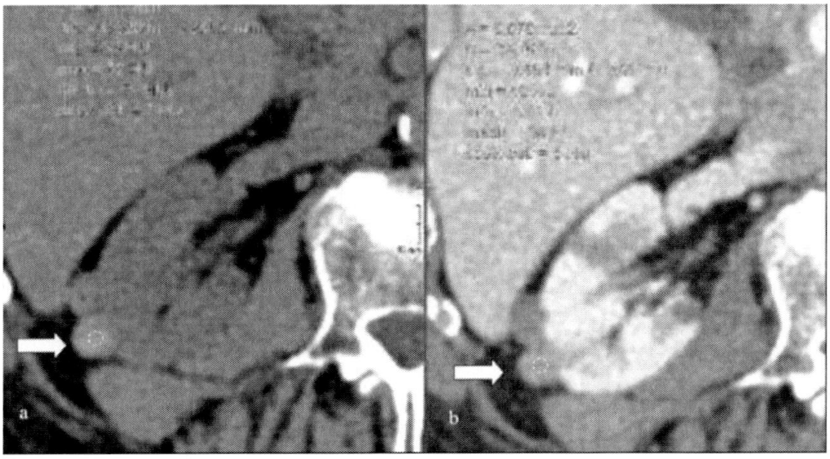

Figure 4. Benign hyperattenuating cystic. (a) Axial unenhanced CT image shows a subcentimetre, exophytic, hyperattenuating renal mass in the right kidney which had a mean attenuation of 30 HU. (b) Axial contrast-enhanced CT scan shows no significant enhancement (attenuation, 33 HU).

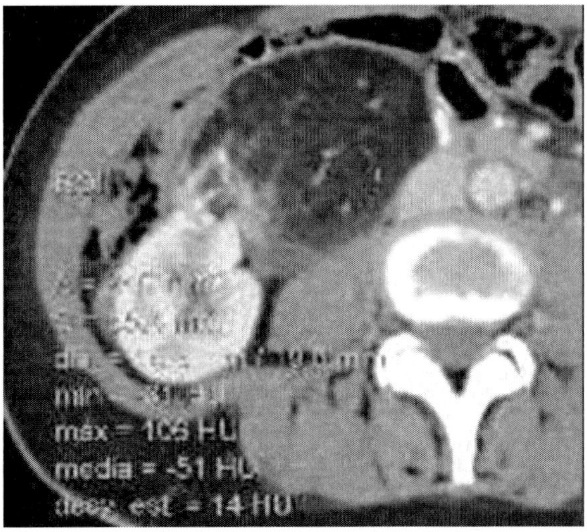

Figure 5. Angiomyolipoma. Axial contrast-enhanced CT shows an exophytic renal mass which is composed primarily of fat (attenuation, -51HU).

Nephrographic phase images are also useful in assessment of renal vein and inferior vena cava [9, 30].

- The excretory phase is usually performed in combination with the corticomedullary or nephrographic phase and is acquired after a 5- to 8- minute delay. It results in opacification of the renal collecting system being useful to demonstrate its relationship with the tumor (Figure 9). The collecting system is best visualized using coronal multiplanar reformation and volume rendering to simulate a conventional excretory urography [27].

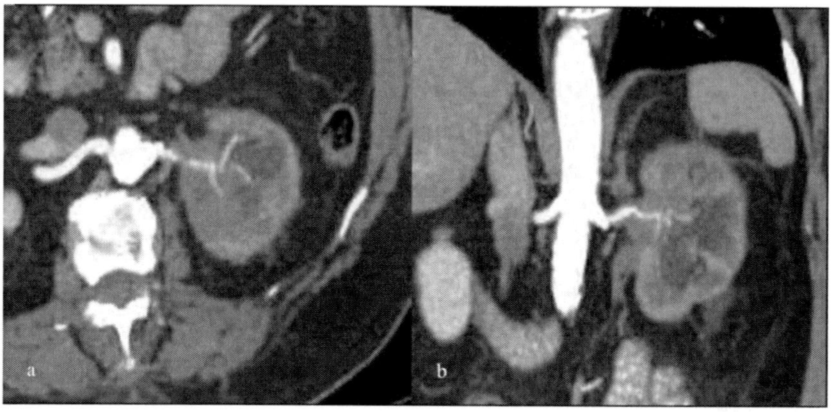

Figure 6. Clear cell RCC. (a) Axial and (b) Reformat coronal contrast-enhanced corticomedullary CT scan demonstrate a left kidney contains a poorly defined parenchymal mass with no alteration of the renal contour. The mass involves the renal sinus and it is enveloping the renal artery.

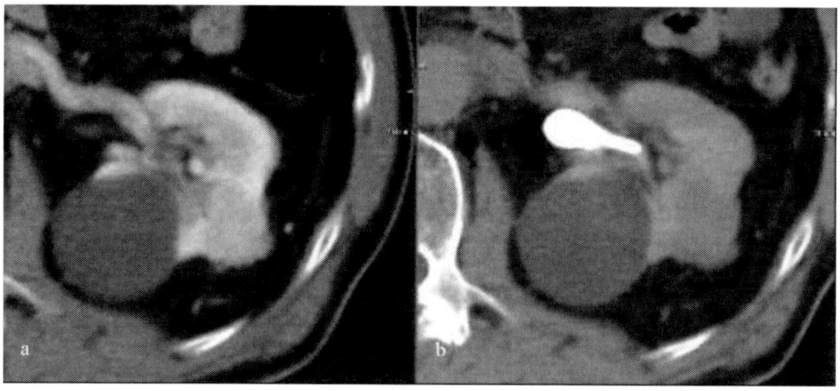

Figure 7. (a) Axial contrast-enhanced CT scan obtained during corticomedullary phase shows a cortical renal mass. The mass shows a degree of enhancement similar to that of renal parenchyma. (b) Axial contrast-enhanced CT image obtained during excretory phase. The mass is more conspicuous since it has become hypoattenuating to the renal parenchyma.

Adequate hydration of the patient, considering medical conditions such as cardiac or renal impairment, is necessary to guarantee optimal excretion of contrast media and minimize its nephrotoxic effects [38].

Considering both, lesion detection and characterization, data set reconstruction also plays a role. In this regard, thinner overlapping reconstructions resulted in an increase in the percentage of small lesions detected, markedly improved ability to distinguish cystic from solid lesions among those measuring 5–10 mm, and decreased the percentage of indeterminate lesions (typically <1.5mm interval and 10-50% overlap) [27, 39]. Some small masses are better visualized in the coronal plane. By displaying the kidney coronally, both shape and enhancement of a mass may become more apparent [29]. The combination between three-dimensional CT and CT angiography may potentially provide the best information needed to plan the surgical procedure. The three-dimensional CT images can be viewed in multiple planes and orientations depicting accurately the tumor and its relationship to the renal surface, the excretory system (Figure 10), and adjacent organs.

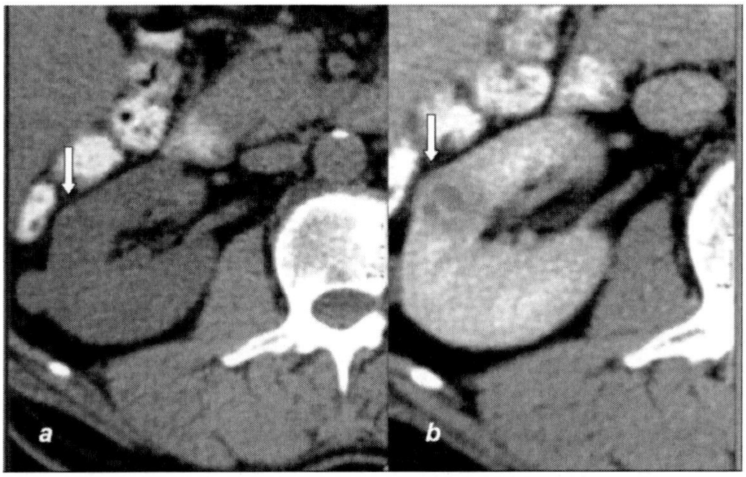

Figure 8. (a) Incidentally papillary RCC detected as subtle renal hump at unenhanced CT. (b) Axial contrast-enhanced CT image obtained during nephrographic phase confirms that bulge is due to well-defined renal mass.

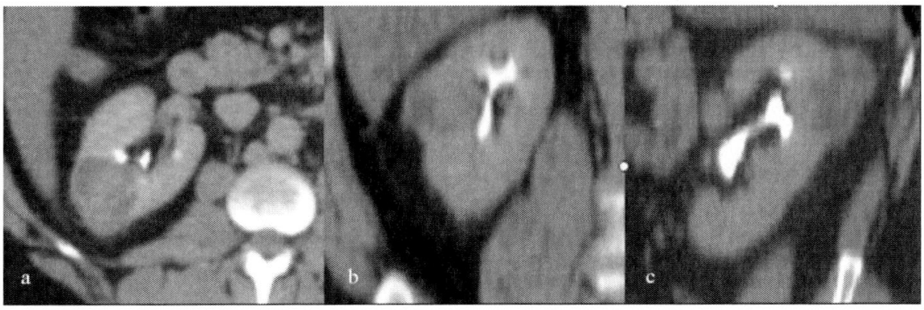

Figure 9. Papillary RCC. Axial (a), coronal (b), and sagittal (c) contrast-enhanced CT scan obtained during the excretory phase show well-defined enhancing renal mass which not compresses adjacent collecting system elements.

A three dimensional CT angiogram (Figure 11) can be created to delineate the renal arterial and venous anatomy [40]. The most important criterion in the diagnosis and characterization of the renal masses is to determine the vasculature of the lesion, that is, whether or not the lesion enhanced with contrast medium [41].

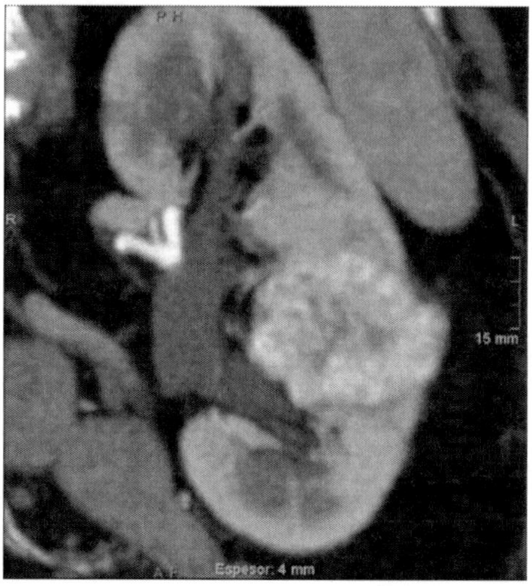

Figure 10. Reconstructed coronal CT scan during corticomedullary phase demonstrates the collecting system and a well-defined enhancing mass occupying the inter-polar aspect to the left kidney.

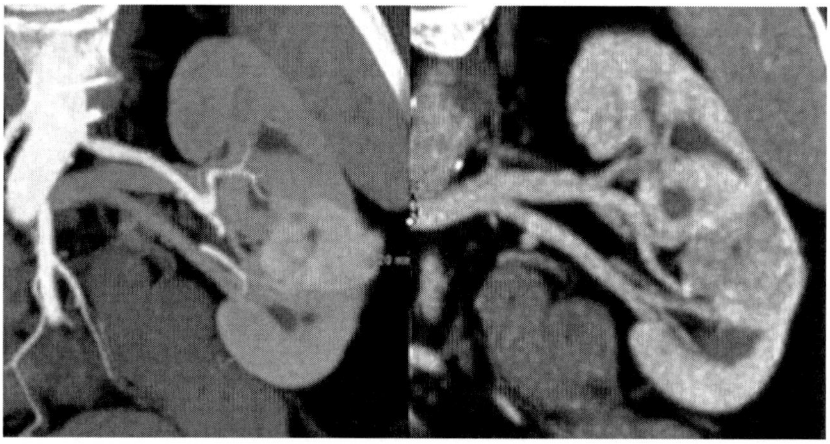

Figure 11. Small left renal mass that bulking to the renal hilium. Reconstructed coronal MIP images demonstrate the arterial anatomy during the corticomedullary phase (a) and the venous anatomy during the nephrographic phase (b).

The enhancement is defined as an increase in attenuation by 20 HU or more on contrast-enhanced images compared with unenhanced images (Figure 12). Lesser degrees of change in attenuation value may be attributable to pseudo-enhancement [24] which can occur especially in small renal masses as a result of intense enhancement of adjacent normal renal parenchyma and should always be considered, particularly with endophytic masses. Thus, measurement of enhancement in heterogeneous masses must be carefully performed, quantifying at each time the same area of the mass so that enhancement determination is reliable. Recently updated European Clinical Guides set enhancement threshold at 15 HU [42].

2.2.2. CT Imaging Features

Renal masses can be subdivided into cystic and solid masses. Simple cystic renal masses are composed of spaces filled of fluid that not enhance. The cystic mass that has enhancing soft-tissue components, thickened wall or septa, can be benign or malignant.

The Bosniak renal cyst classification is a useful guide to the management of cyst renal mass since it separates renal cyst into five categories based on their CT imaging appearance, in an attempt to predict the risk of malignancy (Table 1) (Figure 13) [43]. When the predominant part of a renal mass enhances it is considered solid and likely neoplastic. However, different entities such as vascular anomalies, aneurysms, and focal inflammatory processes should be excluded before a neoplasm is considered [44].

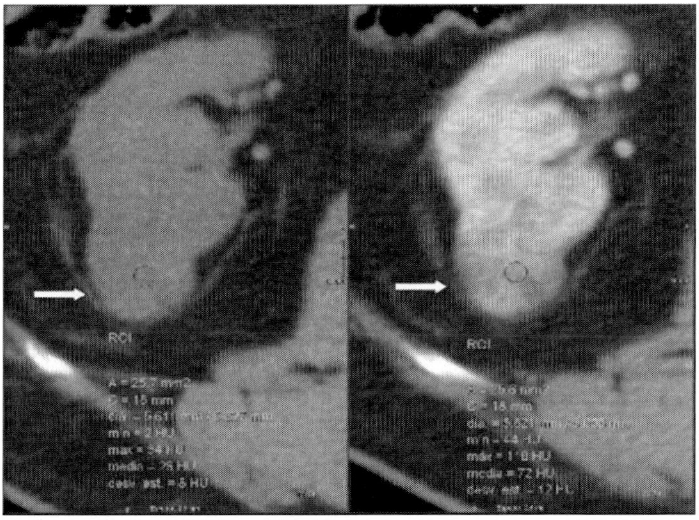

Figure 12. (a) Axial unenhanced CT scan shows an exophytic cortical mass with attenuation of 29 HU. (b) Axial corticomedullary phase CT scan shows the mass with attenuation of 72 HU which is an enhancement of 43 HU.

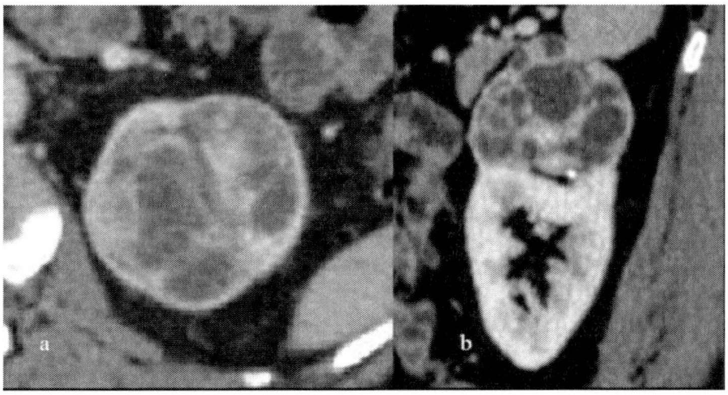

Figure 13. Bosniak category IV cystic mass. Axial (a), and sagittal (b) contrast-enhanced CT scan obtained during the nephrographic phase show a complex cystic mass that contains a grossly thickened and enhancing wall, and enhancing soft-tissue components.

Although enhancing hyper-attenuating renal masses in adults more often are malignant, benign neoplasms such as angiomyolipomas or oncocytomas may also show this pattern.

Regarding this condition, macroscopic fat seen on unenhanced images is virtually pathognomonic for angiomyolipoma (attenuation of -10HU or less). Nevertheless, approximately 4-5% of angiomyolipomas either not contain any fat cells or contain an insufficient amount of fat cell ("fat-poor angiomyolipomas"). Therefore, attenuation on unenhanced and homogeneous enhancement on contrast enhanced CT images are features that may be shared by AML and the more indolent types of RCCs (e.g., papillary and cromophobe RCC). In these cases MRI can be performed (Figure 14) [24, 41, 44].

On CT scan the diagnosis of oncocytoma may be suggested if a central stellate scar ("spoke-wheel pattern") is identified within another wise homogeneous tumor. However, the classic central scar, which was long thought to represent oncocytoma, is present in less than half of cases. Thus, oncocytomas cannot be reliably differentiated from RCC by imaging [24, 33].

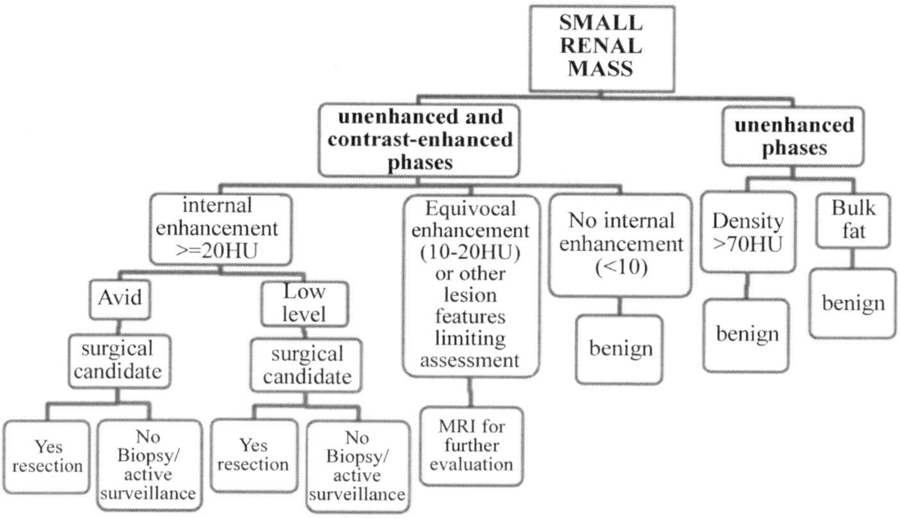

Figure 14. Diagnostic algorithm small renal mass. Adapted table Kang et al.

2.3. Magnetic Resonance Imaging

MRI most often complements CT in renal mass characterization, although it may also be used as the initial dedicated study for evaluation of a renal mass under current American College of Radiology guidelines [25]. The lack of ionizing radiation and superior soft tissue contrast compared to CT are the main advantages of MRI. In addition, MRI can better detect cystic and solid areas inside a tumor and the presence of fat or blood derivatives. Disadvantages include high cost, limited availability, and expertise. The potentially long duration of the procedure makes it unavailable for some patients suffering from claustrophobia [45]. Nephrogenic systemic fibrosis (NSF) is a rare and serious syndrome that involves fibrosis of skin, joints, eyes, and internal organs. It must be taken in account that recent evidence suggests that NSF is associated with exposure to gadolinium (with gadolinium-based MRI contrast agents being frequently used as contrast agents for MRI) in patients with severe kidney failure [46].

Table 1. The Bosniak classification of renal cysts

Bosniak Category	Features	Work up
I	Benign simple cyst with a hairline thin wall that does not contain septa, calcification or solid components. It measures as water density and does not enhance with contrast material. calcifications, or solid components	
II	A benign cyst that might contains a few hairline thin septa. Fine calcifications might be present in the wall or septa. Uniformly high-attenuation lesions less than 3 cm that are sharply marginated, and not enhanced.	
IIF	These cysts might contain more hairline thin septa. Minimal enhancement of a hairline thin septum or wall can be seen and there might be minimal thickening of the septa or wall. The cyst might contains calcification that might be nodular and thick but there is no contrast enhancement. There are no enhancing soft tissue elements. Totally intrarenal non-enhancing high-attenuation renal lesions of < = 3cm are also included in this category. These lesions are generally well marginated.	Surgery or follow up.
III	These lesions are indeterminate cystic masses with thickened irregular wall or septa in which enhancement can be seen	Surgical therapy recommended.
IV	These lesions are clearly malignant cystic lesions that contain enhancing soft-tissue components.	

MDCT and MRI provide equal accuracy in staging RCCs. However, MRI offers problem-solving capability in some scenarios where CT may be limited in identifying enhancing soft tissue and can achieve an accurate diagnosis of a cyst or solid mass. Moreover, it is regarded as the most accurate imaging modality to assess the extent of venous thrombus because of its multiplanar capability and excellent tissue contrast (Figure 15) [25].

MRI is used when optimal CT cannot be obtained (e.g., in cases of allergy to iodinated contrast media). MRI of the kidney is most commonly performed at high field MRI scanner (1.5-3 T) with better performance in terms of signal-to-noise ratio (SNR). The examinations are performed with a phased-array body coil with the patient supine.

Performing scan with rapid sequences within a breath-hold is preferred in order to avoid worsening of image quality due to respiratory motion of the kidneys.

Coronal localizer should be included in every examination since it provides an anatomic overview of the abdomen and allows depiction of contour abnormalities at the renal poles. Axial dual-echo in-phase and opposed-phase gradient-echo (GRE) T1-weighted images are helpful in identification of macroscopic and microscopic fat in a renal tumor. T2-weighted with and without fat suppression is helpful for evaluating the overall anatomy, renal collecting system and complexity of a cystic renal lesion. Fat suppression is especially useful for revealing perinephric edema and fluid collections [33, 45].

A homogeneous hyperintense lesion with a thin wall on T2-weighted images can be accurately characterized as a simple cyst. Septa and solid nodules can be readily seen within cysts on T2-weighted images due to their relatively low signal intensity compared with the fluid contents within the cysts.

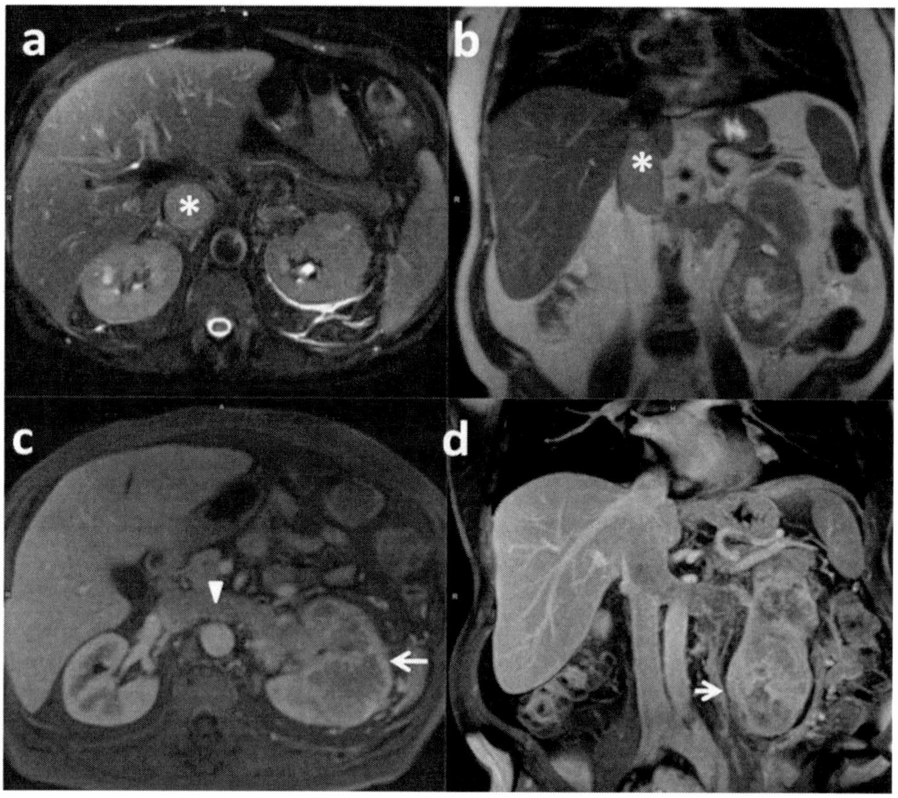

Figure 15. MR images in a 63-year-old man with a malignant cortical left renal tumor showing venous invasion. (a) Axial fat-saturated fast spin-echo T2-weighted and (b) coronal T2-weighted single-shot fast spin-echo sequences show marked expansion of the inferior vena cava from tumor thrombus(*). Axial (c) 3D GRE fat-suppressed T1-weighted MR images after Gd-based agent injection during cortico-medullary and (d) coronal 3D GRE fat-suppressed T1-weighted MR images in nephrographic phase show a left renal mass (short arrow) with tumor thrombus extending into the left renal vein (arrowhead).

Complicated renal cysts with intra-cystic hemorrhage (Figure 16) or proteinaceous contents may have heterogeneous or low signal intensity on T2-weighted images, whereas solid tumors have variable signal intensity.

Three-dimensional (3D) fat-suppressed GRE T1-weighted images are obtained prior to and following the intravenous administration of gadolinium chelate contrast (0.1 mmol/kg) of extracellularly distributed.

Contrast material–enhanced images are obtained during the corticomedullary, nephrographic, and excretory phases.

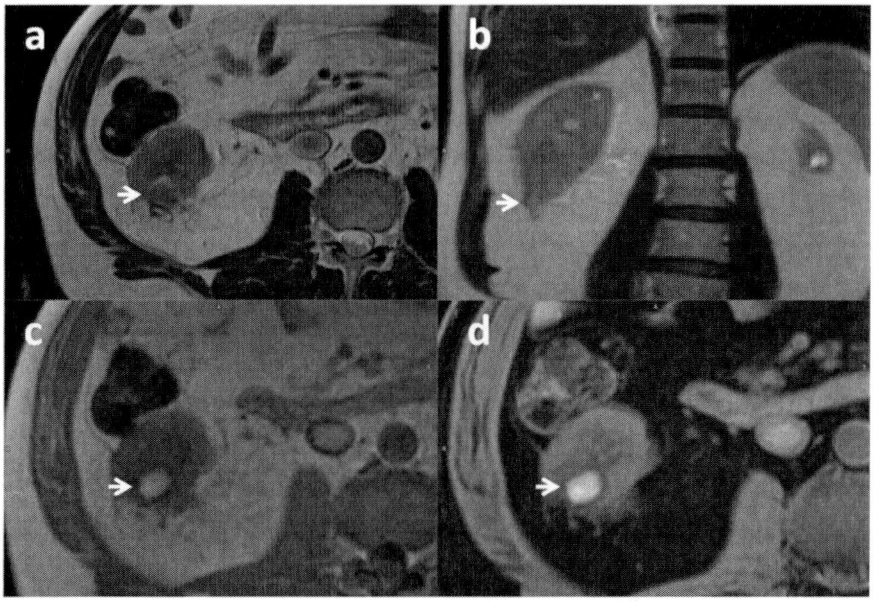

Figure 16. Complex hemorrhagic cyst in a 66-year-old man. Axial (a), coronal (b) T2-weighted and T1-weighted MR images without (c) and with fat-suppression (d) show small nodule (arrow) hypointense in T2 weighted images and hyperintense on T1-weighted images due to hemorrhagic content.

The presence of enhancement within a renal lesion after the administration of gadolinium-based contrast material is the most reliable criterion for distinguishing solid masses from cysts at MRI [3]. Comparison of pre- and post-contrast T1-weighted images is the key to the detection and characterization of renal lesions [20, 45, 47, 48].

To achieve a better representation of the spatial relationship of the renal mass to adjacent anatomic structures, multiplanar reconstruction may be necessary. MR angiography sequence during the arterial phase may be performed for better visualization of accessory renal vessels and facilitation of surgical planning.

Coronal T1-weighted images also may be obtained during the excretory phase with administration of diuretics from which maximum intensity projection images are useful for evaluating the overall anatomy and the renal collecting system [20, 33]. Diffusion-weighted imaging (DWI) of the kidneys is an area of growing interest. DWI derives its contrast from the movement of water molecules in the tissue microenvironment and thus provides an insight into tissue cellularity and architecture. DWI can improve diagnostic confidence and the use of apparent diffusion coefficient (ADC) values seem to be useful even in renal masses characterization, since malignant lesions (RCC) tend to show lower ADC values than benign solid (e.g., oncocytomas) and cystic lesions [45, 47, 48]. DWI may particularly be helpful in lesion detection and evaluation when gadolinium based contrast medium cannot be administered.

As in other organs, lack of standardization in the technique has limited the reproducibility of results. Although investigators have examined the use of ADC values to predict RCC subtypes and separate benign from malignant lesions, their use is limited [24].

Carcinoma clear cell RCC appears typically isointense or slightly hypointense on T1-weighted images and tends to be mildly hyperintense on T2-weighted images [45, 48]. Clear cell carcinomas can also be predominantly cystic with only scant areas of solid enhancing component which are essential for diagnosis [49]. Papillary RCC accounts for approximately 10%–15% of all RCCs and may be multifocal [50]. At MRI, they typically demonstrate homogeneous low signal intensity on T2-weighted images. Chromophobe renal tumors account for approximately 4%–11% of RCCs [51, 52]. The imaging features of chromophobe RCC can be identical to those of clear cell RCC [24, 47].

2.4. Positron Emission Tomography (PET/CT)

The efficacy of PET in renal malignancy remains under investigation.

Oncological PET imaging with F-18 deoxyglucose (FDG) is used as an adjunct to CT and MRI and mainly involves the post therapy staging. FDG PET/CT can be particularly helpful for guiding biopsy to the most metabolically active tumor tissue, identifying metastatic disease (Figure 17) and monitoring response to therapy [20, 53, 54]. FF-18FDG PET has limitations in kidney tumors, mainly due to the fact that excreted FDG present in the urinary tract interferes with image reading and the generally moderate FDG uptake by primary renal tumors.

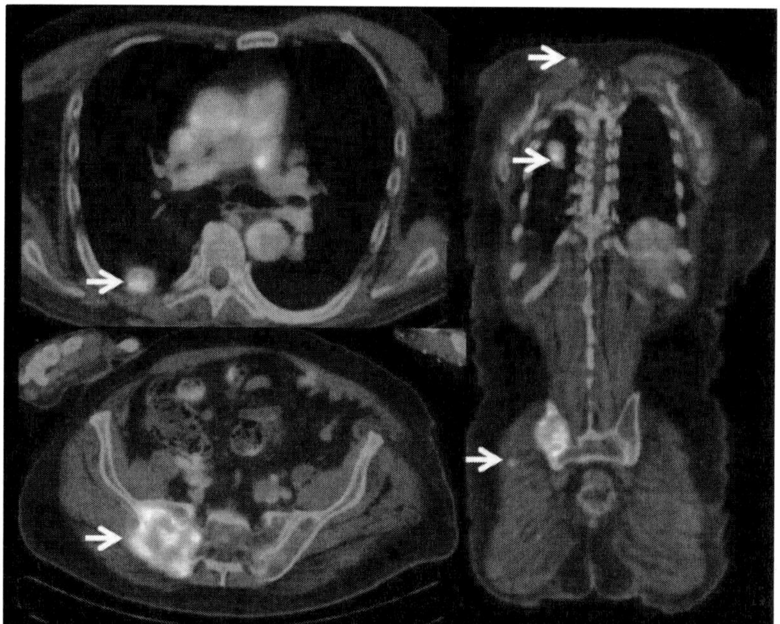

Figure 17. Follow-up 65-year-old man with a history of nephrectomy for clear cell carcinoma. PET-CT demonstrates increased metabolic activity (arrows) in the lung, right iliac bone and muscle due to metastases.

For this reason, alternative tracers have been suggested, in particular radiopharmaceuticals directed toward tumor-associated antigens. C-acetate is taken up by both the clear cell and papillary histologic subtypes of RCC [55]. Further, the 124I-labeled monoclonal antibody G250 can be used to target an epitope of the carbonic anhydrase IX antigen found in the clear cell histologic subtype of RCC and has potential for noninvasive characterization of RCC [53, 56]. New radiotracers and further advancement in PET/CT techniques are expected to further improve the performance of PET/CT [56].

2.5. Renal Biopsy

Although needle biopsy of renal tumors used to be rejected due to concerns about safety, accuracy and tumor seeding, it is currently considered as an accurate and safe technique (risk of tumor seeding less than 0.01%) [57], which avoids unnecessary nephrectomies [58].

European guidelines, updated in 2014, recommend the use of percutaneous renal tumor biopsies: 1- for histological diagnosis of "indeterminate" renal masses; 2- to select patients with small renal masses for surveillance approaches; 3- to obtain histology before ablative treatments; 4- to select the most suitable form of targeted pharmacologic therapy in the setting of metastatic disease [42].

The aims of biopsy are to determine malignancy and histologic type in order to support treatment decisions. Percutaneous sampling of renal masses can be performed under local anesthesia in most of cases and can be performed with either ultrasound or CT guidance (Figure 18). 18-gauge needles are considered ideal for renal tumor core biopsies, as they are associated with low morbidity and provide sufficient tissue for diagnosis in the majority of biopsies [42, 59, 60]. A coaxial technique is currently considered as the best, since it allows multiple biopsies in an attempt to avoid the potential risk of tumor seeding [42, 59].

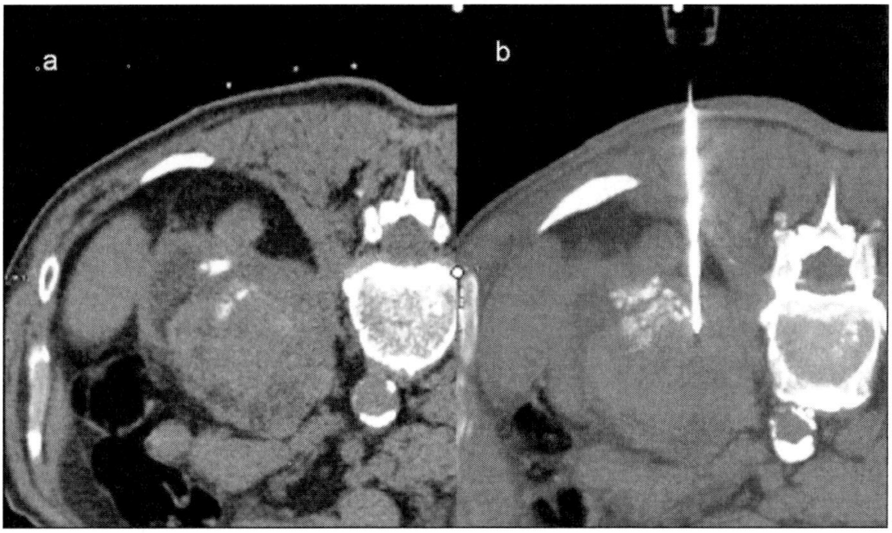

Figure 18. Biopsy of solid renal mass. (a) Unenhanced CT obtained prior to biopsy shows a renal mass. (b) CT-guided percutaneous biopsy, shown on transverse CT image, was performed with patient in the prone position by using an 18-gauge needle.

Regarding non diagnostic biopsy, strong consideration should be given to repeat biopsy. A multidisciplinary approach leading to a final decision should be considered [58, 60]. Spontaneously resolving subcapsular/perinephric hematoma and hematuria are the most frequently reported complications and bleeding is generally self-limiting, whereas major complications are unusual [42, 61].

Further clinical research is needed to solve the current limitations of renal tumor biopsy and to increase their application in clinical practice. Histologic, molecular, and genetic data from renal tumor biopsy could be integrated with clinical information in algorithms and protocols to be used for management of the disease counseling and treatment decision making [62].

3. Histologic Types and Differential Diagnosis

3.1. Histologic Types

The 2004 World Health Organization classification for renal neoplasms recognizes several distinct histologic subtypes of RCC, based on morphological and immunohistochemical features. These subtypes include clear cell RCC (CcRCC), papillary RCC (pRCC), chromophobe, hereditary cancer syndromes, multilocular cystic RCC, collecting duct carcinoma, medullary carcinoma, mucinous tubular and spindle cell carcinoma, neuroblastoma-associated RCC, Xp 11.2 translocation-TFE3 carcinoma and unclassified lesions.

The most common subtype is Clear cell carcinoma (70%), followed by papillary (10-15%) and chromophobe (4-6%) [16, 17]. Epidemiology, histopathology, clinical and biologic behavior and imaging manifestations are different for every histologic variant [18].

Pretreatment determination of tumor subtypes is important for patients who are either poor surgical candidates or who have metastatic disease since subtypes respond differently to molecularly targeted therapies. Recent improvements in CT and MR imaging techniques allow both morphologic evaluation and assessment of the physiologic characteristic of tumors which may assist in imaging diagnosis.

3.2. Common Histologic Subtypes of RCC

3.2.1. Clear Cell RCC

Clear cell type (CcRCC) is the most common histologic subtype accounting for 70% of all RCCs. It originates from the renal cortex and typically shows an expansive growth pattern.

CcRCC typically shows hypervascularity on contrast enhanced studies, including MDCT and MRI. It commonly appears heterogeneous at imaging due to the presence of hemorrhage, necrosis and cyst (Figure 19) [7]; cystic change is seen in up to 15% of cases and calcification is seen in 10-15% of tumors. The degree of contrast enhancement may help distinguish CcRCC from the other tumors subtypes. CcRCC can also be predominantly cystic with only scant areas of solid enhancing component. Identification of the presence of contrast enhancement is essential for diagnosis [49].

Renal vein tumor thrombus can be seen with aggressive higher-stage tumors. The MRI appearance of CcRCC varies depending on the presence of fat, hemorrhage and necrosis.

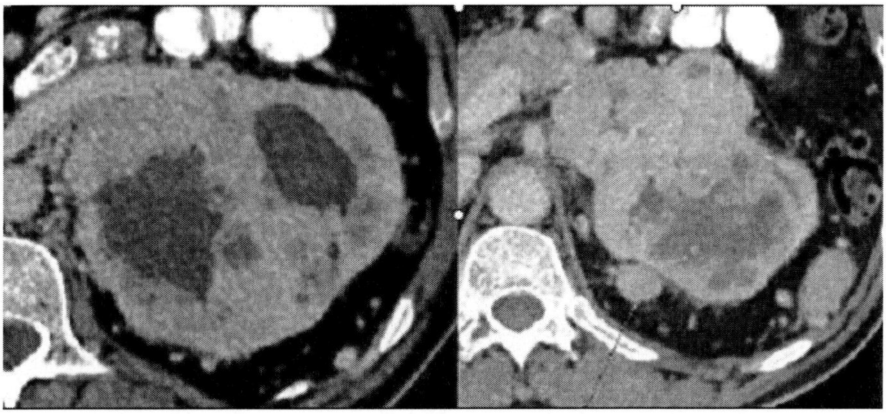

Figure 19. Clear cell renal carcinoma. Axial contrast-enhanced CT images obtained during the nephrographic phase show an expansive renal mass that contains enhancing solid soft-tissue and low-attenuation areas that may represent cystic o necrotic changes.

CcRCC is typically isointense similar to that of the renal parenchyma or slightly hypointense on T1-weighted images and mildly hyperintense on T2-weighted images.

Loss of signal intensity within the solid portions of CcRCCs on opposed-phase images compared with in-phase images is due to cytoplasmic fat and has been observed in up to 60% of these tumors [45, 48]. Central necrosis is common and is typically seen as a homogeneous hypointense area in the center of the mass on T1-weighted images.

Post-contrast images demonstrate lack of enhancement in areas of necrosis and marked enhancement in the viable components of the tumor. Intratumoral hemorrhage may occur and has a variable appearance depending on the stage of degradation of the component blood products. A hypointense rim or pseudocapsule may be seen on both T1- and T2-weighted images and is thought to be related to compression of the adjacent renal parenchyma by the expanding tumor. Interruption of pseudo-capsule correlates with advanced stage (i.e., invasion of perirenal fat) and higher nuclear grade [48].

3.2.2. Papillary RCC

Papillary RCC (PRCC) is the second common histologic subtype, comprising up to 10-15% of RCCs. It is divided into two histologic types: basophilic and eosinophilic [50]. Type I (basophilic) papillary tumors are associated with better prognosis and lower stage [63]. There are not large studies that show any specific features that help differentiate between type I and type II. Bilateral and multifocal tumors are more common, especially with hereditary syndromes. PRCC is typically less vascular than other types of RCC (Figure 20). They are more often homogeneous or present peripheral enhancement on contrast-enhanced CT or MRI and usually shows fewer degrees of contrast enhancement than CcRCC in all phases of postcontrast imaging.

Large tumors show heterogeneity due to necrosis, hemorrhage and calcification. The relative hypovascularity of PRCC can cause it to be mistaken for a renal cyst. In that case the ultrasonography can be helpful to distinguish cyst from solid renal mass. At MR, PRCCs typically demonstrate homogeneous low signal intensity on T2-weighted images, with homogeneous and poor enhancement on post-contrast images (Figure 21) [45].

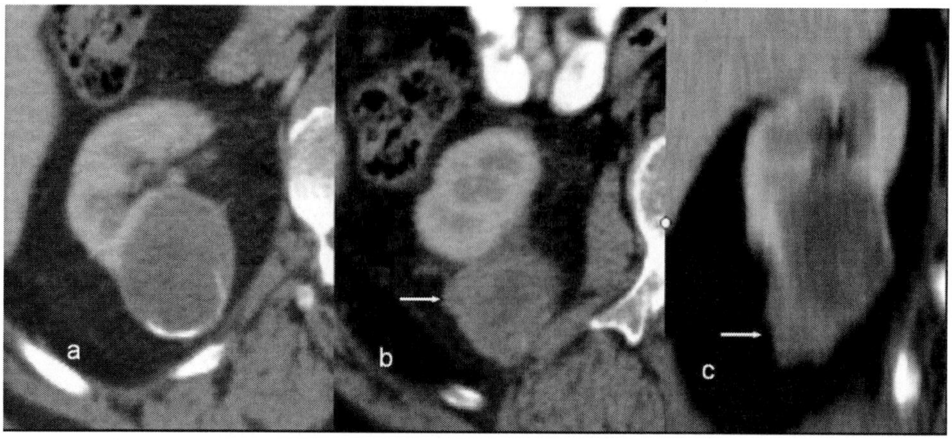

Figure 20. Papillary RCC. Axial (a-b), and reconstructed coronal MIP (c) contrast-enhanced CT scan obtained during the nephrographic phase show a periphericaly calcified cyst left renal containing a solid low-enhancing nodule that is adjacent to the wall.

Large tumors may show heterogeneity due to necrosis, hemorrhage and calcification [47, 63, 64]. A fibrous capsule is typically present in this type of tumor.

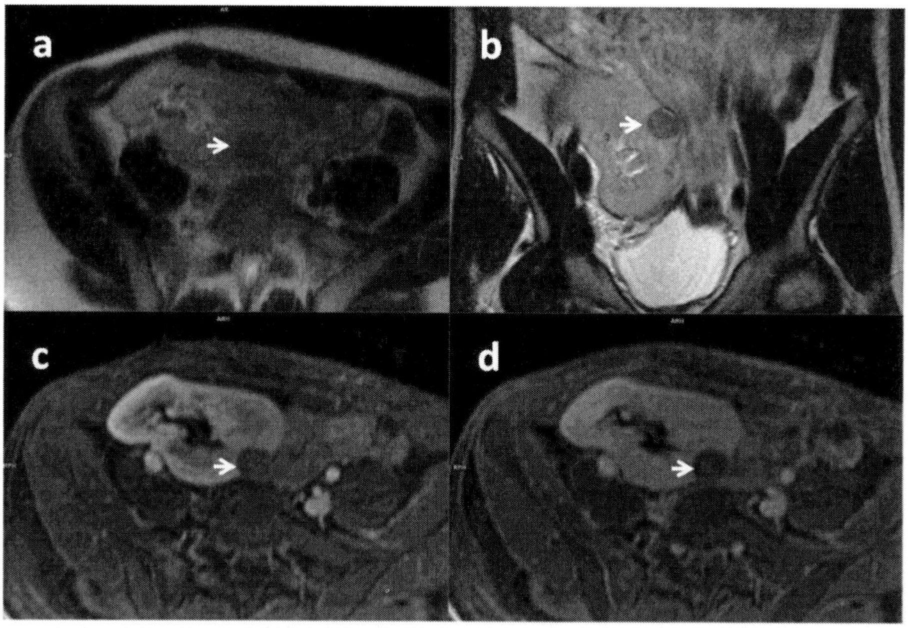

Figure 21. Papillary type I RCC in a 21-year-old man with renal transplantation. (a, b) Axial and Coronal fast spin-echo T2-weighted MR images show a small mass (arrow) in the posterior aspect of the renal graft. The mass is homogeneously hypointense relative to the adjacent renal parenchyma. (c, d) Axial 3D GRE fat-suppressed T1-weighted MR images during cortico-medullary and nephrographic phases after intravenous gadolinium-based contrast agent administration. The nodule (arrow) enhances less than the normal parenchyma.

3.2.3. Chromophobe RCC

Chromophobe RCC is the third most common histologic subtype, accounting for less than 5% of RCCs. This type shows variable degrees and patterns of enhancement [42] although usually appears as a well circumscribed homogeneous mass at CT and MRI, despite their large size. The wheel pattern of contrast enhancement classically associated with oncocytomas has been described in association with Cromophobe RCC (Figure 22).

Oncocytomas and Chromophobe RCC share similar oncogenic and histologic features and some imaging findings. MRI may show a hypointense mass on T2-weighted images and cystic changes within a solid tumor [47].

The images features of cromophobe RCC can be identical to those of clear cell RCC [24, 48]. It usually appears uniformly hyperechoic at ultrasonography.

3.3. Differential Diagnosis

Preoperative characterization of benign and malignant renal masses is imperfect, and approximately 10%–17% of renal masses that are surgically excised are benign [65]. In all cases, an exhaustive differential diagnosis should be carried out, even when a definitive diagnosis is not achieved.

If a benign neoplasm is suspected, a prompt sparing preoperative biopsy or observation should be performed depending on tumor size, location and patient condition. If lymphoma appears in the differential diagnosis, a biopsy may be warranted to avoid unnecessary surgery.

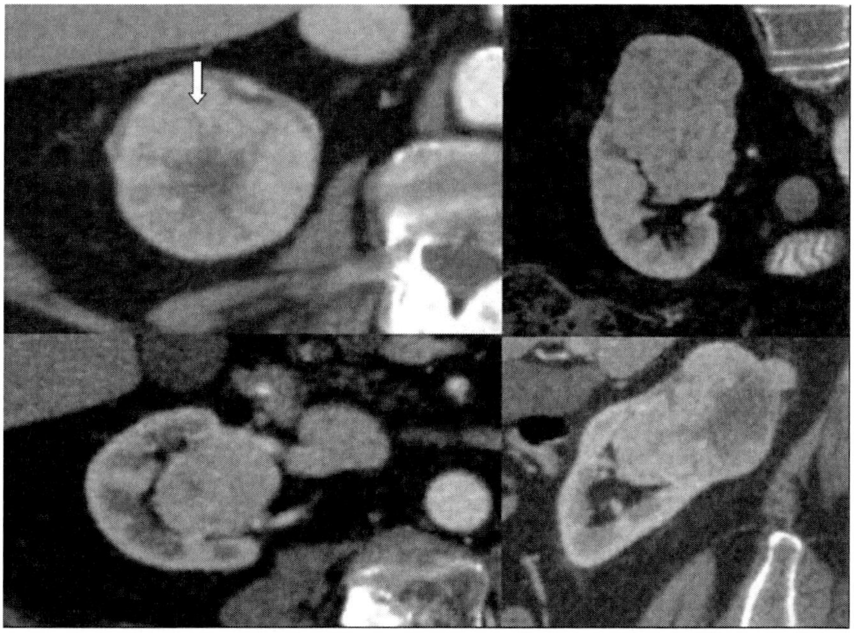

Figure 22. Cromophobe RCC. Contrast-enhanced CT images obtained during the nephrographic phase demonstrate a large, well-defined, homogeneous enhancing mass with stellate central scar (arrow).

3.3.1. Lipid-Poor Angiomyolipoma

Angiomyolipomas (AML) represent approximately 2%–6% of the benign solid masses excised from the kidney in surgical series [66]. CRCC and AML with minimal fat are both solid renal tumors that can contain microscopic fat on chemical shift imaging creating a diagnostic challenge [45]. Moreover, AML do not need to be surgically removed in most cases, thus discrimination between both entities is crucial.

At MRI, decreased signal intensity of the mass at opposed-phased imaging compared with in-phase imaging has been proposed for adequate differentiation between lipid-poor AML and other renal neoplasms. However, caution must be exercised when the diagnosis of angiomyolipoma is made based on this phenomenon alone since a loss of signal intensity on opposed-phase images can also be seen in clear cell RCC with small amounts of fat [44, 45, 67, 68].

One clue that can be useful to distinguish both types is that AML with minimal fat is typically hypointense on fat suppressed T2-weighted images [45]. Furthermore, CcRCC tend to be larger and more likely to demonstrate necrosis, while both CcRCC and AML can demonstrate significantly lower ADC values than renal cortex. It has been published that CcCCR is more likely to show heterogeneity on diffusion weighted images and several peaks in the ADC histogram, whereas AML is more likely to show homogeneous signal on DWI and a single dominate peak on histogram analysis [69].

It can also be difficult to differentiate AML from papillary RCC given that both types of lesions tend to demonstrate lower signal intensity than renal parenchyma on T2-weighted images.

Papillary RCC is typically a hypo vascular neoplasm and shows mild contrast enhancement, whereas AML with minimal fat are generally hyper vascular and show marked enhancement [24]. Nevertheless, it is difficult to differentiate a papillary RCC from an AML with minimal fat on the basis of enhancement. Observation of an enhancing hyper-attenuating renal mass that appears hypointense on T2-weighted images and is not suppressed on frequency selective fat suppressed images or opposed phases gradient echo images, should lead to contemplate the performance of percutaneous biopsy prior to surgical excision [45, 47, 48].

3.3.2. Oncocytoma

Its classic radiologic description is that of a well marginated avidly enhancing solid renal mass with a central stellate scar ("spoke-wheel" pattern), though these features can appear in RCC as well. No diagnostic imaging criteria are able to accurately and consistently differentiate these benign tumors from RCC [45]. Oncocytomas are typically depicted by spherical and well-defined masses. T

he finding of segmental "enhancement inversion" [70] (i.e., segmental enhancement inversion describes changes in the pattern of heterogeneous enhancement within a renal mass: areas that enhance avidly on early phase imaging will de-enhance on delayed imaging, whereas areas that appear hypovascular on early imaging will progressively enhance on delayed) (Figure 23) in combination with other imaging parameters might prompt consideration of oncocytoma and subsequent biopsy. Investigators have suggested that renal masses showing a central scar hyperintese on T2-weighted images, the absence of central area signal intensity inversion or the presence of a signal drop on chemical shift imaging may be helpful to exclude the diagnosis of oncocytoma [24, 45].

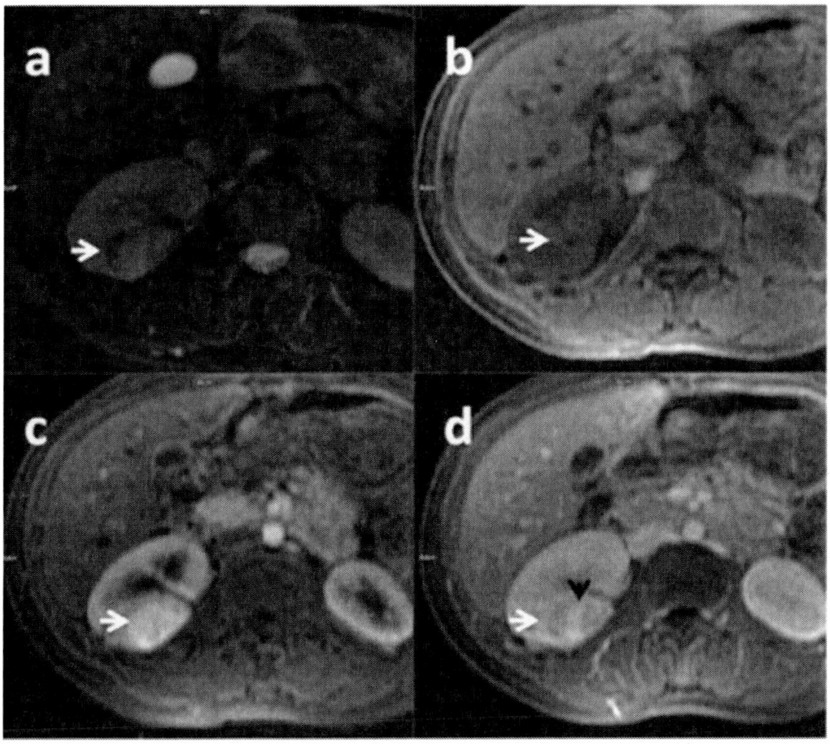

Figure 23. Renal oncocytoma in a 28-year-old woman. (a) Axial fat-saturated fast spin-echo T2-weighted MR image shows a small solid well-defined renal mass (arrow) in the lower pole of the right kidney. (b, c, d) Axial 3D GRE fat-suppressed T1-weighted MR images before (b) and after Gd-based agent injection during cortico-medullary (c) and nephrographic (d) phases. The renal mass (arrows) presents diffuse contrast enhancement on cortico-medullary phase. Nephrograpic phase shows triangular region (black arrowhead) is more enhancing than rest of tumor. This finding (coincident with a linear area of less enhance in the corticomedullary phase) suggest segmental enhancement inversion.

4. Unusual Imaging Manifestations

Unusual radiologic features can be shown by RCC in certain cases. For instance, the possibility of tumor multifocality or adrenal metastases from a high-grade small renal tumor, as well as the association of RCC with lymphoma, must be taken into consideration by the radiologist who should also be aware of the necessity of following up a multiseptated cystic mass found at US or a Bosniak category II F renal cyst, given that these lesions can be an early manifestation of cystic carcinoma.

Occasionally, other rare imaging manifestations of RCC may occur such as an arteriovenous communication within the tumor or retroperitoneal lymph node metastases as the firsts sign of an otherwise undetectable renal cancer.

Recognizing these unusual manifestations by the radiologist improves the diagnosis process and leads to develop in specific scenarios an appropriate follow up and treatment strategy [71].

5. Staging

The formal staging system is the TNM system of the American Joint Committee on Cancer. Since cancer-specific survival for patients treated with surgery is highly correlated with the tumor stage, accurate staging is crucial for preoperative planning and prognosis [33]. The American Joint Committee on Cancer released a new staging system for renal cancer in January 2010 (Table 2, 3) [72].

The changes made in the new edition AJCC TNM classification were:

1. Subdivision of T2 tumors into T2a (lesions>7cm but < or = 10 cm) and T2b (lesions >10cm)
2. Reclassification of ipsilateral adrenal involvement as T4 (contiguous involvement) or M1 (non-contiguous involvement)
3. Reclassification of renal vein involvement as T3a
4. Reclassification of any nodal involvement as N1

Table 2. The TNM classification

T-Primary Tumour
TX: Primary tumor cannot be assessed T0: No evidence of primary tumor T1: Tumor < 7 cm in greatest dimension, limited to the kidney T1a Tumor < 4 cm in greatest dimension, limited to the kidney T1b Tumor > 4 cm but < 7 cm in greatest dimension T2: Tumor > 7 cm in greatest dimension, limited to the kidney T2a Tumor > 7 cm but < 10 cm in greatest dimension T2b Tumors > 10 cm limited to the kidney T3: Tumor extends into major veins or perinephric tissues but not into the ipsilateral adrenal gland and not beyond Gerota's fascia T3a Tumor grossly extends into the renal vein or its segmental (muscle-containing) branches or tumor invades perirenal and/or renal sinus (peripelvic) fat but not beyond Gerota's fascia T3b Tumor grossly extends into the vena cava below the diaphragm T3c Tumor grossly extends into vena cava above the diaphragm or invades the wall of the vena Cava T4: Tumor invades beyond Gerota's fascia (including contiguous extension into the ipsilateral adrenal gland)
N-Regional Lymph Nodes
NX: Regional lymph nodes cannot be assessed N0: No regional lymph node metastasis N1: Metastases in regional lymph node (s)
M-Distant Metastasis
M0: No distant metastasis M1: Distant metástasis

Table 3. American joint committee RCC stage grouping

TNM stage	
Stage I	T1 N0 M0
Stage II	T2 N0 M0
Stage III	T1 or T2 N1 M0
	T3 N0-N1 M0
Stage IV	T4 Any N M0
	AnyT Any N M1

An overall staging accuracy of 91% by preoperative CT has been reported in the past.

Historically, radical nephrectomy (RN) was considered to be the only curative treatment for RCC but over the last decade partial nephrectomy (PN) is being increasingly used in the management of RCC. The following information is critical for the surgeon:

1. Size and number of lesions.
2. Location of the tumor.
3. Involvement of renal sinus and perinephric fat
4. Involvement of renal vein an IVC
5. Involvement of adjacent organs
6. Presence of distant metastases
7. Renal vascular supply

5.1. Size and Number of Lesions

Tumor size is an important criterion which helps in deciding partial *vs* radical nephrectomy. Initially partial nephrectomy was reserved for tumors smaller than 4 cm in the greatest dimension. In patients with tumors greater than 7 cm may be amendable to partial nephrectomy (PN) [72]. In patients with multiple renal lesions who are potential candidates for PN it is important to report the total number of suspicious renal lesions (Figure 24).

5.2. Location of the Tumor

As a result of the expanding indications for partial nephrectomy and the need for standardized reporting of outcome, several groups have made the effort to develop methods of preoperative scoring to quantify renal tumor size, location and depth based on preoperative imaging findings (preoperative Aspects and Dimensions Used for Anatomic Assessment score, renal Nephrometry Score and Centrality Index) [73].

The following are the key imaging features which should be reported: the localization of the tumor (upper pole, lower pole or mid pole; anterior or posterior; near the medial or lateral rim of kidney); exophytic or endophytic tumor (>50% or <50%); involving the sinus; involving the collecting system.

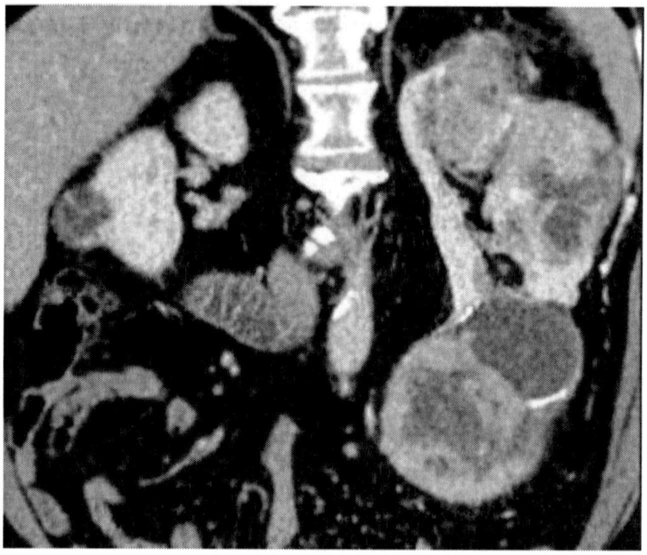

Figure 24. Reconstructed coronal contrast-enhanced CT scan shows large, heterogeneous renal masses of varying size in a sporadic bilateral synchronous multifocal RCC case.

5.3. Assessment of Renal Sinus and Perinephric Fat Invasion

Currently, there are no reliable indicators for perinephric tumor spread on CT and some considerations may be pointed. Under and over-staging of perinephric invasion are the most common staging errors at CT [32].

Perinephric stranding may be present in absence of tumor spread. The presence of an intact pseudo-capsule (i.e.; compressed normal renal parenchyma) suggests a lack of perinephric fat invasion. The pseudo-capsule is detected on MRI by T2-weighted imaging [9]. MDCT plays an important role in the diagnosis of renal sinus fat invasion and it has relatively high sensitivity but poor specificity. However, the clinical usefulness of MDCT is limited due to the low prevalence of this condition being then associated to a low positive predictive value. A tumor size larger than 50 mm, decreased perfusion of the diseased kidney, an irregular tumor margin and lymph node metastasis are predictive factors of renal sinus fat invasion (Figure 25) [74, 75] and intraoperative ultrasound may be useful in such circumstance [9]. Diagnostic accuracy of MR for assessing renal sinus invasion remains unclear [9, 33].

5.4. Venous System Invasion and Thrombus Tumor

Evaluation of the venous system in patients with renal malignancy is crucial for treatment planning. Previously performed with conventional venography, this evaluation is now being done with noninvasive cross-sectional imaging [33].

MRI was traditionally the gold standard for assessing vascular invasion but there is increasing evidence that advent MDCT is an effective imaging modality for showing tumor thrombus level [9] and highly accurate in the detection of spread of RCC into the venous system (Figure 26) [76].

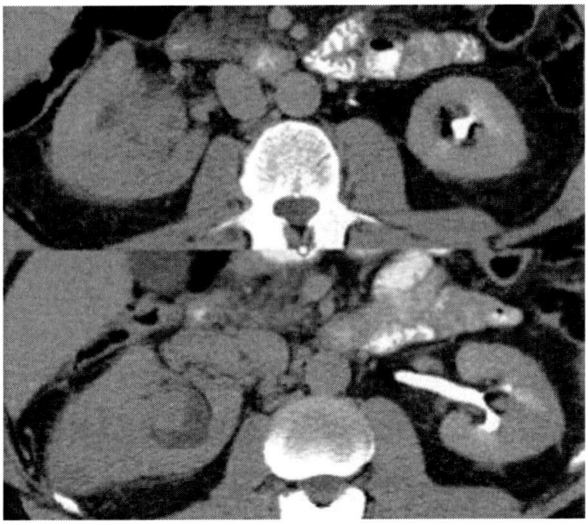

Figure 25. Non- enhancing kidney. Axial contrast-enhanced CT during excretory phase shows a renal mass in the middle and upper portions of the left kidney involving the renal sinus. Neither enhancement nor contrast material excretion is present in the right kidney.

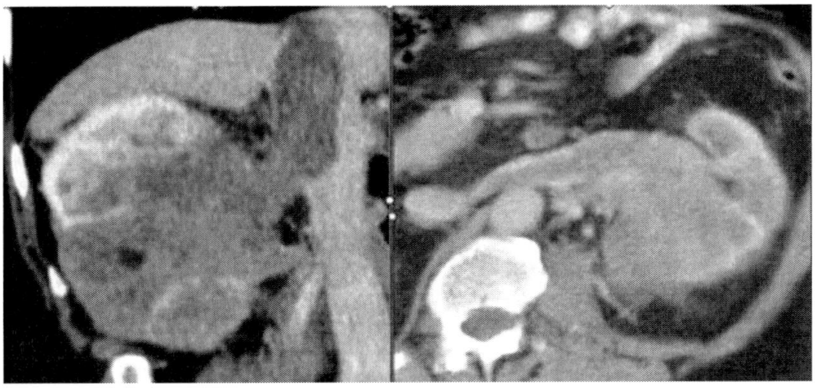

Figure 26. (a) Coronal contrast-enhanced nephrographic-phase CT scan shows enlargement of right renal vein and inferior vena cava due to intravenous extension of tumor originating in the right kidney. (b) Axial contrast-enhanced CT scan shows a tumor thrombus in the left renal vein.

Accurate assessment of the upper extent of caval thrombus is crucial in determining the surgical approach and risk of complications. Extent of involvement has been defined with several thrombus levels: level 0, renal vein; level I, <2 cm above renal vein; level II >2cm above renal vein but below hepatic veins; level III, at the hepatic veins but below the diaphragm; level IV, above the diaphragm. Levels 0-II are usually approached with anterior subcostal or midline abdominal incision and levels III-IV may require sternotomy [9, 77].

A thrombus involving the renal vein or inferior vena cava may represent tumor thrombus or a bland blood clot or both. The presence of enhancement within the thrombus indicates tumor thrombus [33].

In some cases, the tumor thrombus may extend beyond the margin of the wall of inferior vena cava indicating invasion of the wall. Invasion of the IVC wall has shown to be a significant prognostic factor and must be assessed by the radiologist in order to determine the extent of IVC resection and reconstruction, use of neo-adjuvant therapy and identify those patients who can be treated without surgery.

Occasionally, pseudo-thrombosis can be seen on CT as an IVC filling defect caused by laminar flow of enhanced blood from renal veins streaming parallel to the column of unopacified blood returning from the lower body, or as a result from poorly enhanced blood. Delayed images to show resolution of the filling defect are usually sufficient to confirm the artefactual nature [78].

5.5. Nodal Involvement

Identification of cases of clinical node positive disease or other high risk findings alters the planned surgical procedure and is critical to the urologist [74]. On cross-sectional imaging, assessment of lymph nodes relies on anatomic size criteria and it is limited for detecting normal-sized lymph nodes. Studies show CT had 83% sensitivity and 88% specificity for detecting metastatic lymphadenopathy using a 1 cm cut off size. However, it is well known that this size based evaluation is associated with high false positive and false negative rates. Some data suggest that about 50 percent of patients with radiography enlarged nodes in the 1 to 2 cm size range do not harbor metastases [9, 74].

5.6. Invasion of Adrenal Gland and Adjacent Organs

Adrenalectomy was historically simultaneously carried out with nephrectomy in RCC surgery. However, the reported low incidence of adrenal invasion by RCC and the morbidity of adrenal insufficiency had led to question this traditional procedure [9, 74]. Abnormality in size, shape and density of the adrenal gland, presence of adrenal nodule, direct tumor infiltration, displacement or abnormal location of adrenal and not visualization of the adrenal gland are some of the imaging features which may predict adrenal involvement.

If preoperative CT or MRI findings show equivocal or abnormal imaging findings in the adrenal gland the adrenalectomy is indicated [79].

While CT scan has high negative predictive value, its positive predictive value is relatively low [9]. However, imaging outcomes are likely to improve with technical advances. The demonstration of adjacent organs or structures involvement confers a poor prognosis. CT scan has a limited positive predictive value for detecting invasion into adjacent organs, as has been noted regarding adrenal spread, but it has 100% specific. Involved structures are most commonly the colon, pancreas, diaphragm, liver, spleen, and bowel mesentery. However, any suspicious finding should be reported to the surgeon so the possibility of a more extensive surgery, which may require of multidisciplinary approach [9, 74].

5.7. Metastatic Disease

The size of the primary tumor seems to correlate with the likelihood of renal tumor metastases. As a general rule, incidentally detected small renal tumors are unlikely to present with metastases.

Multi phasic images obtained in the arterial and portal venous phase allow accurate detection of metastases, which common sites comprise the lung, lymph nodes, bone, liver (Figure 27) and brain.

It is important to carefully identify the full extent of metastases since patients with oligo-metastases may still be considered for aggressive curative resection.

CT of the abdomen and pelvis and a chest radiograph are studies in the initial workup. Other procedures that may be useful to assessing for distant metastases include a chest CT, MRI and PET. PET may be more sensitive than radionuclide scan for detection of bone metastases

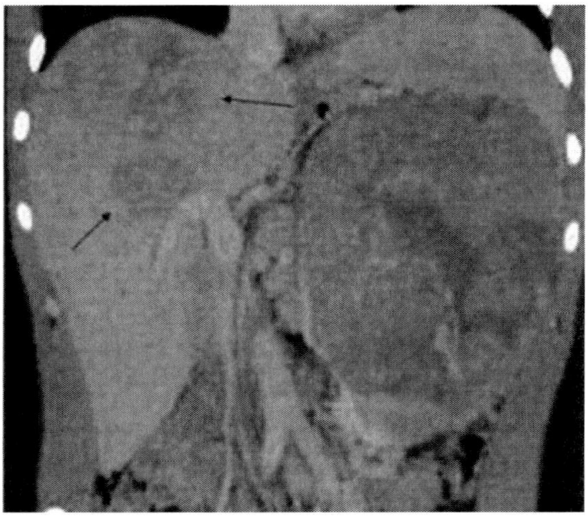

Figure 27. Liver metastases of RCC. Coronal CT scan reveals two hypovascular hepatic metastases.

6. Surveillance and Follow up

6.1. Active Surveillance

Surgical resection is considered to be the only effective curative treatment for clinically localized renal tumor. Classically it comprises total nephrectomy but in recent years partial nephrectomy has been shown to be equally effective in selected groups.

Furthermore, active surveillance might be an alternative in those patients presenting with small renal masses who appear to have no local tumor progression and a decreased risk of metastatic disease [41].

Active surveillance is defined as the initial monitoring of tumor size by serial abdominal imaging, ultrasound, CT or MRI, with delayed intervention reserved for those tumors that show clinical progression during follow up [42].

6.2. Post Operative Surveillance

In order to monitor or identify postoperative complications, renal function, local recurrence, recurrence in the contralateral kidney and development of metastases, surveillance after treatment must be carried out. Although most of them take place within 3 years after surgery [80] late tumor recurrences many years after initial treatment occasionally occurs.

The lung is the most vulnerable site for distant recurrence, affecting 50% to 60% of patients. Other common sites include bone, the nephrectomy site, brain, liver, and the contralateral kidney. Greatest tumor diameter, TNM staging and nuclear grade are important factors in determining the likelihood of recurrence [81]. Planning follow-up on the basis of risk of progression and the type of treatment performed seem reasonable and strict follow up schedules may be required depending on the availability of new effective treatments.

Available guidelines from the American College of Radiology [82] and the European Association of Urology [42] are not categorical in their recommendations and neither is there uniformity in the strategies (Table 4) [83].

Table 4. Recommended regimens follow-up of renal carcinoma

	American College of Radiology	European Association of Urologist
After nephrectomy	– T1: chest radiograph every 6–12 months for 3 years, and at year 5. – T2: chest radiograph every 6–12 months for 3 years, then annually until year 5; CT of abdomen year 2 and 5 or annually until year 5. – T3/T4: chest radiograph every 6–12 months for 3 years, then annually until year 5; CT of abdomen every 3–6 months for 3 years, then annually until year 5.	– Low risk: chest radiograph or ultrasound at 6, 12, 24, 36, and 48 months and CT of chest and abdomen at year 5. – Intermediate risk: CT of chest and abdomen at 6, 24, and 60 months; chest radiograph or ultrasound at 12 and 48 months. – High risk: CT of chest and abdomen at 6, 12, 24, 36, 48, and 60 months.
After ablative therapy	1, 3, 6, and 12 months (with unenhanced and contrast-enhanced abdominal CT). Later follow-up not specified. Chest imaging not commented on.	– Low or intermediate risk: CT of chest and abdomen at 6, 24, and 60 months; chest radiograph or ultrasound at 12 and 48 months. – High risk: CT of chest and abdomen at 6, 12, 24, 36, 48, and 60 months.
Receiving chemotherapy	Not specified	Not specified
Hereditary renal cancers	Not specified	– Mild phenotype: imaging every 2–3 years. – Aggressive phenotype: imaging every 3–6 months. Imaging methods not further specified.
Active surveillance	Not specified	Not specified

CT with contrast of the chest and abdomen is the investigation of choice in case of high/intermediate risk of relapse, although the significant morbidity associated with the radiation exposure involved in repeated CT scans should be taken into account. It should include arterial phase images since pancreatic and liver metastases may be hyper-vascular and can be missed if only portal venous phase images are obtained [9].

Gadolinium-enhanced MRI of the abdomen and pelvis may be performed in patients with impaired renal function, contraindications to iodinated contrast or in case of pregnancy.

For low risk disease CT abdominal can be used infrequently.

Chest imaging is recommended, being chest radiography still supported by some organizations (Table 4), for thoracic surveillance in low risk groups, despite the fact it is far less sensitive than chest CT in the early detection of potentially treatable lung nodules. Chest CT should be considered for those patients in higher risk, which is based on the size of the primary lesion [83].

Brain scans and bony evaluation should be used only in selected cases and usually in patients with relevant symptoms outside the thorax and abdomen.

Abdominal ultrasound may be used but only in the low-risk disease group. Moreover, 18F-FDG PET plays a limited role [83].

The follow-up strategy after nephron-sparring surgery is similar to nephrectomy, though especial attention should be put on the remnant kidney where local recurrence rates are 4-6%. These tend to appear a maximum of 6-24 months after surgery in patients with stage T3 disease and later than 48 months in stage T2 disease [39]. Abdominal studies should be undertaken after administration of IV contrast medium [81] regardless the chosen protocol given that normal enhancement is a key diagnostic sign. Abnormal renal enhancement is an indication of recurrence near the surgical resection site or *a de novo* renal tumor.

The resection site can also show unusual appearances soon after surgery, due to the presence of thrombogenic material or the use of radiofrequency cauterization used to aid local homeostasis. A subtle margin of enhancement can be observed and occasionally a frank masslike effect which can persist for up to 12 months or even longer [83].

Depending on the availability of new effective treatments, stricter follow up schedules may be required, particularly because there is a higher local recurrence rate after cryotherapy and radiofrequency ablation. Although there is no agreement about the timing of the first scan after treatment (from immediately after ablation to up to 1 month) early scanning seems important given that most of inadequate treatments were noted within 3 months of ablation in one study [84]. There are no formal recommendations but abdominal surveillance should be undertaken using a dedicated renal mass protocol CT (or MRI) with unenhanced and contrast-enhanced studies, because abnormal enhancement is a key indicator of residual or recurrent local disease [83].

Those patients with end stage renal disease due to acquired cystic disease of the kidney or von Hippel-Lindau syndrome deserve more specialized follow-up. One of the features of RCC is that it can have an unpredictable time course with recurrence-free intervals of up to 30 years, thus prolonged periods of follow up may therefore be needed [39].

There are no formal recommendations yet, but patients with a proven high-risk tumor should be imaged more regularly (e.g., with a CT or MRI scan every 3–6 months), whereas those with a low-risk tumor should be imaged every 2–3 years [85].

There is no agreement regarding the optimal duration of follow-up and it has been considered that follow-up with imaging is not cost-effective after 5 years. However, late metastases are more likely to be solitary and justify more aggressive therapy with curative intent. PET, PET-TC and bone scintigraphy are not the standard of care in RCC surveillance, due to their limited specificity and sensitivity.

6.3. Evaluation of Tumor Response to Targeted Therapy

Several criteria may be helpful in evaluating response to targeted therapy in metastatic RCC patients (table 5). The Response Evaluation Criteria in Solid Tumor classification (RECIST 1.1) is the most frequently used method to evaluate tumor response and it is based on lesion change size [86].

However, RECIST has substantial limitations since the news therapies (e.g., antiangiogenic) are a mechanism of action cytostatic which leads to disease stabilization without tumor regression. New criteria that did not rely only on change in tumor size were needed to assess tumor response to treatment so more emphasis has been placed on functional criteria (e.g., changes in attenuation) than morphologic criteria.

The "functional" molecular imaging techniques to depict physiologic process within tumors (e.g., dynamic contrast-enhanced CT or MR imaging, PET) are being incorporated into the new classifications based on attenuation, structure and morphology criteria to assess response of metastatic disease (Choi, Modified Choi) [87]. Morover, complications related to drugs toxicity can also be detected on follow-up imaging [9].

Table 5. Response evaluation criteria in solid tumors

	RECIST criteria 1.1*	CHOI criteria	Modified CHOI**	WHO Criteria***
CR	Disappearance of all target lesions		Disappearance of all lesions	
SD	<30% size reduction an <10% size increase	<10% size reduction or <15% enhancement reduction	<10% size reduction and <15% enhancement reduction	
PR	> 20% increase in the SLD taking as reference the smallest SLD recorded since the treatment started (nadir) and minimum 5 mm increase over the nadir or appearance of new lesions;	>10% size reduction or >15% enhancement reduction	>10% size reduction and >15% enhancement reduction	≥50% decrease from baseline, confirmed at ≥4 wk.
PD	PR, ≥30% decrease from baseline, confirmed at 4 wk.	>10% size reduction enhancement reduction criteria not fulfilled and new disease	>10% size, reduction enhancement reduction criteria not fulfilled and new disease	≥25% increase of one or more lesions or appearance of new lesions; NC, neither PR nor PD criteria met

*RECIST: Response Evaluation Criteria in Solid Tumors.

**CHOI: Choi et al. criteria.

***WHO=World Health Organization criteria.

Abbreviations: CR=complete response; SD=stable disease; PR=partial response; PD=progressive disease. SLD=sum of longest diameters of target lesion.

7. Advances on Imaging

7.1. Dual Energy CT

Dual-energy CT refers to the use of CT data representing two different energy spectra to display anatomy and pathology in addition to differentiating and classifying tissue composition.

Dual-energy CT data can be obtained and viewed using various hardware and software applications capable of material-specific classification and image display. Although image acquisition with dual-energy CT is similar to that with single-energy CT, comprehensive post-processing is able to generate not only images that are similar to single-energy CT (SECT) images, but a variety of other images, such as virtual unenhanced (VUE), virtual monochromatic (VMC) and material-specific iodine images [88-90]. Dual-energy CT provides radiologists with promising technology that has the potential to improve detection and characterization of renal lesions, while decreasing radiation dose exposure to patients [90]. A daily challenge for the radiologist is the differential diagnosis between benign high-attenuation cysts (Bosniak category II cystic mass) and solid enhancing lesions (most importantly renal cell carcinoma) on contrast-enhanced images. Differentiating a small or minimally enhancing neoplasm from a hyperattenuating cyst may be difficult on conventional CT images acquired with a single energy and a single contrast-enhanced scanning phase. The use of VUE and iodine images, which are post-processed from a dual-energy acquisition, may help differentiate enhancing renal lesions from non-enhancing lesions. Iodine-specific maps may demonstrate iodine in tissues (e.g., a solid lesion) or its absence (e.g., a hyperattenuating cyst) to aid lesion characterization. Enhancement may also be quantified in lesions that are suspicious for malignancy.

As renal cysts are avascular, color-coded iodine-specific images show a cyst as devoid of iodine signal. This is opposite to what is found in enhancing solid renal masses, which demonstrate iodine signal within the lesion [89, 90].

Color-coded iodine overlay images can provide benefits over conventional greyscale imaging for the evaluation of enhancement in sub-centimeter lesions, as well as in eliminating the potential errors in region of interest (ROI) positioning on renal tumors that are isodense to the renal parenchyma on the unenhanced image.

Preliminary evidence suggests that iodine quantification may be superior to standard attenuation measurements, especially in discriminating minimally enhancing tumors, such as papillary subtypes of renal cancer, from high-attenuation cysts.

Processed VUE images may provide supplementary information about fat, hemorrhage, and calcification in a lesion, similar to TUE images [91].

Iodine maps may also help differentiate a bland thrombus in the renal vein from a tumoral thrombus by qualitatively and quantitatively depicting iodine in the thrombus.

On the other hand, dual-energy CT is attractive because iodine maps (which are created with data from dual-energy CT) may be used to evaluate and quantify tumor viability [92]. The color scales in iodine maps indicate the amount of iodine-vascularity in lesions. Although this approach requires validation and standardization, it is promising and provides whole-body coverage in one acquisition.

In a recent study, it was observed that iodine maps obtained immediately after radiofrequency ablation showed better lesion conspicuity and internal homogeneity of the ablation zone, an additional benefit for assessing safety margins after radiofrequency ablation [93].

Some other important advantages are Low-energy (kilo-electron voltage) images generated from dual-energy CT that permit the use of low dose of iodine at chest and abdominal CT and by following a low-dose-contrast material protocol, in which we administer 50–70 mL of 370 mg I/mL contrast material, on a case-by-case basis for those undergoing dual-energy CT [90].

There are some workflow challenges with this new technique, some of which are related to the availability and costs of CT scanners. To date, dual-energy CT can only be read on workstations with dedicated post-processing software, but in the near future, reading on picture archiving and communication system (PACS) workstations will become available [91].

Patients with a large body habitus may exceed the maximum table weight (with both dual-energy CT systems) and tube FOV (with dual-source dual-energy CT), which may result in excessive artifacts and poor material separation. Therefore, educating technologists on the importance of careful protocol selection on the basis of the clinical indication and organ of interest and on proper patient positioning during imaging is critical [90]. Despite the progressive spread of dual-energy CT capability, it is still not widely available and some clinical applications are in early stages.

7.2. Advances on MR Applications

The risk of nephrogenic systemic fibrosis (NFS) in patients with severely compromised renal function (estimated glomerular filtration rate <30 mL/min/ 1.73 m) has given a new boost in the development of MRI techniques without the use of gadolinium-based contrast agent to perform MR angiography and MR perfusion.

Arterial Spin Labeling (ASL) is an MR technique using the water in arterial blood as an endogenous contrast agent to evaluate perfusion non-invasively. Several investigations have demonstrated it is a promising procedure in characterizing tumor perfusion. Quantitative images of blood flow can be generated and thus used as quantitative markers of response to therapy (e.g., anti-angiogenic therapy) [48].

8. Termal Ablation of RCC

Currently, the majority of all renal tumors will be being detected incidentally. Moreover, they are often diagnosed in elderly patients with preexisting medical comorbidities in whom the risk of surgical complications due to underlying medical problems has led to an increased interest in minimally invasive, ablative modalities as an alternative to extirpative surgical intervention for selected patients [94].

To preserve renal function and avoid unnnecesary surgical removal of the entire kidney to treat a small renal tumor, nephron-sparing surgery (NSS) has replaced radical nephrectomy for patients in whom complete removal of the tumor is possible without compromising the remnant portion of the kidney [95].

Concurrent advances in thermal ablation (TA) technology and refinement of this technique have established a role of TA in the treatment of renal masses [96]. The most extensively used techniques are Radiofrequency ablation (RFA) and Cryoablation [97]. The increasing acceptance of RFA and cryoablation for kidney tumors is based upon favorable outcomes in initial studies, a low incidence of serious complications, less immediate morbidity and mortality than with surgery, lower cost and the ability to treat patients in the outpatient setting [98, 99]. However, no randomized comparisons have been performed between the outcome of ablative techniques and radical nephrectomy or partial nephrectomy [100].

8.1. Indications

The indications for RFA and cryoablation to treat RCC have not been definitively established. Factors that can lead to consideration of an ablative approach rather than surgery include:

- A small (less 4 cm in diameter) incidentally detected RCC.
- A patient who is considered a poor surgical candidate, based upon older age or significant comorbidity.
- The need for nephron-sparing treatment. This includes patients with a single kidney, bilateral RCCs or a genetic predisposition to multiple tumors (e.g., von Hippel-Lindau syndrome).
- As well as patient preference [101].

8.2. Contraindications

Relative contraindications may include a poor life expectancy of less than 1 year, multiple metastases or difficulty for successful treatment due to size or location of tumor.

In general, large tumors (i.e., There is no absolute size limit of a renal mass that would exclude a patient from radiofrequency ablation; however, the likelihood of complete ablation is higher for smaller tumors <5 cm) or tumors in the hilum or central collecting system are not typically recommended for percutaneous tumor ablation but the only absolute contraindications include irreversible coagulopathies or severe medical instability [20].

8.3. Technical Considerations

Successful percutaneous tumor ablation requires killing all viable malignant cells including a 5 to 10 mm "ablative" margin of surrounding tissue [102].

Although radiofrequency and cryoablation devices can be introduced intra-operatively with US guidance during an open procedure, the most experience with and the maximum benefit from these techniques have been with percutaneous imaging guided procedures. The laparoscopic route is only suggested for tumors at risk due to their topography, particularly in anterior position, justifying direct visual control during thermal ablation.

Apart from its less invasive character, the advantages of the percutaneous approach are less pain, immediate verification (which is possible using CT, MRI or ultrasound), a shorter period of hospitalization and reduced overall cost. CT guidance is currently best for localizing the tumor and controlling the procedure [103].

The technique of placing the electrode is analogous to that of performing percutaneous imaging guide biopsy of renal mass. After local anesthesia is applied, the applicator is advanced into the center of tumor under CT, US or MRI guidance.

In radiofrequency ablation, a high frequency is emitted through an electrode placed within the targeted tissue generating a frictional heat which results in cancer cell destruction when the temperatures exceed 60°C. Cryoablation uses liquid nitrogen or argon introduced into a probe in a controlled fashion, destroying the tumor by cellular damage resulting from freezing, apoptosis, coagulation necrosis and immunologic action, with the formation of an "ice ball" that can be visualized. Hypothermic ablation decreases tissue temperature to −40°C [104]. It has been recommended that a biopsy should be performed to establish a histological diagnosis either prior to or at the time of therapy and the correct knowledge about tumor histology is of paramount importance for further clinical management of these patients [94].

8.4. Complications

The rate of major complications is generally in the range of 0 to 6% [103] and can be classified as major or minor based on the classification of the Society of Interventional Radiology, with major complications requiring treatment or hospitalization and minor complications needing only conservative monitoring.

Major complications are ureteric stricture, acute tubular necrosis resulting in permanent renal failure, calyceal cutaneous fistula, renal abscesses and thermal injury to adjacent organs. Minor complications include lateral cutaneous nerve paresthesia, skin burn, self-limiting subcapsular hematoma and self-limiting pneumothorax [104]. Perirenal hematoma is the most common complication, in 0 to 30% of cases depending on the series, and particularly concerns procedures performed using cryotherapy. Gross hematuria at the end of the procedure, pain and neuromuscular weakness are usually temporary and uncommon. Tumor dissemination along the applicator path is exceptional, as only two cases have been reported in the literature [105]. Despite taking aseptic measures, the risk of infection is not negligible, being in the order of 0 to 2% in radiofrequency ablation.

A self-limited post-ablation syndrome manifested by fever and flu-like symptoms has been reported in up to one-third of patients following RFA and cryoablation [105, 97].

In conclusion, complications following renal ablation are infrequent. Collaboration between urologists and radiologists can optimize peri and post-procedural outcomes.

8.5. Surveillance after Ablation

It is essential for patients to be monitored by imaging for remnants or recurrences.

A clear increase in the volume of the site treated by heat ablation appears early in the following week and the first 2 months after the procedure.

Then, the scar volume gradually decreases over 1 to 2 years. In a CT scan, the density of the treated area, is and remains spontaneously denser than the adjacent renal parenchyma. No contrast uptake should be identified. A thin ring of peripheral enhancement can be seen on late acquisitions throughout follow-up with no suspicious character, probably related to inflammatory changes.

In MRI, the treated site is heterogeneous, generally with a T1 hypersignal and a T2 hyposignal without contrast uptake. A spontaneously dense peripheral halo with a T1 hyposignal has been reported in nearly 75% of cases; it appears during the first months and often persists.

In both CT and MRI, edema of peripheral fat is almost systematic, especially with exophytic tumours.

MRI has no particular advantage over CT apart from not requiring injection of an iodinated contrast agent; it should therefore be preferred in cases of renal impairment. The presence of focal nodular contrast enhancement is still the only validated marker of living residual or recurrent tumor tissue and involves acquisition first without injection of contrast agent and then with this injection.

In the CT scan, enhancement is evaluated qualitatively and quantitatively, any contrast enhancement of the radiofrequency site of more than 10 HU or 15 HU must be considered significant, thus suggestive of a residual or recurrent local tumor.

In MRI, because of the T1 hypersignal from the ablation site, subtraction techniques must be widely used to detect or eliminate focal enhancement. Quantitatively, enhancement is considered significant if it exceeds 15% on the dynamic sequence.

There is no recommendation on follow-up in terms of examination dates, but there is some consensus in the literature. Follow-up is generally frequent during the first year following the ablation, with examinations gradually more widely spaced at 2, 6, 12, 18 and 24 months. An annual follow-up is then recommended for 5 years or even longer [103].

8.6. Outcomes

Long-term follow-up data are very limited, but results suggest that the recurrence-free survival rate is approximately 90 percent at five years [106].

Smaller lesion size, exophytic tumor location, and a single ablation zone were associated with primary treatment effectiveness [107].

In addition to its oncological efficacy, the low morbidity of percutaneous thermal ablation is a major asset for the treatment of kidney cancer in patients who are poor candidates for surgery because of their comorbidities [108].

Percutaneous image-guided thermal ablation is increasingly be used to treat stage T1a renal malignancies and has been adopted as an alternative treatment by the American Urological Association in patients with major comorbidities or who are at high surgical risk [104]. However, the long-term efficacy of these approaches remains to be established [20].

Multiple modalities are available, but the most common are RF and cyroablation which are likely similar in efficacy but still lack sufficient long-term data. These technologies are continuously improving and it is expected that as a result, patient selection and satisfaction will continue to expand [20].

Conclusion

The new functional imaging techniques provide both excellent anatomic and functional details which are able to depict smaller renal tumors and offer applicability to subtyping the tumors. They have considerably improved our ability of noninvasive diagnosis, staging, follow-up and reliable evaluate treatment response of RCC.

The new imaging techniques offer information unavailable to date.

On the other hand, ablative technologies, with percutaneous imaging guided procedures, have emerged as a potential alternative to surgery in select patients without compromising the oncologic outcome.

References

[1] Heidenreich, A[1]., Ravery, V. (2004) European Society of Oncological Urology. Preoperative imaging in renal cell cancer. *World J. Urol.* 22(5):307-15.

[2] American Cancer Society (2013) *Cancer facts and figures 2013*. American Cancer Society. http./www.cancer.org/acs/groups/content/@epidemiologysurveilance/documents/document/acspe-036845.pdf. Accessed 15 June 2013.

[3] Ljungberg, B., Cowan, N. C., Hanbury, D. C., et al. (2010) European Association of Urology Guideline Group. EAU Guidelines on renal cell carcinoma: The 2010 update. *European Urology*. 58:398-406.

[4] Motzer, R. J., Russo, P., Nanus, D. M., et al. (1997) Renal cell carcinoma. *Curr. Prob. Cancer* 21(4):185-232.

[5] Mathew, A[1]., Devesa, S. S., Fraumeni, J. F. Jr, et al. (2002) Global increases in kidney cancer incidence, 1973-1992. *Eur. J. Cancer Prev.* 11(2):171-8.

[6] Vargas, H. A[1]., Chaim, J., Lefkowitz, R. A., et al. (2012). Renal cortical tumors: use of multiphasic contrast-enhanced MR imaging to differentiate benign and malignant histologic subtypes. *Radiology* 264(3):779-88.

[7] Prasad, S. R., Humphrey, P. A., Catena, J. R., et al. (2006) Common and uncommon histologic subtypes of renal cell carcinoma: imaging spectrum with pathologic correlation. *Radiographics* 26(6):1795-806; discussion 1806-10. Review.

[8] Sanz-Ortega, J., Olivier, C., Pérez Segura, P., et al. (2009) Hereditary renal cancer. *Actas Urol. Esp.* 33(2):127-33. Review.

[9] Ganeshan, D., Morani, A., Ladha, H., et al. (2014) Staging, surveillance, and evaluation of response to therapy in renal cell carcinoma: role of MDCT. *Abdom. Imaging*. 39(1): 66-85.

[10] Reddan, D. N[1]., Raj, G. V., Polascik, T. J. (2001) Management of small renal tumors: an overview. *Am. J. Med.* 110(7):558-62.

[11] Rendon, R. A[1]., Stanietzky, N., Panzarella, T., et al. (2000) The natural history of small renal masses. *J. Urol.* 164(4):1143-47.

[12] Brown, C. L., Hartman, R. P., Dzyubak, O. P., et al. (2009) Dual-energy CT iodine overlay technique for characterization of renal masses as cyst or solid: a phantom feasibility study. *Eur. Radiol.* 19(5):1289-1295.

[13] Mitterberger, M., Pelzer, A., Colleselli, D., et al. (2007) Contrast enhanced ultrasound for diagnosis of prostate cancer and kidney lesions. *Eur. J. Radiol.* 64:231-238.

[14] Pischon, T[1]., Lahmann, P. H., Boeing, H., et al. (2006) Body size and risk of renal cell carcinoma in the European Prospective Investigation into Cancer and Nutrition (EPIC). *Int. J. Cancer.* 1;118(3):728-38.

[15] Bluth, E. I., Bush, W. H., Amis, E. S., et al. (2000) Indeterminate renal masses: American College of Radiology. ACR Appropriateness Criteria. *Radiology.* 215 (suppl.):747-75.

[16] Hoffmann, U., Edwards, J. M., Carter, S., et al. (1991) Role of duplex scanning for the detection of atherosclerotic renal artery disease. *Kidney Int.* 39:1232-1239.

[17] Xu, Z. F[1]., Xu, H. X., Xie, X. Y., et al. (2010) Renal cell carcinoma: real-time contrast-enhanced ultrasound findings. *Abdom. Imaging* 35:750-756.

[18] Nicolau, C[1]., Buñesch, L., Paño, B., et al. (2014). Prospective evaluation of CT indeterminate renal masses using US and contrast-enhanced ultrasound. *Abdom. Imaging.* 11 [Epub. ahead of print].

[19] Nagaraj-Setty Holalkere, Daichi Hayashi and Ali Guermaz. Renal Cell Carcinoma. En: E. Quaia (ed.). *Radiological Imaging of the Kidney.* Berlin: Springer; 2011.543-556.

[20] Bach, A. M[1]., Zhang, J. (2008). Contemporary radiologic imaging of renal cortical tumors. *Urol. Clin. North Am.* Nov;35(4):593-604.

[21] Setola, S. V., Catalano, O., Sandomenico, F., et al. (2007). Contrast-enhanced sonography of the kidney. *Abdom. Imaging.* 32(1):21-8.

[22] Bhosale, P. R[1]., Wei, W., Ernst, R. D., et al. (2014). Intraoperative sonography during open partial nephrectomy for renal cell cancer: does it alter surgical management? *AJR Am. J. Roentgenol.* 203(4):822-7.

[23] Gill, I. S., et al. (2012) Rationale for percutaneous biopsy and histologic characterization of renal tumours. *Eur. Urol.* 62:491-504.

[24] Kang, S. K[1]., Huang, W. C., Pandharipande, P. V., et al. (2014) Solid renal masses: what the numbers tell us. *AJR Am. J. Roentgenol.* 202(6):1196-206.

[25] American College of Radiology. ACR appropriateness criteria: indeterminate renal masses.American College of Radiology website. www.acr.org/~/media/ACR/Documents/Appcriteria/Diagnostic/IndeterminateRenalMasses.pdf. Published 1996. Updated 2010.

[26] Alshumrani, G[1]., O'Malley, M., Ghai, S., et al. (2010). Small (< or = 4 cm) cortical renal tumors: characterization with multidetector CT. *Abdom. Imaging.* 35(4):488-93.

[27] Johnson, P. T[1]., Horton, K. M., Fishman, E. K. (2010) How not to miss or mischaracterize a renal cell carcinoma: protocols, pearls, and pitfalls. *AJR Am. J. Roentgenol.* 194(4):W307-15.

[28] Smith-Bindman, R. (2010) Is computed tomography safe? *N. Engl. J. Med.* 363:1-4.

[29] Prakash, P., Kalra, M. K., Kambadakone, A. K., et al. (2010). Reducing abdominal CT radiation dose with adaptive statistical iterative reconstruction technique. *Invest. Radiol.* 45:202-210.

[30] Zhang, J., Lefkowitz, R. A., Bach, A. (2007) Imagin of kidney cancer. *Radiol. Clin. N. Am.* 45:119-147.

[31] Pooler, B. D[1]., Pickhardt, P. J., O'Connor, S. D., et al. (2012) Renal cell carcinoma: attenuation values on unenhanced CT. *AJR Am. J. Roentgenol.* 198(5):1115-20.

[32] Silverman, S. G., Lee, B. Y., Seltzer, S. E., et al. (1994) Small (<3-cm) renal masses correlation of spiral CT features and pathologic findings. *AJR Am. J. Roentgenol.* 163: 597-605.

[33] Sheth, S., Scatarige, J. C., Horton, K. M., et al. (2001). Current concepts in the diagnosis and management of renal cell carcinoma: role of multidetector ct and three-dimensional CT. *Radiographics.* 21 Spec. No: S237-54. Review.

[34] Cohan, R. H., Sherman, L. S., Korobkin, M., et al. (1995) Renal masses: assessment of corticomedullary-phase and nephrographic phase. *Radiology* 196;445-451.

[35] Birnbaum, B. A., Jacobs, J. E., Ramchandani, P. (1996) Multiphasic renal CT: comparison of renal mass enhancement during the corticomedullary and nephrographic phases. *Radiology* 200:753-758T scans. *Radiology* 195:445-451.

[36] Yuh, B. I., Cohan, R. H. (1999). Different phases of renal enhancement: role in detecting and characterizing renal masses during helical CT. *AJR Am. J. Roentgenol.* 173:747-755.

[37] Szolar, D. H., Kammerhuber, F., Altziebler, S., et al. (1997) Multiphasic helical CT of the kidney: increased conspicuity for detection and characterization of small (<3-cm) renal masses. *Radiology.* 202:211-217.

[38] Coppenrath, E. M[1]., Mueller-Lisse, U. G. (2006). Multidetector CT of the kidney. *Eur. Radiol.* 16(11):2603-11.

[39] Ng, C. S., Wood, C. G., Silverman, P. M. (2008). Renal Cell Carcinoma: Diagnosis, Staging, and Surveillance. *AJR* 191:1220-1232.

[40] Smith, P. A., Marshall, F. F., Corl, F. M., et al. (1999). Planning nephron-sparing renal surgery using 3D helical CT angiography. *J. Comput. Assist. Tomogr.* 23:649-654.

[41] Stakhovsky, O., Yap, S. A., Leveridge, M. (2011). Small renal mass: what the urologist needs to know for treatment planning and assessment of reatment results. *AJR.* 196: 1267-1273.

[42] Ljungverg, Bensalah K., Bex, A., et al. (2013) *Guidelines on renal cell carcinoma.* European Association of Urology.

[43] Bosniak, M. A. (1997) the use of the Bosniak classification system for renal cyst s and cystic tumors. *J. Urol.* 157(5):1852-3.

[44] Silverman, S. G., Mortele, K. J., Tuncali, K., et al. (2007) Hyperattenuating renal masses: etiologies, pathogenesis, and imaging evaluation. *Radiographics.* 27(4):1131-43. Review.

[45] Allen, B. C., Tirman, P., Clingan, M. J., et al. (2014) Characterizing solid renal neoplasms with MRI in adults. *Abdom. Imaging.* 38:358-387.

[46] Thomsen, H. S. (2009) Nephrogenic systemic fibrosis: history and epidemiology. *Radiol. Clin. North Am.* 47(5):827-31.

[47] Pedrosa, I[1]., Sun, M. R., Spencer, M., et al. (2008). MR imaging of renal masses: correlation with findings at surgery and pathologic analysis. *Radiographics.* 28(4):985-1003.

[48] Chong, S., Kappil, M., Azar, S. F., et al. (2014) MR imaging in the characterization of small renal masses. Willatt, J. M., Hussain, H. K. *Abdom. Imaging.* 39(4):761-9.

[49] Yamashita, Y., Watanabe, O., Miyazaki, T., et al. (1994). Cystic renal cell carcinoma: imaging findings with pathologic correlation. *Acta Radiol.* 35:19-24.
[50] Leroy, X., Zini, L., Leteurtre, E., et al. (2002) Morphologic subtyping of papillary renal cell carcinoma: correlation with prognosis and differential expression of MUC1 between the two subtypes. *Mod. Pathol.* 15:1126-1130.
[51] Motzer, R. J., Bander, N. H., Nanus, D. M. Renal-cell carcinoma. *N. Engl. J. Med.* 1996;335:875-875.
[52] Reuter, V. E., Tickoo, S. K. (2004). *Adult renal tumors.* Philadelphia, Pa: Lippincott Williams and Wilkins.
[53] Zukotynski, K[1]., Lewis, A., O'Regan, K., et al. (20129 PET/CT and renal pathology: a blind spot for radiologists? Part 1, primary pathology. *AJR Am. J. Roentgenol.* 199(2): W163-7.
[54] Bouchelouche, K[1]., Oehr, P. (2008) *Positron emission tomography and positron emission tomography/computerized tomography of urological malignancies: an update review.* Jan; 179(1):34-45.
[55] Oyama, N., Okazawa, H., Kusukawa, N., et al. (2009) Cacetate PET imaging for renal cell carcinoma. *Eur. J. Nucl. Med. Mol. Imaging*; 36:422-427.
[56] Divgi, C. R., Pandit-Taskar, N., Jungbluth, A., et al. (2007) Preoperative characterization of clear-cell renal carcinoma using iodine-124-labelled antibody chimeric G250 (124I-cG250) and PET in patients with renal masses: a phase I trial. *Lancet Oncol.* 8:304-310.
[57] Herts, B. R., Baker, M. E. (1995) The current role of percutaneous biopsy in the evaluation of renal masses. *Semin. Urol. Oncol.* 13:254-61.
[58] Maturen, K. E., Nghiem, H. V., Caoili, E. M., et al. (2007). Renal mass core biopsy: accuracy and impact on clinical management. *AJR Am. J. Roentgenol.* Feb; 188(2):563-70.
[59] Lebret, T., Poulain, J. E., Molinie, V., et al. (2007). Percutaneous core biopsy for renal masses: indications, accuracy and results. *J. Urol.* 178(4 Pt 1):1184-8; discussion 1188.
[60] Leveridge, M. J., Finelli, A., Kachura, J. R., et al. (2011). Outcomes of small renal mass needle core biopsy, non-diagnostic percutaneous biopsy, and the role of repeat biopsy. *Eur. Urol.* 60:578-584.
[61] Aribas, B. K., Arda, K., Aktas, E., et al. (2011) Percutaneous US-guided needle biopsies of solid renal masses. *Neoplasma.* 58(2):146-52.
[62] Volpe, A., Finelli, A., Gill, I. S., et al. (2012) Rationale for percutaneous biopsy and histologic characterisatin of renal tumours. *European urology.* 32:491-504.
[63] Roy, C., Sauer, B., Lindner, V., et al. (2007) MR Imaging of papillary renal neoplasms: potential application for characterization of small renal masses. *Eur. Radiol.* 17:193-200.
[64] Yoshimitsu, K., Kakihara, D., Irie, H., et al. (2006) Papillary renal carcinoma: diagnostic approach by chemical shift gradient-echo and echo-planar MR imaging. *J. Magn. Reson. Imaging.* 23:339-344.
[65] Fujii, Y., Komai, Y., Saito, K., et al. (2008). Incidence of benign pathologic lesions at partial nephrectomy for presumed RCC renal masses: Japanese dual-center experience with 176 consecutive patients. *Urology.* 72(3):598-602.
[66] Milner, J., McNeil, B., Alioto, J., et al. (2006). Fat poor renal angiomyolipoma: patient, computerized tomography and histological findings. *J. Urol.* 176(3):905-909.

[67] Kim, J. K., Kim, S. H., Jang, Y. J., et al. (2006). Renal angiomyolipoma with minimal fat: differentiation from other neoplasms at double-echo chemical shift FLASH MR imaging. *Radiology*. 239(1):174-180.

[68] Tanaka, H., Yoshida, S., Fujii, Y., et al. (2011) Diffusion-weighted magnetic resonance imaging in the differentiation of angiomyolipoma with minmal fat from clear cell renal cell. *Int. J. Urol*. 18(10):727-730.

[69] Hindman, N[1]., Ngo, L., Genega, E. M., et al. (2012). Angiomyolipoma with minimal fat: can it be differentiated from clear cell renal cell carcinoma by using standard MR techniques? *Radiology*. 265(2):468.

[70] Kim, J. I., Cho, J. Y., Moon, K. C., et al. (2009). Segmental enhancement inversion at biphasic multidetector CT: characteristic finding of small renal oncocytoma. *Radiology*. 252(2):441-8.

[71] Prando, A., Prando, D., Prando, P. (2006) Renal cell carcinoma: unusual imaging manifestations. *Radiographics*. 26(1):233-44.

[72] Kim, S. P., Alt, A. L., Weight, C. J., et al. (2011) Independent validation of the 2010 American Joint Committee on Cancer TNM classification for renal cell carcinoma: results from a large, single institution cohort. *J. Urol*. 85(6):2035-9.

[73] Karellas, M. E[1]., O'Brien, M. F., Jang, T. L., et al. (2010) Partial nephrectomy for selected renal cortical tumours of $\geq$ 7 cm. 106(10):1484-7.

[74] Chapin, B. F., Delacroix, S. E. Jr, Wood, C. G. (2011) Renal cell carcinoma: what the surgeon and treating physician need to know. *Am. J. Roentgenol. AJR*. 196(6):1255-62. doi: 10.2214/AJR.10.6249. Review.

[75] Kim, C., Choi, H. J., Cho, K. S. (2014) Diagnostic value of multidetector computed tomography for renal sinus fat invasion in renal cell carcinoma patients. *Eur. J. Radiol*. Jun;83(6):914-8.

[76] Stern Padovan, R., Perkov, D., Smiljanic, R., et al. (2007). Venous spread of renal cell carcinoma: MDCT. *Abdom. Imaging* 32(4):530-7.

[77] Schimmer, C., Hillig, F., Riedmiller, H., et al. (2004). Surgical treatment of renal cell carcinoma with intravascular extension. *Interact. Cardiovasc. Thorac. Surg*. 3:395-397.

[78] Catalano, C., Fraioli, F., Laghi, A., et al. (2003). High-resolution multidetector CT in the preoperative evaluation of patients with renal cell carcinoma. *AJR Am. J. Roentgenol*. 180(5):1271-7.

[79] O'Malley, R. L[1]., Godoy, G., Kanofsky, J. A., et al. (2009). The necessity of adrenalectomy at the time of radical nephrectomy: a systematic review. *S. J. Urol*. 181 (5):2009-17.

[80] D. S. Sandock, A. D. Seftel, M. I. Resnick A. (1995). New protocol for the followup of renal cell carcinoma based on pathological stage. *J. Urol*., 154(1):28-31.

[81] E. J. Chae, J. K. Kim, S. H. Kim, *et al.* (2005). Renal cell carcinoma: analysis of postoperative recurrence patterns. *Radiology*, 234(1):189-196.

[82] American College of Radiology. ACR appropriateness criteria: follow-up of renal cell carcinoma. American College of Radiology Website. www.acr.org/secondarymainmenu categories/quality_safety/app_criteria/pdf/expertpanelonurologicimaging/ follow up of renal cell carcinoma doc5.aspx. Published 1996. Updated 2009. Accessed November 9, 2011.

[83] Patel, U[1], Sokhi, H. (2012). Imaging in the follow-up of renal cell carcinoma. *AJR Am. J. Roentgenol*. 98(6):1266-76.

[84] Matin, S. F., Ahrar, K., Cadeddu, J. A., et al. (2006) Residual and recurrent disease following renal energy ablative therapy: a multi-institutional study. *J. Urol.* 176:1973-1977 [Erratum in J. Urol. 2008;179:24106].

[85] Choyke, P. L., Glenn, G. M., Walther, M. M., et al. (2003). Hereditary renal cancers. *Radiology* 226:33-46.

[86] Eisenhauer, E. A., Therasse, P., Bogaerts, J., et al. (2009). New response evaluation criteria in solid tumor: revised RECIST guideline (version 1.1). *Eur. J. cancer* 45(2): 228-247.

[87] Nathan, P. D., Vinayan, A., Stott, D., Juttla, J., Goh, V. (2010). CT response assessment combining reduction in both size and arterial phase densitive correlates with time in progression in metastases in metastatic renal cancer patients treated with targeted therapies. *Cancer boil ther.* 9(1):15-19.86.

[88] Hartman, R[1]., Kawashima, A., Takahashi, N., et al. (2012). Applications of dual-energy CT in urologic imaging: an update. *Radiologic Clinics of North America.* 50(2):191-205.

[89] Graser, A., Johnson, T. R., Hecht, E. M., et al. (2009; Dual-energy CT in patients suspected of having renal masses: can virtual nonenhanced images replace true nonenhanced images? *Radiology* 252(2):433-440.

[90] Kaza, R. K[1]., Platt, J. F., Cohan, R. H., et al. (2012) Dual-energy CT with single- and dual-source scanners: current applications in evaluating the genitourinary tract. *Radiographics* 32(2):353-69.

[91] Agrawal, M. D., Pinho, D. F., Kulkarni, N. M., et al. (2014) Oncologic applications of dual-energy CT in the abdomen. *Radiographics.* 34(3):589-612.

[92] Mileto, A., Marin, D., Nelson, R. C., et al. (2014) Dual energy MDCT assessment of renal lesions: an overview. *Eur. Radiol.* 24(2):353-62.

[93] Apfaltrer, P., Meyer, M., Meier, C., et al. (2012) Contrast-enhanced dual-energy CT of gastrointestinal stromal tumors: is iodine-related attenuation a potential indicator of tumor response? *Invest. Radiol.* 47(1):65-70.

[94] Tracy, C. R., Raman, J. D., Donnally, C., Trimmer, C. K., Cadeddu, J. A. (2010) Durable oncologic outcomes after radiofrequency ablation: experience from treating 243 small renal masses over 7.5 years. *Cancer* 116:3135-3142.

[95] Tobias Klatte, Nils Kroeger, Uwe Zimmermann, Martin Burchardt, Arie S. Belldegrun, Allan J. Pantuck- The contemporary role of ablative treatment approaches in the management of renal cell carcinoma (RCC): focus on radiofrequency ablation (RFA), high-intensity focused ultrasound (HIFU), and cryoablation. *World J. Urol.* (2014)32: 596-605.

[96] Scott M. Castle, Michael A. Gorin, Vladislav Gorbatiy, Raymond J. Leveillee. Preoperative patient counseling for diagnostic renal biopsy and complications with renal radiofrequency ablation. *World J. Urol.* (2013)31:1105-1110.

[97] M. Saksena, D. Gervais (2009). Percutaneous renal tumor ablation. *Abdom. Imaging* 34: 582-587.

[98] McAchran, S. E., Lesani, O. A., Resnick, M. I. (2005) Radiofrequency ablation of renal tumors: past, present, and future. *Urology* 66:15-22.

[99] Onishi, T., Nishikawa, K., Hasegawa, Y., et al. (2007) Assessment health-related quality of life after radiofrequency ablation or laparoscopic surgery for small renal

carcinoma: a prospective study with medical outcomes Study 36-Item Health Survey (SF-36). *Jpn. J. Clin. Oncol.* 37:750-754.

[100] Van Poppel, H., Becker, F., Cadeddu, J. A., Gill, I. S., Janetschek, G., Jewett, M. A., Laguna, M. P., Marberger, M., Montorsi, F., Polascik, T. J., Ukimura, O., Zhu, G. (2011) Treatment of localised renal cell carcinoma. *Eur. Urol.* 60:662-672.

[101] R. Houston Thompson, Tom Atwell, Grant Schmit, Christine M. Lohse, A. Nicholas Kurup, Adam Weisbrod, Sarah P. Psutka, Suzanne B. Stewart, Matthew R. Callstrom, John C. Cheville, Stephen A. Boorjian, Bradley C. Leibovich. Comparison of Partial Nephrectomy and Percutaneous Ablation for cT1 Renal Masses. *Eur. Urol.* In press (doi: 10.1016/j.eururo.2014.09.011.).

[102] Nahum Golberg, S., Dupuy, D. E. (2001) Image-guided radiofrequency tumor ablation: challenges and oportunities-part. *I. J. Vasc. Interv. Radiol.* 12:1021.

[103] F. Cornelisa, P. Balageasa, Y. Le Brasa, et al. (2012) G. Rigoua, J. R. Boutaulta, M. Bouzgarroua, N. Greniera. Radiologically-guided thermal ablation of renal tumours. *Diagnostic and Interventional Imaging*. 93, 246-261.

[104] Wah, T., Irving, H., Gregory, W., et al. (2014) Radiofrequency ablation (RFA) of renal cell carcinoma (RCC): experience in 200 tumours. *BJU Int.* 113(3):416-428.

[105] J. Martin, S. Athreya. (2013) Meta-analysis of cryoablation versus microwave ablation for small renal masses: is there a difference in outcome? *Diagn. Interv. Radiol.* 19:501-507.

[106] Levinson, A. W., Su, L. M., Agarwal, D., et al. (2008) Long-term oncological and overall outcomes of percutaneous radiofrequency ablation in high risk surgical patients with a solitary small renal mass. *J. Urol.* 180(2):499-504.

[107] T. D. McClure, D. S. Chow, N. Tan, J., et al. (2014) Intermediate Outcomes and Predictors of Efficacy in the Radiofrequency Ablation of 100 Pathologically Proven Renal Cell Carcinomas. *J. Vasc. Interv. Radiol.* 25(11):1682-8.

[108] P. Balageas, F. Cornelis, Y. Le Bras, et al. (2013) Ten-year experience of percutaneous image-guided radiofrequency ablation of malignant renal tumours in high-risk patients. *Eur. Radiol.* 23:1925-1932.

In: Renal Cell Carcinoma
Editors: J. M. Fernández-Gomez, J. García-Rodríguez
ISBN: 978-1-63482-495-8

Chapter 5

Surveillance of Small Renal Masses

J. A. Portillo, PhD[1,*], M. Domínguez, MD[1], A. Azueta, MD[2], P. Lastra, MD[3], E. Ramos, MD[1] and J. L. Gutiérrez, PhD[1]

[1]Department of Urology, Marqués de Valdecilla University Hospital, Santander, Spain
[2]Department of Pathology, Marqués de Valdecilla University Hospital, Santander, Spain
[3]Department of Radiology, Marqués de Valdecilla University Hospital, Santander, Spain

Abstract

The frequent use of abdominal imaging tests has resulted in an increased diagnosis of small renal masses (SRMs), defined as those measuring ≤4 cm. Although their natural history is not exactly known, there are data in the literature that lead us to believe that they are generally not very aggressive tumours. Therefore, the current trend is to perform partial nephrectomy (PN) following the recommendations of the European Association of Urology (EAU) (grade of recommendation A and level of evidence 1b) and American Urological Association (AUA) guidelines (grade of recommendation A). However, there are disquieting data on locally advanced, poorly differentiated and metastatic SRMs.

Moreover, in many cases the patients are elderly and have comorbidities that call into question the efficacy and cost-effectiveness of surgically treating them or using ablative methods. Radical nephrectomy (RN) can sometimes speed chronic renal failure and shorten survival. Percutaneous renal biopsy in these circumstances can have an important role in determining tumour aggressiveness and can help obtain reliable data for implementing active surveillance (AS) more safely or for treating the patient. However, the interpretation of the biopsy is not always easy due to the lack of extracted material, the difficulty in safely assigning a histological pattern and the heterogeneity of the

* Corresponding author: Jose A. Portillo, Avda del Faro 1-Bl.2-3ºb, 39012 Santander-Spain. E-mail: josepm117@gmail.com.

tumour, which can lead to difficulty determining its aggressiveness. Tumour markers can play a role in determining a better or poorer tumour prognosis.

If AS is chosen, imaging tests should be performed periodically. An increase in lesion size is the decisive factor that changes the approach to treating the patient. Although an array of other prognostic factors have been proposed that could lead us to change the expectant criterion, currently there are no reliable data beyond the increase in tumour size. We should also not forget the impact on the quality of life of patients who undergo AS.

In this chapter, we discuss the current evidence for practicing AS in SRMs, the prognostic growth factors and their progression, the indications for renal biopsy, the difficulty in interpreting them and a method for performing AS.

Keywords: small renal masses, biopsy renal masses, surveillance

Introduction

Renal cell carcinomas (RCCs) represent 2-4% of all cancers (4% in men and 3% in women) and are one of the most lethal of the genitourinary apparatus along with muscle-infiltrating bladder carcinoma. Up to 25-35% of RCCs are metastatic at diagnosis.

However, the incidence has been increasing for years due to the massive implementation of abdominal imaging tests, especially ultrasonography. It is estimated that the diagnosis increases by 2% annually. Other factors contributing to the increase in the incidence of RCC are obesity, hypertension and smoking. A high body-mass index and high blood pressure independently increase the long-term risk of renal cancer in men.

In contrast, a reduction in blood pressure lowers the risk. Tobacco smoke is clearly involved in the etiology of RCC [1, 2]. The incidence of localized RCC tumours has increased from 7.6 in 1999 to 12.2 (per 100,000 individuals) in 2008 [3]. The most significant increase has occurred in patients between 70 and 90 years of age.

As a result of this increase in the diagnosis of RCC, a significant change has been observed in the initial stages. There is a clear movement from advanced T2-T4 stages to others in which the tumour is located in the kidneys. In addition, the size of the tumours is much smaller, which is why the term "small kidney masses" (SRMs) has been increasingly used in recent years. The first step is to accurately define what we call SRMs. How small is small? From the reviewed literature, the majority of authors refer to tumours measuring ≤4 cm (or just <4 cm) as small, a size that is known as T1a from the 2002 Classification of Malignant Tumors, which is the current classification system in use. However, with the increase in the use of ultrasonography (US), computed tomography (CT) and magnetic resonance imaging (MRI), many tumours classified as SRMs are even smaller than 2.5 cm. Should all lesions measuring ≤4 cm be managed the same way, regardless of their size and/or location? Is a 1-cm lesion the same as a 3-cm lesion? The threshold only changes in von Hippel-Lindau disease, in which more aggressive approaches are taken starting from 3 cm than possible observation [4]. The Surveillance, Epidemiology and End Results (SEER) database of the National Cancer Institute programme showed an increase of 7.1-10.8 cases of the SRMs per 100,000 US inhabitants between 1983 and 2002, which represents a 52% increase [5].

The incidence of tumours measuring ≤2 cm has also increased from 0.2 to 0.8 cases per 100,000 US inhabitants; the incidence of tumours measuring between 2 and 4 cm has increased from 1 to 3.3 cases per 100,000 inhabitants [6].

Between 1988 and 2002, renal tumour size at diagnosis has gone from 6.68 cm to 5.86 cm worldwide [7]. During 1993-2004, the size of stage T1 tumours decreased from a mean diameter of 4.1 cm to 3.6 cm [8]. It is also estimated that the incidence of SRMs during 1983-2008 increased by 285% for lesions measuring <2 cm and by 244% for those measuring 2-4 cm [9]. Approximately 80-90% of all solid malignant renal masses correspond to RCC, with its various histological and genetic varieties. There are data showing that 80% of SRMs have an indolent course or have histological characteristics of low aggressiveness, but we do not know with any certainty their biological potential for growth and metastasis.

The natural history of untreated solid renal tumours is still to be defined. However, there are data that show that untreated tumours in elderly individuals have a mean growth of 0.28 cm/year, with a mean follow-up of 34 months [10].

A study also found, however, that up to 25-35% of the tumours did not grow at all over the course of 29 months (on average) [11].

Moreover, by analysing 8,400 patients with SRMs and comparing the various treatments applied (RN, PN and AS), it was observed that RN and PN were associated with a reduction in cancer-specific mortality (CSM), but this difference was not associated with patients older than 75 years [12]. Another study found that in 7,148 patients, AS was correlated with a significantly lower mortality risk when compared with RN or PN [13].

The increasing diagnosis of SRMs should lead us to believe that CSM has decreased, which does not appear to match reality. CSM appeared to be rising between 1983 and 2001 [14]; however, from 2004 to 2008, mortality decreased by 0.6% in women and by 0.4% in men per year. CSM seems to have remained stable or decreased by a trivial amount.

By diagnosing more SRMs, a greater number of surgical (or ablative) procedures have been performed, based on the idea that their extirpation will achieve a better survival outcome. A possible response to these contradictory data is that CSM has not changed for patients with large tumours because the tumours tend to have highly unfavourable histological characteristics and thereby considerable aggressiveness and their incidence has not changed significantly despite the increase in SRMs.

Although observational studies have demonstrated an increase in survival for patients with low-volume disease who have been treated, this improvement could be the result of length-time bias. Advances in the use of vascular endothelial growth factor tyrosine kinase inhibitors and mammalian target of rapamycin inhibitors seem to have increased the survival for patients with advanced disease from 7.3% (1992-1995) to 12.3% (2003-2009) [8].

The increased diagnosis of SRMs, as well as the increased diagnosis in elderly patients and/or those with additional comorbidities, has led to the consideration of AS instead of initial surgical or other ablative treatments.

Immediate surgery is deferred to avoid the potential morbidities of aggressive treatments, opting instead to monitor the SRM with imaging tests. In this context, percutaneous renal biopsy becomes relevant to help us understand the tumour's biological potential and, based on this potential, decide whether or not to treat the patient.

Indications for Renal Biopsy

Until recently, renal biopsy had been seldom used for renal tumour disease due to the lack of tissue obtained, the lack of certainty in determining the histological degree and type, the fear of tumour implants in the trajectory of the puncture and their potential complications, as well as the limited influence on the decision making process based on the results.

However, the current situation has changed, and the diagnostic certainty is approximately 90%. The sensitivity of renal biopsies varies between 86% and 100%, and the specificity varies between 97% and 100% [15].

The risk of tumour implantation in the trajectory of the puncture is almost anecdotal [16]. Currently, biopsy for renal tumour disease appears to have clear indications [17, 18]:

- Determine the histology and degree of differentiation of the SRMs to decide upon the appropriate treatment
- Before ablative treatment.
- During the follow-up of patients treated with ablative therapies.
- Suspected renal lymphoma or xanthogranulomatous pyelonephritis
- Suspected metastatic renal disease spread to lung, liver or other location and for ruling out metastases of another primary tumour.
- Unresectable renal tumour, to apply molecular therapies.

The renal biopsy of SRMs is gaining adherents, its use is increasing and it has been observed that the results of the biopsy can change the treatment of these masses; however, routine biopsy is not indicated, and its role is still controversial. In theory, biopsy should only be performed if, based on its results, one treatment or another will be adopted. Biopsy may also be performed for bilateral masses in which nephron preservation is paramount or in solitary tumours [19].

In addition, there are no exact data on the prognosis for patients whose masses are biopsied. Observational studies are usually focused on the correlation between the biopsy and the surgical specimen. However, we do not know the impact of biopsies on the prognosis of the tumour disease; studies are needed to better clarify its usefulness [20].

In theory, SRM biopsy should help identify lesions with benign histologies, define the histological subtype, determine the Fuhrman grade and obtain tissue for the study of biological markers [21]. At present, there is no standardised method for optimising the results of renal biopsies to reduce the percentage of undiagnosed samples, which in a number of series reaches up to 33% [17, 22].

The AUA guidelines state that the accuracy of renal percutaneous biopsy has improved substantially due to refinements in CT and MRI-guided techniques. However, the procedure is not indicated for patients with comorbidities and who should consider only conservative management options regardless of the biopsy results or who have higher risks of biopsy-related complications [23]. In a series of 294 patients with 314 SRMs, 345 biopsies were performed on these masses, which were either treated surgically or with AS. In 80.6% of the cases, the biopsy was diagnostic (79.4% malignant, 94.1% of them RCC); in 19.4% of the cases, the biopsy was not diagnostic (67 cases). Of these 67 cases, the biopsy was repeated in 12 cases and was diagnostic in 10 cases (8 malignant and 2 oncocytomas).

The authors reached the conclusion that a large tumour size (within the SRM size range) and a suspicion of a solid mass predict a diagnostic biopsy and that a nondiagnostic biopsy should not be considered as the probable absence of malignancy [24].

We increasingly see more authors who believe that renal biopsies should be performed on all patients with SRMs for whom AS is planned, especially if their life expectancy is not short. After what we have learned with AS in prostate cancer in which the biopsy is essential for decision making, it appears to be reasonable to perform AS for kidney disease with the same principles [25]. We might therefore avoid finding metastatic cases in the follow-up, which, although uncommon, are still disquieting. In the only (to date) prospective, phase II clinical trial of AS of 209 SRMs [22] renal tumour biopsy was only performed in 56% of the cases at study entry.

Of considerable importance are the recommendations published by an international consensus panel in 2014 [26]. These guidelines recommend performing biopsies for SRMs when AS is applied but not for watchful waiting (WW). Of course, biopsies should be performed for cases of ablative therapy, if possible before the treatment.

Likewise and whenever feasible, biopsies (of all tumours) should be performed in cases of multiple tumours and for those cases in which there is another primary tumour or when the patient has had other, already treated renal lesions.

Renal Biopsy Technique and Complications

Technical Aspects

In general, the biopsy procedure is performed in an outpatient setting, with the patient remaining under observation to rule out any complications.

A normal coagulation study is required, but antibiotic prophylaxis is not necessary. The approach is percutaneous and image-guided, using US, CT or MRI.

CT provides precise control over the procedure and is the most widely used modality despite the use of ionising radiation (Figure 1). Practically all lesions are visible with this modality, and the control of the needle's trajectory is optimal.

The ultrasound modality has the advantage of high availability and low cost. It provides real-time, multiplanar control, is versatile in terms of the approach and does not use ionising radiation.

Not all lesions are accessible by this modality, and the control of the needle's trajectory can occasionally be limited by interposing structures (Figure 2, 3).

Lastly, MRI is the least employed technique due its lower availability and greater cost.

The modality to employ depends on numerous factors, including those that are available, operator preferences and the approach possibilities depending on the lesion size, location and relationship with adjacent structures. In any case, there is no evidence in the literature that supports the superiority of one modality over the other [24].

The procedure is performed under local anaesthesia or light sedation because patient collaboration is often required in terms of positioning and/or assistance with breathing for an optimal approach, especially if the procedure is performed with ultrasound guidance.

To obtain tissue from a kidney tumour, needles of various thicknesses can be used.

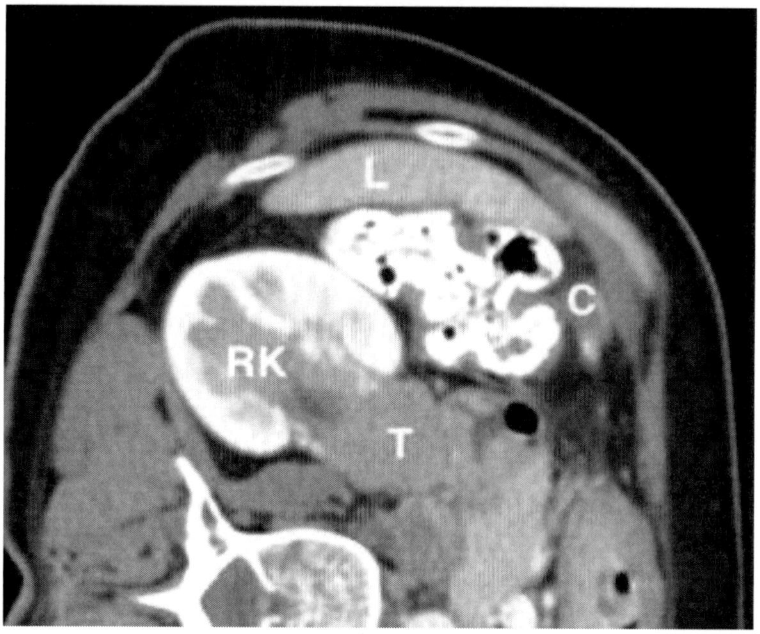

Figure 1. CT Image rotated 90º. Right renal tumour (T), in an eccentric location in the renal sinus. Interposing right colon (C), which appears replete with contrast, between the liver (L) and right kidney (RK).

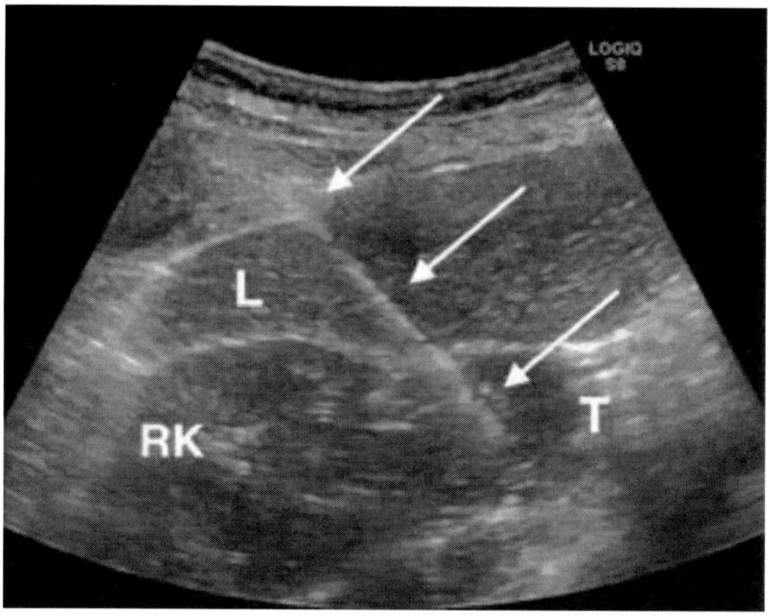

Figure 2. Ultrasound-guided renal biopsy. The biopsy needle (arrows) passes through the hepatic lobe (L) until it reaches the tumour (T) on the right kidney (RK). Positioning the patient in lateral decubitus allows the colon to be moved medially away from the needle's trajectory.

Although there is no clear standardisation, we use the term fine-needle aspiration (FNA) when using small-calibre needles (in general 21G or finer); the sample is then studied using cytology techniques.

With larger calibre needles (20G or thicker) using automatic or semiautomatic devices, the true renal mass biopsy (RMB) is performed, obtaining cores for histological analysis.

To perform the RMB, needles measuring between 7 cm and 15 cm are employed, according to the patient's somatic characteristics and the location of the lesion. The needle thickness is 16-20G, with 18G the most widely used to provide an appropriately thick core, with a good balance between sample quality and risk of complications. A study with biopsies performed *ex vivo* on surgical specimens compared histological results using devices with 14G, 18G and 20G, with greater diagnostic yield (97%) for 18G needles [27].

The diagnostic yield for RMBs is currently high, with a greater than 90% diagnostic accuracy for malignancy [28]. FNA has lower diagnostic yield, and its use is therefore not recommended alone [26].

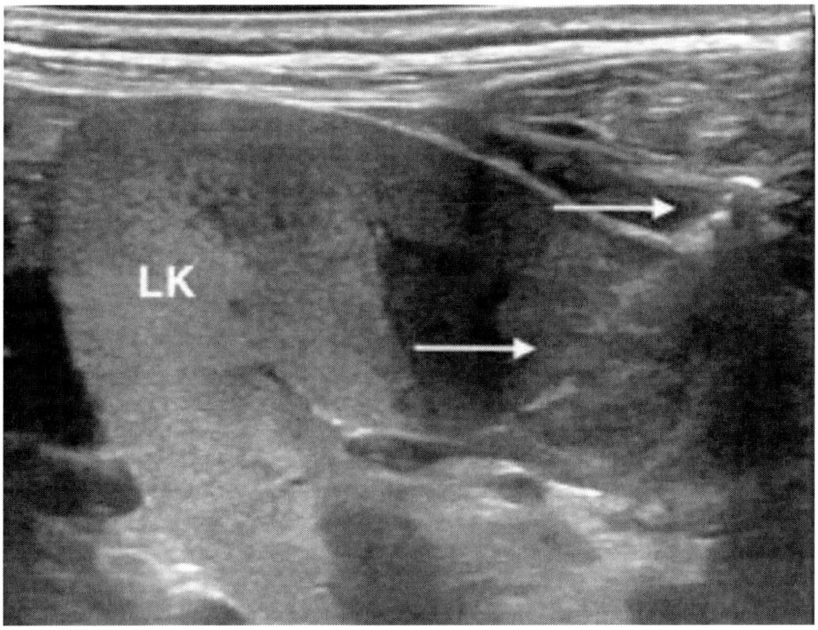

Figure 3. Ultrasound-guided renal biopsy. Ultrasound access to the left kidney (LK), posterior pathway. a) Left intraparenchymal and hypoechoic renal tumour in posterior cortical mesorenal location (between arrows). b) The needle (arrows) passes through the posterior muscle plane until it reaches the tumour.

Complications

In an extensive review of the standard practice of renal biopsies in small renal masses [17] the authors concluded that RMB is a safe, cost-effective technique that has few complications and considerable diagnostic yield.

The technique is also highly useful for individuals who have traditionally been treated with surgery or ablative techniques. Active surveillance can now be a perfectly valid option.

RMB is currently considered a safe procedure, with a very low rate (0-2%) of major, clinically significant complications [29]. The situation is different with renal biopsies of native kidneys of patients with nephropathy and coagulation disorders in whom the index of complications can be higher. A number of authors have found a 5.6% rate of complications and the need for an interventional approach for 1.6% of cases when using 16G needles in these patients [30]. Other authors, however, found rates of up to 13%, although only 3.7% of the cases involved major complications [31].

The most common complication was perinephric haemorrhage, present in a lesser or greater degree as in any other biopsy procedure. In the vast majority of cases, the complication was subclinical, self-limiting and only detectable using post biopsy check-up imaging studies. Although the presence of a certain degree of perinephric haemorrhage can be shown in the majority of biopsies (90%), the percentage of clinically significant haemorrhages (i.e., those that require hospitalisation or transfusion) is exceptionally low (0-1.3%) [32]. Haematuria can also occur, and it is assumed that a certain degree of microscopic haematuria will frequently occur, especially in endophytic lesions. However, gross haematuria is uncommon, as is local or systemic infection.

The formation of an arteriovenous fistula is another reported complication, although it is rare and is commonly related to renal parenchyma biopsies in patients with suspected parenchymal nephropathy.

The formation of pneumothorax is also very uncommon; when it does occur, it generally lacks clinical significance. Its presentation can usually be avoided by using, whenever possible, a subcostal access [33].

Tumour implantation through the biopsy needle trajectory is another reported complication and is especially feared, despite the fact that the available literature shows that the complication is rare (less than 0.01%) [8, 29]. This complication might not be well studied, however, due to the lack of long follow-ups [26].

Renal Biopsy Interpretation

The need for improvements in preoperative risk stratification has led to a resurgence of interest in the use of renal mass biopsy (RMB) to guide the treatment of SRMs [34, 35]. Recent series have demonstrated safety and diagnostic accuracy with RMB for the detection of malignancy and histological subtype. Even so, RMB continues to have poor accuracy in assessing Furhman grade in cRCC [15, 24, 36].

Obtained Material

The representativeness of the obtained material depends on variables such as needle size, size of the tumour, location, morphological characteristics of the mass, conservation of the structure and experience level of the involved personnel.

The representativeness of the biopsy in SRMs represents 80.6% [37]. Not all non-diagnostic biopsies are the same; the findings will vary from necrotic tissue to normal renal parenchyma. In cases of high suspicion of malignancy, we can repeat the biopsy after a minimum of three months, which increases the ability to reach a diagnosis in these patients in up to 85% of cases [15, 24]. Thus, a non-diagnostic biopsy should not be considered definitively negative [28].

Best Technique for RMB

Currently, core biopsies are recommended to obtain the most information about SRMs. FNA has been shown to be inferior to core biopsies in diagnostic yield.

One way to increase the diagnostic ability is to combine a core biopsy and FNA, which results in a correct diagnosis between 96.5% and 100% [38].

FNA can obtain multiple samples without increasing the number of complications, but it has less diagnostic power as a stand-alone tool [39].

Tumour Size

Lechevallier et al. [40] reported a 37% biopsy failure rate in lesions ≤ 3 cm compared with a 9% failure rate for lesions > 3cm. Leveridge et al. [24] found a positive association between tumour size and biopsy success on multivariable analysis. However, Wang et al. [28], in a study of 110 RMBs in SRMs, reported no diagnostic difference between lesions of < 2.5 cm or larger. Similarly, Barwari et al. [41] could not find an association between tumour size and biopsy yield in a series of 100 RMBs during laparoscopic renal cryoablation for lesions <4.5 cm.

Number of Cores

There is uncertainty regarding the number of cores that must be taken to be representative of an SRM. Estimates range from 1 core [15] to four cores [28]. Increasing the number of cores taken improves the diagnostic accuracy [42], especially if samples from central and peripheral areas are obtained. However, the location may be a secondary issue.

Some authors have found some intratumoural genetic heterogeneity [43] but renal neoplasms have little histologic heterogeneity [29], which could explain the similar results of all series regardless of the number of cores obtained. A study on 88 RMBs reported obtaining 96.6% sufficient material for diagnosis with two or more cores [44].

Similarly, Wang et al. [28] reported on 110 RMBs with at least two cores sampled, achieving diagnoses in 91% of cases via percutaneous biopsy. Tsivian et al. [26] reports that a minimum of two cores should be taken during RMB to maximise the diagnostic potential. We can conclude that for successful RMB diagnosis, the quality of the obtained tissue is more important than the number of cores.

Diagnostic Accuracy for Malignancy

The main indication for biopsy is still to categorise renal masses, and to determining whether a lesion is benign or malignant as well as its histologic type and grade. It is remarkable that there have been no errors in identifying renal neoplastic processes [40].

The diagnostic accuracy of RMB in differentiating malignant from benign lesions ranges between 86 and 100%, with a specificity close to 100% in most series [45-47] (Figure 4).

The false negative rate of renal tumour biopsies is about 1% [8]. Sampling errors, tumour necrosis and tumour heterogeneity are responsible for the false negative rate with RMB.

A second biopsy after an initial nondiagnostic biopsy increases the rate of diagnosis up to 85% [24]. A nondiagnostic result in RMB seems to be more frequent with smaller masses and those of a cystic nature [39].

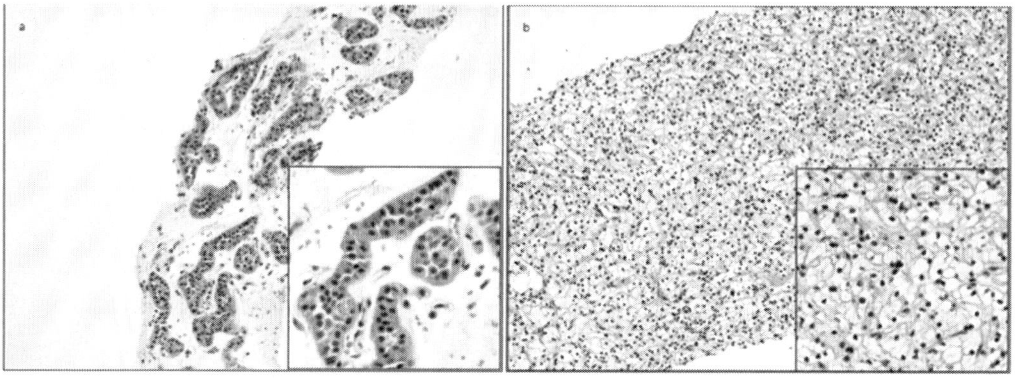

a b

Figure 4. Core biopsy. A: oncocytoma. B: Clear-cell renal cell carcinoma. Haematoxylin and eosin staining x20. Inset x40.

Diagnostic Accuracy for Histological Subtyping

The rates of accurate histological subtyping in the recent literature review were 86-98% [45] and the reported interobserver agreement is high [48]. While in most cases correct histological subtyping can be performed on a unique core biopsy, some instances remain problematic.

For example, hybrid tumours that combine areas of different histological architecture pose a challenge to accurately defining the malignant subtype. With percutaneous biopsy, histologic subtype identification is possible in 88% to 93 % of cases and grade determination is in the range of 63.5% to 68% [24, 47].

In most series, core biopsies of SRM reveal the same incidence of the various histological subtypes as with larger diameter neoplasms [49]. The diagnosis from a core biopsy and a nephrectomy specimen matches in about 93.5% of cases in terms of histologic subtype and 76% in terms of grade. However some authors have observed more papillary renal cell carcinomas in SRMs (15.8% vs. 9.4%) [50].

As mentioned previously, a biopsy is the best method for an accurate diagnosis, but it also has its limitations, especially in the case of inconclusive biopsies. One way to improve the results of the biopsy is with the use of immunohistochemistry.

Unfortunately, there are as yet no histological subtype-specific markers, thus the immunophenotype is determined by the rate of positivity of the various antibodies [51]. Most diagnostic biopsies are challenging with eosinophilic cell neoplasms, and the tumours with these cells often express various markers. This situation also occurs in other variants of RCC and thus immunohistochemistry can be used, but we must always keep in mind that they should be considered as indicative markers (Figure 5).

FISH (fluorescence in situ hybridization) is a less commonly used method that is recommended in cases when reasonable doubts remain.

The use of FISH obtains a 7% increase in diagnoses. Another possible tool is molecular analysis, which offers an increase of 11.7% in diagnoses [52].

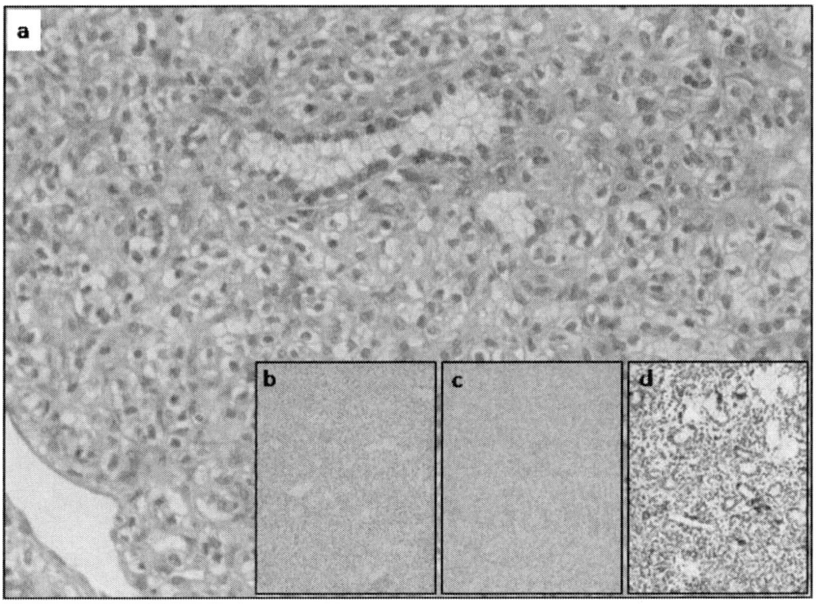

Figure 5. Usefulness of immunohistochemistry in diagnostic challenge. a) HE of challenge case of clear-cell (tubulo) papillary renal carcinoma vs. Clear-cell renal cell carcinoma, b) Racemase, c) CD10, d) CK7.

Diagnostic Accuracy in Grading

After stage, the nuclear grade is the most important prognostic feature of cRCC [53].

The results in the literature indicate suboptimal performance of RMB for grading these tumours. Due to the sampling nature of biopsies and the lack of homogeneity of tumour grades, identifying an area of low-grade (LG) cancer does not necessarily exclude the presence of high-grade (HG) morphology in the remainder of the lesion (Figure 6). This finding is a high positive predictive value for HG and a lower value for LG.

These occurrences may have accounted for the findings of Harris et al. [54] who suggest under-grading of cRCC on biopsies compared to the final pathology. In their study, Ball et al. [36] stated that the median amount of LG tissue found in HG specimens was 38.9%, thus tumours that contain HG elements may be undergraded on RMB. Moreover, grading accuracy might be improved by using a two-tier system that reduces the inter-observer variability inherent to cRCC grading [15].

Of special importance is the recently published study by Dominguez et al. [46], which compared the results of in-bench renal biopsies (2 central and 2 peripheral) upon removing the renal mass with the surgical specimen (47 tumours, 21 SRMs).

The authors concluded that, in their experience, biopsies are useful in 100% of cases for the diagnosis of benignity and 97.2% for the diagnosis of malignancy. In terms of the Fuhrman grade, the sensitivity and specificity were 100% and 50-57% for grades I-II and 50-57% and 100% for degrees III-IV, respectively.

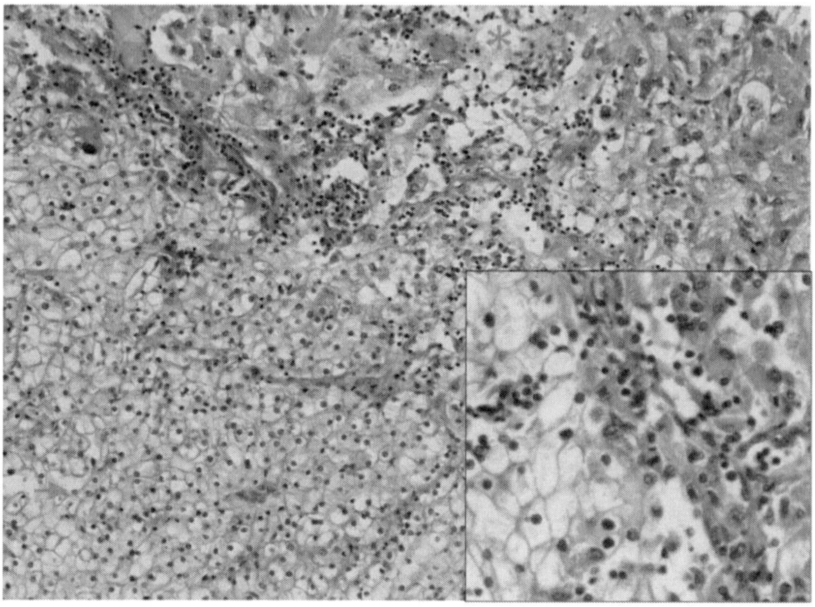

Figure 6. Clear-cell renal cell carcinoma showing heterogeneity with low Fuhrman grade (arrow) and high Fuhrman grade (asterisk). Haematoxylin and eosin staining x20. Inset x40.

Prognostic Factors of SRM Aggressiveness

The main problem when treating SRMs is determining their possible malignancy and metastatic capacity as precisely as possible. To this end, it is of vital importance that we understand the histological characteristics and evolution of those tumours measuring ≤4 cm that were extirpated either by RN or PN.

However, there are few published series that have removed these renal masses, and these series only did so in cases in which the tumour progressed in size.

For example, in 1997 Vega et al. [55] observed that of 286 RNs for RCC, 11 were tumours measuring <3 cm (measured after the nephrectomy), and 2 of these developed metastases during the follow-up.

Tumour Size, Growth and Metastatic Capacity

At present, only tumour size and growth rate seem to have a certain prognostic value.

The role of radiological images obtained by ultrasonography, CT and MRI is to determine not only the tumour size but also its relationship with the breast and excretory pathway, the presence of positive nerve ganglia and potential metastases. Ultrasonography is probably the first imaging technique with which SRMs are detected. CT is the technique of choice, in most cases, for assessing SRMs. An increase in enhancement of >20 HU should warrant further investigation. This increase can help differentiate between RCCs and other histological types of renal tumours. However, it is not yet capable of identifying the presence of oncocytomas or even small angiomyolipomas that contain virtually no fat. MRI has shown similar detection, diagnostic and staging capabilities. When compared with CT imaging, MRI offers the advantages of higher contrast resolution, the absence of ionizing radiation and its possible use in patients with contraindications for iodinated contrast [56].

It is generally accepted that the possibilities of the tumour being malignant, having a higher histological grade, being a clear kidney cell carcinoma (cRCC) (rather than one with less aggressive histology) and that it has synchronous metastases increase as the SRM tumour size grows [57]. Data published in 2003 estimate that if the SRM measures <1 cm then the probability of benignity is 43-46%; if it measures 1-1.9 cm then the probability is 22-30%; if it measures 2-2.9 cm then the probability is 19-23%; and if it measures 3-3.9 cm then the probability is 16-20%. In addition, a high histological grade was found in 15.9% of the tumours that measured <4 cm [58]. These data were corroborated in 2012 in a study that reported that the incidence of benign lesions among SRMs measuring between 2 cm and 4 cm was 4.8%; when the size was <1 cm, the incidence was approximately 42.8% [59]. Elderly patients seem to have a higher propensity (3.5 fold) for harbouring a benign lesion than younger patients.

Classifications of the renal masses have been attempted based on anatomical data. For example, the Preoperative Aspects and Dimensions Used for an Anatomical (PADUA) classification analyses the following characteristics: exophytic vs. endophytic; face, polar and rim location; relationship with renal sinus and urinary collecting system; tumour deepening; and maximum diameter. Using these characteristics, the PADUA classification seeks to predict the risk of complications secondary to nephron-sparing surgery and thereby help in making decisions on alternatives (AS?) [60]. The classification was applied to 164 patients treated with PN. The authors concluded that all the previously mentioned characteristics are correlated with the risk of complications, except for size and location (anterior or posterior). Following the criteria of the PADUA classification, these anatomical characteristics have been correlated with tumour histology. These results have been partially validated by other authors with 1,129 T1 RCCs, of which 754 were SRMs-pT1a, as has been recently published [61]. In a multivariate analysis, the predictors of malignancy and high grade were age, sex, exophytic tumour and tumour size (both for T1 and T1a). Affecting the collecting system was a predictor of high-grade tumour for T1a.

Another attempt to characterise renal masses and correlate the radiological images (CT and/or MRI) with surgical difficulty was performed by Kutinov and Uzzo [62]. The authors designed the RENAL Nephrometry Score, which includes the maximum diameter of the tumour, whether it is exophytic or endophytic, its proximity to the collecting system and renal sinus, whether it is anterior or posterior and its location in relation to the renal poles. Depending on the score, renal masses are classified as low (score 4-6), moderate (score 7-9) or high (score 10-12) surgical difficulty. After retrospectively assessing 50 cases, the authors concluded that the nephrometry score could help in choosing among PN, open PN and laparoscopic RN.

Of possibly greater interest are the data published by Kutinov et al. [63] two years later. When the authors applied the same RENAL nephrometry score, they found that it could help predict whether the renal masses were high-grade or had a malignant histology. Considering that we are witnessing an era in which there is a clear tendency to treat SRMs with an expectant approach, the ability to know the histological characteristics of these masses can be of considerable usefulness. However, given that the cohort of cases analysed by the authors extends to tumours of any stage, validation of this nomogram in SRMs is needed. Bragodia et al. [64] applied this nomogram to 252 SRMs in 250 patients who underwent PN. The authors concluded that the nomogram does not discriminate well between benign and malignant SRMs, although it could be useful for identifying high-grade tumours.

In contrast, Koo et al. [65] stated that the RENAL nephrometry score is not reliable for preoperatively predicting the histological grade of SRMs but that is was reliable for determining the malignancy of solid masses in general. More studies are needed to resolve these conflicting results in the study of the possible aggressiveness of SRMs.

Although series with SRMs generally have very high cancer-specific survival (CSS), there are published series of patients in AS who despite having a mass measuring ≤4 cm have progressed and have even developed metastases. Youssif et al. [66], in a study of 35 patients with 44 SRMs, observed a mean mass growth of 0.24 cm/year and a volume increase of 2.7 cc/year; 2 of the patients developed metastases (both measuring 2.7 cm in diameter). There was no correlation between initial tumour size and size growth rate or initial tumour volume and volume growth rate.

In an extensive series of 173 tumours in 154 patients who underwent AS [67], the mean size of the tumours was 2.45 cm (22 of the tumours were T1b); with a mean follow-up of 24 months, the mean growth of the mass was 0.285 cm. The interesting finding of this series was that the authors observed faster growth rates in the smaller masses. Of the 173 masses, 39% (68 of 173) were applied some surgical treatment; 84% of the masses were RCCs. Only 6% (3 tumours) were >T1, and 2 patients developed metastases (1.3%).

Data from the National Swedish Kidney Cancer Quality Register published in 2011 [68] in a series of 918 patients with T1a masses showed that locally advanced growth, lymph node and distant metastases and high tumour grade were correlated with tumour size. Some 5.6% of the SRMs were actually pT3a or greater; 19.9% were grade 3 or 4, and 7% were metastatic.

Mason et al. [69] studied 84 SRMs in 82 patients in whom the mean annual growth of the tumour was 0.25±0.49 cm. With a 36-month follow-up, only 3 patients progressed. The authors established that an initial size >2.45 cm was the cutoff predictor for growth. Nine masses did not progress, and 1 patient had metastases and died due to the cancer.

Patel et al. [70], compared AS with RN and PN in a total of 234 T1a masses. In the 71 patients with 93 SRMs treated with AS, the authors observed that 53% of the SRMs did not grow.

Surgery was performed for 14 patients due to the growth of their SRM or for other reasons. Only 1 patient had an SRM that metastasised (1.4%). The oncological result when comparing the 3 treatments showed no difference at all.

In a multicentre study with 2197 patients with stage T1a RCC removed surgically and a mean follow-up of 56.2 months, Steffens et al. [71] observed that after the surgery, 8% of the RCCs were actually pT>3a, 6.2% were poorly differentiated and 3.5% metastasised. The characteristics of a poor prognosis were microvascular involvement and invasion of the collecting system. Five-year survival was 93.8% for the true pT1a RCCs and 79.4% for those >4 cm. The disquieting message of this study is that we are mistaken in 8% of cases and that 3.5% are metastatic.

In a series of 2,058 patients with RCC removed surgically, Zastrow et al. [72] found that tumour size was significantly correlated with synchronous metastatic disease. However, no significant correlation was found for SRMs measuring <4 cm, despite the fact that 2.8% of these tumours were metastatic (1.6% if the SRMs measured <3 cm), which should not be considered an insignificant risk. The authors concluded that true metastatic risk starts at 5 cm.

In a comprehensive review of the series published up to 2012, Smaldone et al. [73] conducted a meta-analysis of 936 SRMs followed with AS in 880 patients corresponding to 18 retrospective studies. Of these, only 284 SRMs in 259 patients were valid for the analysis. Some 75.6% of the patients (mean age, 66.6±12.3 years) had an elective indication, 10.9% had a relative indication and 13.5% had an absolute indication. The mean size of the SRMs was 2.3±1.3 cm, and the mean volume was 15.1±60 cm^3. At the end of the observation, the mean size was 3±1.6 cm and the mean volume was 29.5±109.3 cm^3. With a mean follow-up of 33.5±22.6 months, the mean growth rate was 0.31±0.38 cm/year and the mean volume growth rate was 6.3 ± 27.4 cm^3/year. Some 22.9% of the SRMs had zero net growth. Of the SRMs from which histological data was obtained, 88% were malignant, 80.5% of which were low-grade. Clear cell tumours represented 64.1% of the SRMs, and papillary disease represented 17.1%. Among the benign lesions, oncocytomas (10.3%) and angiomyolipomas (1.7%) were the most common. Of the 284 SRMs, 129 (45.4%) were operated on after a mean follow-up 30.5 months; 155 were kept under AS. The causes for the surgery were patient preference (57.2%), improved general condition of the patient (7.1%), tumour growth (35.7%) and other causes (1.2%). Of the 880 initial patients, 18 experienced metastases (2.04%) and in all of them the tumour had grown in size.

Brunocilla et al. [74], with a very long follow-up (91.5 m), recently observed progression in size in 13 of 62 patients who underwent AS, with surgery performed in 16 cases and 1 case progressing to metastatic disease.

Reviewing the data from all of these series on SRMs treated with AS or with surgery, we observe that in almost all series there are cases of metastatic disease, which, although in low proportions, should lead us to reflect [10, 22, 66-76]. Although there appears to be a relationship between tumour growth and metastatic disease, we should search for other molecular factors that lead us to suspect the greater aggressiveness of SRMs. We can see in Table 1 a number of series with data on SRM growth and the rate of metastatic cases.

In order to correlate tumour size with CSS and the development of synchronous metastases, Ingimarsson et al. [77] analysed the prognosis of 794 RCCs operated on between

1971 and 2005. The probability of synchronous metastases increased nonlinearly with the increase in tumour size (11%, 25%, 35% and 50% for tumours measuring ≤4, 4.1-7, 7.1-10 and >10 cm, respectively). In a multivariate analysis, tumour size was an independent prognosis factor for CSS but not for synchronous metastases.

Table 1. Description of some SRMs series, detailing the tumor growth, treatmentsapplied and the number of metastases

Authors Year	Nº PAT./ Nº SRMs	Mean F. Up in Months	Mean age	Mean size SRMs	Mean Increase size	Treatments	MTXS
Chawla 2006 [10]	234	34 M.	¿?	2.6 CM	0.28 CM/Y	¿?	3 (1.2%)
Youssef 2007 [66]	35/44	47.6 M.	71.8 Y	2.2 CM	0.24 CM/Y 8 PATIENTS	3 RN 5 PN	2 (5.7%)
Crispen 2009 [67]	154/173	24 M.	71Y	2.45CM	0.285 CM	68 Tumours	2 (1.3%)
Rosales 2010 [75]	212/223	35 M.	71Y	2.8 CM	0.34 CM	11 Surgery	4 (1.9%)
Mason 2011 [69]	82/84	36 M.	74 Y	2.3 CM	0.25 CM/Y 3 Patients	12 Surgery	1 (1.2%)
Jewett 2011 [22]	127/151	28 M.	73 Y	2.1 CM	0.13 CM/Y 27 Patients	3 RN 4 PN 1 RF 1 CRY	2 (1.1%)
Patel 2012 [70]	71/93	34 M.	71.9 Y	2.2 CM	0.21 CM/Y 14 Patients	2 RN 7 PN 3 RF 2 HIFU	1 (1.4%)
Leonard 2013 [76]	83/86	27.8 M.	70.6 Y	2.36 CM	0.48 CM/Y 36 Patients	1 PN 5 RF 2 CRY	1 (1.2%)
Brunocilla 2014 [74]	62/64	91.5%	75 Y	2 CM	0.4 CM/Y 13 Patients	4 RN 12 PN	1 (1.6%)

RN: Radical Nephrectomy. PR: Parcial Nephrectomy. RF: Radiophrequency. CRY: Cryotherapy.

Molecular Markers

A key epigenetic disorder involved in the initiation and progression of cancer is aberrant methylation in a gene's promoter region. Hypermethylation is associated with transcriptional repression and is an important mechanism for inactivating suppressor genes in neoplastic cells. Ibragimova et al. [78] have determined the genome-wide promoter methylation profiles of 47 pT1 and 2 pT2 RCCs, 25 oncocytomas and 4 in normal renal tissue. They identified gene promoter hypermethylation signatures that differentiate RCC and papillary carcinoma from other tumours and normal renal tissue.

The genes identified as differentially methylated implicate pathways involved in metabolism, tissue response to injury, epithelial to mesenchymal transition, cancer and stem cell regulation in the biology of RCC. The authors state that differential methylation signatures could be useful for early detection and differential diagnosis for prognosis stratification, as well as for identifying novel gene and pathway targets for therapeutic intervention.

The most inactivated gene in cRCC is the von Hippel-Lindau gene (VHL) on 3p25-26. VHL inactivation is considered the first step of cRCC development, playing the role of gatekeeper tumour suppressor; VHL is inactivated in 80% of sporadic cRCCs [79]. There appears be a correlation between VHL disorders and advanced disease states and between common VHL mutations and a greater Fuhrman nuclear grade. Metastatic tumours have double the mutations in exon 3 than nonmetastatic tumours. Even VHL disorders can help stratify tumours as having a poor, intermediate or good prognosis [80]. The absence of detectable VHL and low carbonic anhydrase IX (CAIX) mutations is correlated with advanced stages and the presence of metastases. An intermediate prognosis group consists of those who have a VHL or CAIX mutation, and a good prognosis group has both detectable mutations. Chromosomal disorders can also be correlated with the clinicopathological parameters of the tumour and its prognosis. The loss of 3p and 13q is correlated with recurrence-free survival (RFS), and the loss of 3p is present in low stages and low-grade tumours [22]. The loss of 9p is an independent factor of metastases and poor prognosis and was also found to be predictive of recurrence in nonmetastatic RCC and in tumours of considerable size. The loss of 4p and 14q is associated with advanced stages, high grades, large tumour size, poorer prognoses and a tendency to metastasis [81, 82].

Proteomic studies in RCC have been performed on tumour tissues, blood and urine. An abundance of thrombospondin-1 and enolase-2 proteins has been found in the serum of patients with cRCC when compared with that of controls [83]. In addition, changes in glycolysis, propanoate, pyruvate, urea and arginine/proline metabolism and p53 pathways have been observed more often in the urine of patients with RCC than in patients in the control group. It has also been determined that ribosomal s6 protein kinase 4 (RSK4) is overexpressed in RCC compared with normal tissue. After studying its expression in 101 patients with RCC, RSK4 was correlated with various RCC subtypes (especially in the 2 papillary types), high stages, high Fuhrman nuclear grades, the presence of positive nerve ganglia and metastatic disease [84]. In short, molecular biology can facilitate decision making in SRMs by helping to identify cases that tend towards a more aggressive evolution and even to metastasis.

Indications for Active Surveillance

Until recently, RN was the first option in treating RCC, even for SRMs. Over time, it was observed that radical surgery could predispose patients to a certain degree of renal failure, a greater risk of cardiovascular disease and lower survival unrelated to renal tumour disease.

The technical improvements in partial surgery, the emergence of ablative techniques (radio frequency, cryotherapy, high-intensity focused ultrasound) and especially the implementation of laparoscopic and robotic techniques has led to SRMs being treated less frequently with RN. Even simple enucleation has the same oncological result at 5 and 10 years of follow-up when compared with PN, as observed in the results of a non-randomised, retrospective, comparative study with 1519 patients and a mean tumour size of 3.4±1.6 cm [85].

Current management options for SRMs are divided into interventional and conservative. Nephron-sparing surgery, radical surgery and image-guided tumour ablation are commonly used techniques. The use of minimally invasive surgery is increasing in the management of larger tumours with technically challenging anatomical locations.

It is well known that nephron-sparing surgery for SRMs results in equivalent oncologic outcomes, with benefits in renal function outcomes and for nononcologic morbidity and mortality [20]. In 2009, the AUA guidelines established PN as a standard of care for treating T1a tumours.

The likely reason for the existence of the concept of AS is its apparently successful application in prostate cancer. The observation that tumours with low Gleason scores (6) in the surgical specimens do not metastasise and the developments in interpreting mpMRI images have rendered unnecessary thousands of aggressive treatments and lead to treating only when progression is observed in the PSA and/or when there are changes in the histological characteristics of the rebiopsy. We have seen how a procedure initially applied to elderly men has been carried over to younger individuals with disease criteria of a supposedly nonaggressive tumour. We should also consider impairments in the sexual arena and the risk of incontinence with surgery and reserve aggressive treatment for when particular criteria makes us suspect a greater aggressiveness. In other words, AS is actually delaying the treatment to a more appropriate time when aggressive treatment outweighs the tumour aggressiveness.

In principle, the reasoning behind performing AS in renal tumour disease is based on several factors mentioned above: the majority of SRMs have low malignant potential and a benign histology is found in approximately 20% of cases. Of the remaining, only 20-25% have histological characteristics of aggressiveness. Moreover, for elderly patients with SRMs, the probability of dying from the renal tumour is low compared with the probability of dying from some other cause. Lastly, AS does not rule out performing more aggressive treatment if the condition changes [57, 86]. We should not forget to mention renal function preservation and preventing the complications of surgery and ablative techniques.

According to the EAU guidelines [18], population-based analyses show a significantly lower CSM for patients treated with surgery compared with nonsurgical management. However, the same benefit for CSM is not confirmed in analyses that focus on older patients (>75 years). Therefore, AS has its greatest indication in this patient group.

AS should also be reserved for patients in whom intervention would represent a high risk and/or when the SRMs appear to be benign or have low cell differentiation. In these circumstances, a renal biopsy can have considerable value for determining the biological aggressiveness in the most reliable manner possible.

In general, AS in SRMs should be performed electively based on age, comorbidities, solitary renal or bilateral renal masses, a combination of these factors or when surgery is declined (including ablative therapy).

The 5-year CSS of patients with surgically treated T1a masses remains close to 95% [87], but this treatment has not been compared with AS in a randomised manner. In the only prospective, phase II clinical trial of AS for SRMs, the renal masses progressed locally in 25 patients (14%). Two patients (1.1%) who had tumour sizes of 2.4 cm and 2.7 cm went on to develop metastatic disease [22].

In a meta-analysis performed by Zini et al. [88] on 10,291 SRMs from the SEER database, AS was applied to 4.2%; the remainder underwent surgery. A better prognosis was observed in the patients who underwent surgery, with a benefit of 5.2%, 6.5% and 9.4% at 1, 2 and 5 years, respectively. The same benefit persisted in the analysis matched for age, tumour size and date of diagnosis or date of nephrectomy. The authors concluded that AS should not be recommended to patients with no comorbidities and to generally healthy patients for whom surgery is not contraindicated. However, Patel et al. [70] found no differences relative to CSS when comparing AS, RN and PN, which leads us to believe that there can be other types of patients who can benefit from AS, as occurs with AS in prostate cancer. Gill et al. [89] limit AS to tumours measuring <1 cm, regardless of life expectancy, in line with the high possibility that the tumours are benign.

The lack of optimal kidney transplant donors in recent years has led to the implantation of kidneys with certain diseases, which was unthinkable a few years ago. A study was recently published on the implantation of 11 kidneys with SRMs, whose mean size was 1.48 cm (including one that was 4.3 cm). All cases underwent ex vivo tumourectomy with a preoperative pathologic analysis: 5 RCCs, 2 chromophobes and 1 lipoma. With a mean follow-up of 32.34 months, none of the patients presented tumour recurrence, and all had proper renal function [90]. It appears that the low risk of recurrence and metastasis should be balanced with the high risk of mortality in kidney transplantation waiting lists.

When treatments applied to patients with SRMs are analysed, we must consider that there could be socioeconomic factors that determine the treatment to be performed. National public (and private) health services can be different, and at times the treatment choices for SRMs are based on whether the patient must pay part of their treatment or not. Therefore, we must take this factor into account when comparing treatments [76]. Other socioeconomic factors, such as race and sex, can also influence the decision. For example, blacks and women of any race are less likely to undergo RN or PN. In general, elderly patients, women and those at with few economic resources tend to undergo conservative treatments [91].

A recent study brought to light the "surgeon" factor, which can influence the decision for AS. Surgeons who do not perform laparoscopy are more likely to recommend AS than those who do perform laparoscopy and/or robotic surgery [92].

The AUA guidelines recommend that patients undergo cross-sectional abdominal scanning (CT or MRI) within 6 months of starting AS to establish a growth rate. A panel of experts recommended continued imaging (US, CT or MRI) at least annually thereafter [23]. With these imaging techniques, SRM growth and the possible onset of satellite lesions in the same or contralateral kidney can be monitored with very high safety. As we have seen in the various analysed series, the growth rate of SRMs is 0.2-0.4 cm/year. In addition, up to 22.9% of SRMs showed zero net growth [73].

In general, patients with SRMs who undergo some type of conservative treatment (PN or ablative therapy) also undergo many more radiological tests in the follow-up than if they had undergone RN. This increase in testing (especially CT and MRI) leads to increased financial expenditure as observed with thermal ablation [93].

Identifying the lowest cost treatment makes sense, given that conservative treatment with ablative therapies and even AS in selected cases can obtain a very similar oncological result for SRMs. To this end, Bhan et al. [94] proposed comparing radiofrequency, cryoablation and AS from an economic standpoint. The authors reached the conclusion that AS with delayed percutaneous cryoablation, if needed, could be a safe and cost-effective alternative to immediate cryoablation.

An important factor that should be assessed is the quality of life of patients who undergo any type of AS or WW. However, there is practically no information on the QoL of these patients. There are 2 factors of concern: illness uncertainty and disease progression. Parker et al. [95] performed a prospective study to analyse illness uncertainty in 264 patients with T1-T2 renal tumours who underwent WW for various reasons; however, the authors only reported the data from the first 100 patients. After a 24-month follow-up, they came to the conclusion that greater illness uncertainty was associated with poorer general QoL scores in the physical domain; poorer cancer-related QoL in the physical, psychosocial and medical domains; and greater distress. The authors recommended focusing on psychosocial interventions to improve the QoL of patients in WW. A multi-institutional study assessed the QoL of 327 patients treated with AS or surgery. It concluded that patients who are operated on early have greater QoL, and this benefit appears to persist at 1 year of surgery. Depression and anxiety do not seem to affect those treated with AS [96].

Further studies are warranted, especially on patients in AS to assess whether their QoL is significantly affected by this monitored waiting period, knowing that they have a cancer but that it is not yet going to be treated. Such studies are already underway with prostate cancer subjected to surveillance.

Conclusion

The progressive increase in the diagnosis of SRMs and the existing evidence that the smaller the size the greater the probability of benignity, low growth and low aggressiveness justify considering AS a valid initial option. At present, only tumour size and growth seem to be true prognostic factors. For patients with short life expectancies AS should be the first treatment option. Although PN is the treatment of choice for younger individuals, renal biopsy can have a fundamental role in understanding the biology of the tumour and helping in the decision-making process for patients not disposed to aggressive treatments as a first choice. Given that ablative therapies and PN obtain favourable results, the patient should know all options and participate in the decision-making process. In this context, QoL should also be considered, and the patient should know that AS does not mean not treating but rather delaying the treatment until there are changes in the behaviour of the SRM, subject to strict follow-up with cross-sectional images.

References

[1] Chow, W. H., Gridley, G., Fraumeni, J. F., Järcholm, B. Obesity, hypertension, and the risk of kidney cancer in men. *New Engl. J. Med.* 2000;343(18):1305-11.

[2] Renehan, A. G., Tyson, M., Egger, M., Heller, R. F., Zwahlen, M. Body-mass index and incidence of cáncer: a systematic rewiev and meta-analysis of prospective observational studies. *Lancet* 2008;371(9612): 569-78.
[3] Alasker, A., Williams, S. K., Ghavamian, R. *Curr. Urol. Rep*. 2013;14:13-8.
[4] Duffey, B. G., Choyke, P. L., Glenn, G., et al. The relationship between renal tumor size and metástasis in patients with von Hippel-Lindau disease. *J. Urol*. 2004;172(1): 63-5.
[5] Ries, L. A. G., Melbert, D., Krapcho, M., et al. *SEER Cancer Statistics Review*, 1975-2004. Bethesda: National Cancer Institute, 2006. Available at: http://seer.cancer.gov/csr/1975-2004/, based on November 2006 SEER Data submission, posted to the SEER web site. Accessed January 2007.
[6] Hollingworth, J. M., Miller, D. C., Daignault, S., Hollenbeck, B. K. Rising incidence of small renal masses: a need to reassess treatment effect. *J. Natl. Cancer Inst*. 2006;98: 1331-4.
[7] Nguyen, M. M., Gill, I. S., Ellison, L. M. The evolving presentation of renal carcinoma in the United States: trends from the surveillance, epidemiology, and end results program. *J. Urol*. 2006;176:2397-2400.
[8] Fracchia, J. A., Glickman, L. I., Javit, D., Westcott, M., Armenakas, N. A. Contemporary management of small renal tumors. *J. Comm. Supp. Oncol*. 2014;12(6): 212-21.
[9] Kane, C. J., Mallin, K., Ritchey, J., et al. Renal cell cáncer stage migration: analysis of the National Cancer Data Base. *Cancer* 2008;113:78-83.
[10] Chawla, S. N., Crispen, P. L., Hanlon, A. L., Greenberg, R. E., Chen, D. Y., Uzzo, R. G. The natural history of observed enhancing renal masses: meta-analysis and review of the world literatura. *J. Urol*. 2006;175:425-31.
[11] Kunkle, D. A., Crispen, P. L., Chen, D. Y., Greenberg, R. E., Uzzo, R. G. Enhancing renal masses with zero net growth during active surrveillance. *J. Urol*. 2007;177:849-53.
[12] Sun, M., Becker, A., Roghmann, F., Tian, Z., Abdollah, F., Karakiewiecz, P. I. Management of localized kidney cáncer: calculating cancer-specific mortality and competing-risks of death tradeoffs between surgery and active surveillance. *J. Urol*. 2013:189-4s, Suppl.7:e672.
[13] Huang, W. C., Pinhiero, L. C., Lowrance, W. T., Russo, P., Elkin, E. B. Surveillance for the management of small renal masses: outcomes in a population-based cohort. *J. Urol*. 2013;189-4s. Suppl.6:e483.
[14] Hollingsworth, D., Miller, D., Daignault, S., Hollenbeck, B. K. Rising incidence of small renal masses: a need to reassess treatment effect. *J. Natl. Cancer Ins*. 2006;98: 1331-4.
[15] Lebret, T., Poulain, J. E., Molinie, V., et al. Percutaneous core biopsy for renal masses: indication, accuracy and results. *J. Urol*. 2007;178:1184-8.
[16] Volpe, A., Kachura, J. R., Geddie, W. R., et al. Techniques, safety and accuracy of sampling of renal tumors by fine needle aspiration and core biopsy. *J. Urol*. 2007; 178:379-86.
[17] Stakhovskyi, O., Sánchez-Salas, R., Barret, E., et al. Renal biopsies for small renal masses. For whom, when and how. *Arch. Esp. Urol*. 2013;66(1):4-15.

[18] Ljungberg, B., Bensalah, K., Bex, A., et al. Guidelines on Renal cell carcinoma. *Uroweb 2014*. Available at: http://www.uroweb.org/gls/pdf/10%20Renal%20Cell%20 Carcinoma_LR.pdf.

[19] Smaldone, M. C., Corcoran, A. T., Uzzo, R. G. Active surveillance of small renal masses. *Nat. Rev. Urol.* 2013;10:266-74.

[20] Bjurlin, M. A., Huang, W. C. Surgery versus surveillance of small renal masses: a call for comparative effectiveness research in the management of kidney tumors. *J. Compar. Effect. Res.* 2013;2(5):401-3.

[21] Gontero, P., Joniau, S., Oderda, M., et al. Active surveillance for small renal tumors: have clinical concerns been addessed so far?. *Int. J. Urol.* 2013;20:356-61.

[22] Jewett, M. A. S., Mattar, K., Basiuk, J., et al. Active surveillance of small renal masses: progression pattern of early stage kidney cáncer. *Eur. Urol.* 2011;60:39-44.

[23] Donat, S. M., Diaz, M., Bishoff, J. T., et al. Follow-up for clinically localized renal neoplasms: AUA Guideline. *J. Urol.* 2013;190:407-16.

[24] Leveridge, M. J., Finelli, A., Kachura, J. R., et al. Outcomes of small reanl mass needle core biopsy, nondiagnostic percutaneous biopsy, and the role of repeat biopsy. *Eur. Urol.* 2011;60:578-84.

[25] Raman, J. D. Percutaneous renal biopsy may aid management of small renal masses on active surveillance. *Can. J. Urol.* 2013;20(2):6742.

[26] Tsivian, M., Rampersaud, E. N., Laguna, M. P., et al. Small renal mass biopsy-how, what and when: report from an intennational consensus panel. *BJU Int.* 2014;113:854-63.

[27] Breda, A., Treat, E. G., Haft-Candell, L., et al. Comparison of accuracy of 14-, 18- and 20-G needles in ex-vivo renal mass biopsy: A prospective, blinded study. *BJU Int.* 2010;105(7):940-5.

[28] Wang, R., Wolf, J. S. Jr, Wood, D. P. Jr, Higgins, E. J., Hafez, K. S. Accuracy of percutaneous core biopsy in management of small renal masses. *Urology* 2009;73:586-91.

[29] Volpe, A., Finelli, A., Gill, I. S., et al. Rationale for percutaneous biopsy and histologic characterisation of renal tumors. *Eur. Urol.* 2012;62:491-504.

[30] Guerrero, F., Villacampa, F., Jiménez, E., et al. Estudio de seguridad de la biopsia renal percutánea con aguja de calibre 16G. *Act. Esp. Urol.* 2014;38(9):584-8.

[31] Fortuño, J. R., de Lamo, S., García, E., Mateos, A. Safety and yield of percutaneous renal biopsy using an automatic 16G needle in native kidneys. *Radiología* 2010;52:153-6.

[32] Ralls, P. W., Barakos, J. A., Kaptein, E. M., Friedman, P. E., Fouladian, G., Boswell, W. D., et al. Renal biopsy-related hemorrhage: frequency and comparison of CT and sonography. *J. Comput. Assist. Tomogr.* 1987;11:1031-4.

[33] Silverman, S. G., Gan, Y. U., Mortele, K. J., Tuncali, K., Cibas, E. S. Renal masses in the adult patient: the role of percutaneousbiopsy. *Radiology* 2006;240:6-22.

[34] Halverson, S. J., Kunju, L. P., Bhalla, R., et al. Accuracy of determining small renal mass management with risk stratified biopsies: confirmation by final pathology. *J. Urol.* 2013;189:441-6.

[35] Tomaszewski, J. J., Uzzo, R. G., Smaldone, M. C. Heterogeneity and renal mass biopsy: a review of its role and reability. *Cancer Biol. Med.* 2014;11:162-72.

[36] Ball, M. W., Bezerra, S. M., Gorin, M. A., et al. Grade heterogeneity in Small Renal Masses: Potential Implications for ranl Mass Biopsy. *J. Urol.* 2014. Jun. 21. pii: S0022-5347(14)03826-9. doi: 10.1016/j.juro.2014.06.067. [Epub. ahead of print].
[37] Algaba, F. Progresos en la patología de las masas renales pequeñas ¿Puede mejorarse la precisión diagnóstica? *Arch. Esp. Urol.* 2013;66:16-22.
[38] Barwari, K., Kummerlin, I. P., Ten Kate, F. J., et al. What is the added value of combined core biopsy and fine needle aspiration in the diagnostic process of renal tumours? *World J. Urol.* 2013;31:823-7.
[39] Ha, S. B., Kwak, C. Current status of renal biopsy for small renal masses. *Korean J. Urol.* 2014;55:568-73.
[40] Lechevallier, E., Andre, M., Daniel, L., Coulange, G. Accuracy of percutaneous biopsy with computerized tomography guidance of small (less tan 4.0cm) renal masses. *Urology* 2004;171:1802-5.
[41] Barwari, K., Beemster, P. W., Hew, M. N., Wijkstra, H., de la Rosette, J., Laguna, M. P. Are there parameters that predict a nondiagnostic biopsy outcome taken during laparoscopic-assisted cryoablation of small renal tumors? *J. Endourol.* 2011;25:1463-8.
[42] Hobbs, D. J., Zhou, M., Campbell, S. C., Aydin, H., Weight, C. J., Lane, B. R. The impact of location and number of cores on the diagnostic accuracy of renal mass biopsy: an ex vivo study. *World J. Urol.* 2013;31:1159-64.
[43] Gerlinger, M., Rowan, A. J., Horswell, S., et al. Intratumoral heterogeneity and branched evolution revealed by multiregioon sequencing. *N. Eng. J. Med.* 2012.8;366 (10):883-92.
[44] Neuzillet, Y., Lechevallier, E., Andre, M., Daniel, L., Coulange, G. Accuracy of percutaneous biopsy with computerized tomography guidance of small (less tan 4.0cm) renal masses. *Urology* 2009;73:586-91.
[45] Veltri, A., Gaetto, I., Tosetti, I., et al. Diagnostic accuracy and clinical impact of imaging-guided needle biopsy of renal masses. Retrospective analysis on 150 cases. *Eur. Radiol.* 2011;21:393-401.
[46] Domínguez, M., Villacampa, F., García, H., Tejido, A., Romero, J., de la Rosa, F. Enseñanzas derivadas del estudio comparativo entre biopsia de masa renal y el análisis del espécimen quirúrgico. *Act. Esp. Urol.* 2014;38(10):655-61.
[47] Volpe, A., Mattar, K., Finelly, A., Kachura, J. R., Evans, A. J., Geddie, W. R., et al. Contemporary results of percutaneous biopsy biopsy of 100 small renal masses: a single center experience. *J. Urol.* 2008;180:2333-7.
[48] Kümmerlin, I., ten Kate, F., Smedts, F., et al. Core biopsies of renal tumors: a study on diagnostic accuracy, interobserver, and intraobserver variability. *Eur. Urol.* 2008;53: 1219-25.
[49] Turun, S., Banghua, L., Zhen, S., Wei, Q. Is tumor size a reliable predictor of histopathological characteristics of renal cell carcinoma? *Urology Annals* 2012;4:24-8.
[50] Schachter, L. R., Cookson, M. S., Chang, S. S., Smith, J. A. jr, Dietrich, M. S., Jayaram, G., et al. Second prize: frecuency of benign cortical tumors and histologic subtypes base don size in a contemporary series: what to tell our patients. *J. Endourol.* 2007;21:1489-91.
[51] Al-Ahmadie, H. A., Alden, D., Fine, S. W., et al. Role of Immunohistochemistry in the avaluation of Needle Core Biopsies in Adult Renal Cortical Tumors; An Ex Vivo Study. *Am. J. Surg. Pathol.* 2011;35:949-61.

[52] Barocas, D. A., Mathew, S., Del Pizzo, J. J., Vaughan, E. D. Jr, Sosa, R. E., Fine, R. G., et al. Renal cell carcinoma sub-typing by histopathology and fluorescence in situ hybridization on a needle-biopsy specimen. *BJU Int.* 2006;99:290-5.

[53] Cheville, J. C., Blute, M. L., Zincke, H., Lohse, C. M., Weaver, A. L. Stage pT1 conventional (clear cell) renal cell carcinoma: pathological features associated with cancer specific survival. *J. Urol.* 2001;166:453-6.

[54] Harris, C. R., Whitson, J. M., Meng, M. V. Under-grading of <4 cm renal masses on renal biopsy. *BJU Int.* 2012;110:794-7.

[55] Vega, A., Gutiérrez, J. L., Martín, B., et al. "Aproximación a los tumores renales menores de 3 cm". *Arch. Esp. Urol.* 1997;50(1):27-31.

[56] Bradley, A. J., Lim, Y. Y., Singh, F. M. Imaging features, follow-up, and management of inicidentally detected renal lesions. *Clin. Radiol.* 2011;66:1129-39.

[57] Smaldone, M. C., Canter, D., Kutikov, A., Uzzo, R. G. Active surveillance of the small renal mass. S. C. Campbell and B. I. Rini (Eds.). *Renal Cell Carcinoma: clinical management, Current Clinical Urology.* Springer Science+Business Media New York 2013; Chapter 10:167-194.

[58] Frank, I., Blute, M. L., Cheville, J. C., et al. Solid renal tumors; an analysis of pathological features related to tumor size. *J. Urol.* 2003;170:2217-20.

[59] Soga, N., Nishikawa, K., Takaki, H., et al. Low incidence of benign lesions in resected suspicious renal masses greater tan 2 cm: single-center experience from Japan. *Int. J. Urol.* 2012;19:729-34.

[60] Ficarra, V., Novara, G., Secco, S., Macchi, V., Porzionato, A., De Caro, R., Artibani, W. Preoperative aspects and dimensions used for an anatomical (PADUA) classification of renal tumours in patients who are candidates for nephron-sparing surgery. *Eur. Urol.* 2009;56:786-93.

[61] Shin, T. Y., Kim, J., Koo, K. C., et al. Assesing the anatomical characteristics of renal masses has a limited effect on the prediction of pathological outcomes in solid, enhancing, small renal masses: results using the PADUA classification system. *BJU Int.* 2014;113;754-61.

[62] Kutinov, A., Uzzo, R. G. The R.E.N.A.L. nephrometry score: a comprehensive standardized system for quantitating renal tumor size, location and depth. *J. Urol.* 2009; 182:844-53.

[63] Kutinov, A., Smaldone, M. C., Egleston, B. L., et al. Anatomic features of enhancing renal masses predict malignant and high-grade pathology: a preoperative nomogram using RENAL nephrometry score. *Eur. Urol.* 2011;60(2):241-8.

[64] Bragodia, A., Harrow, B., Liu, Z. W., et al. Evaluation of anatomic and morphologic nomogram to predict malignant and high-grade disease in a cohort of patients with small renal masses. *J. Urologic Oncology: Sem and Original Investigations;* 2014:32: 37.e17-37.e23.

[65] Koo, K. C., Yoo, H., Shin, T. Y., Kim, J., Choi, Y. D., Rha, K. H., Ham, W. S. External validation of the RENAL nephrometry score nomogram for predicting high-grade renal cell carcinoma in solid, enhancing, and small renal masses. *World J. Urol.* 2014;32: 249-55.

[66] Youssif, T. A., Kassouf, W., Steinberg, J., Aprikain, A. G., laplante, M. P., Tanguay, S. Active surveillance for selected patients with renal masses: updated results with long-term follow-up. *Cancer* 2007;110:1010-3.

[67] Crispen, P. L., Viterbo, R., Boorjian, S. A., Greenberg, R. E., Chen, Y. T., Uzzo, R. G. Natural history, growth kinetics, and outcomes of untreated clinically localized renal tumors under active surveillance. *Cancer* 2009;115:2844-52.
[68] Guethmundsson, E., Hellborg, H., Lundstam, S., Erikson, S., Ljungberg, B. Metastatic potential in renal cell carcinoma <= 7 cm: National Swedish Kidney Cancer Quality Register data. *Eur. Urol.* 2011;60(5):975-82.
[69] Mason, R. J., Abdolell, M., Trottier, G., et al. Growth kinetics of renal masses: analysis of a prospective cohort of patients undergoing active surveillance. *Eur. Urol.* 2011;59: 863-7.
[70] Patel, N., Cranston, D., Akhtar, M. Z., et al. Active surveillance of small renal masses offers short-term oncological efficacy equivalent to radical and partial nephrectomy. *BJU Int.* 2012;110:1270-5.
[71] Steffens, S., Junker, K., Roos, F. C., et al. Small renal cell carcinomas-How dangerous are they really?. Results of a large multicenter study. *Eur. J. Cancer* 2014;50:739-45.
[72] Zastrow, S., Phuong, A., von Bar, et al. Primary tumor size in renal cell cáncer in relation to the ocurrence of synchronous metastatic disease. *Urol. Int.* 2014;92:462-7.
[73] Smaldone, M. C., Kutinov, A., Egleston, B. L., et al. Small renal masses progressing to metástasis under active surveillance: a systematic review and pooled analysis. *Cancer* 2012;118:997-1006.
[74] Brunocilla, E., Borghesi, M., Schiavina, R., et al. Small renal masses initially managed using active surveillance: results from a retrospective study with long-term follow-up. *Clin. Genitourin Cancer* 2014;12(3):178-81.
[75] Rosales, J. C., Haramis, G., Moreno, J., et al. Active surveillance for renal cortical neoplasm. *J. Urol.* 2010;183:1698-702.
[76] Leonard, M., Gillan, A. S., Rai, B. P., et al. Impact of multiple deprivations on detection, progression and interventions in small renal masses (less tan 4 cm) in a population based study. *EJSO* 2013;39:1157-63.
[77] Ingimarsson, J. P., Sigurdsson, M. I., Hardarson, S., et al. The impact of tumour size on the probability of synchronous metástasis and survival in renal cell carcinoma patients: a population-based study. *BMC Urology* 2014;14:72.
[78] Ibragimova, I., Slifker, M. J., Maradeo, M. E., Banumathy, G., Dulaimi, E., Uzzo, R. G., Cairns, P. Genome-wide promoter methylome of small renal masses. *PLoS ONE* 2013;8(10):e77309.
[79] Gossage, L., Eisen, T. Alterations in VHL as potential biomarkers in renal-cell carcinoma. *Nat. Rev. Clin. Oncol.* 2010;7(5):277-88.
[80] Kurban, G., Gedye, C., Morales, C., Yousef, G. M., Almatar, A., Jewett, A. S. Diagnosis and treatment of small renal masses: the role for molecular biology. *Arch. Esp. Urol.* 2013;66(5):505-16.
[81] Klatte, T., Rao, P. N., de Martino, M., et al. Cytogenetic profile predicts prognosis of patients with clear cell renal cell carcinoma. *J. Clin. Oncol.* 2009 Feb.10;27(5):746-53.
[82] Chen, M., Ye, Y., Yang, H., et al. Genome-wide profiling of chromosomal alterations in renal cell carcinoma using high-density single nucleotide plymorphism arrays. *Int. J. Cancer* 2009 Nov.15;125(10):2342-8.
[83] Teng, P. N., Hood, B. L., Sun, M., Dhir, R., Conrads, T. P. Differential proteomic analysis of renal cell carcinoma tissue interstitial fluid. *J. Proteome Res.* 2011.4;10(3): 1333-42.

[84] Fan, L., Li, P., Yin, Z., et al. Ribosomal s6 protein kinase 4: a prognostic factor for enal cell carcinoma. *Br. J. Cancer* 2013;109:1137-46.

[85] Minervini, A., Ficarra, V., Rocco, F., et al. Simple enucleation is equivalent to traditional partial nephrectomy for renal cell carcinoma: results of a non-randomized, retrospective, comparative study. *J. Urol.* 2011;185(5):1604-10.

[86] Wagstaff, P. G. K., Zondervan, P. J., de la Rosette, J. J., Laguna, M. P. The role of imaging in the active surveillance of small renal masses. *Cuur. Urol. Rep.* 2014;15:386.

[87] Campbell, S. C., Novick, A. C., Belldegrum, A., et al. Guideline for management of the clinical T1 renal mass. *J. Urol.* 2009,182(4).1271-9.

[88] Zini, L., Perrote, P., Jeldres, C., et al. A population-based comparison of survival after nephrectomy vs nonsurgical management for small renal masses. *BJU Int.* 2009;103: 899-904.

[89] Gill, I. S., Aron, M., Gervais, D. A., Jewett, M. A. Clinical practice. Small renal mass. *N. Eng. J. Med.* 2010;362:624-34.

[90] Musquera, M., Perez, M., Peri, L., et al. Kidneys from donors with incidental renal tumors: should they be considered aceptable option for transplantation?. *Transplantation* 2013;95:1129-33.

[91] Becker, A., Roghmann, F., Trinh, Q. D., et al. Sociodemographic disparities in the treatment of small renal masses. *BJU Int.* 2013;111:E274-E282.

[92] Jacobs, B. L., Tan, H. J., Montgomery, J. S., et al. Understanding criteria for surveillance of patients with a small renal mass. *Urology* 2012;79:1027-33.

[93] Kowalczyk, K. J., Harbin, A. C., Choueiri, T. K., et al. Use of surveillance imaging following treatment of small renal masses. *J. Urol.* 2013;190:1680-5.

[94] Bhan, S. N., Pautler, S. E., Shayegan, B., Voss, M. D., Goeree, R. A., You, J. J. Active surveillance, radiofrequency ablation, or cryoablation for the nonsurgical management of a small renal mass: a cost-utility analysis. *Ann. Surg. Oncol.* 2013;20:3675-84.

[95] Parker, P. A., Alba, F., Fellman, B., et al. Illness uncertainty and Quality of life of patients with small renal tumors undergoing watchful waiting: a 2-year prospective study. *Eur. Urol.* 2013;63(6):1122-7.

[96] Pierorazio, P., McKierman, J., Allaf, M. Quality of life on active surveillance for a small renal masses versus immediate intervention: interim analysis of the DISSRM (delayed intervention and surveillance for small renal masses) registry. *J. Urol.* 2013; 189-4s. Suppl. 5:e259.

In: Renal Cell Carcinoma
Editors: J. M. Fernández-Gomez, J. García-Rodríguez ISBN: 978-1-63482-495-8

Chapter 6

Surgical Treatment of Renal Carcinoma: An Update

H. Rodriguez Nuñez, MD*, J. A. Gonzalez Dacal, MD, A. Zarraonandia Andraca, MD, M. Ruibal Moldes, MD, and V. I. Garcia Riestra, MD

Urology Service, Department of Urology, University
Hospital of Pontevedra, Pontevedra, Spain

Abstract

During the last two decades, an increase in the incidence of renal cell carcinoma (RCC) has been observed. This is largely the result of an improved detection of localized RCC in asymptomatic patients who undergo imaging for nonspecific abdominal or musculoskeletal complaints. Although surgical removal is the standard of care for renal cancer, actually alternative minimally invasive and conservative treatment options are possible in these patients.

In the present chapter, a review of the indications, techniques and outcomes of surgical treatments for RCC is presented. The scope of this review is to evaluate, based on the evidence acquisition, the current status of minimally invasive surgery (MIS) and the rationale for its use as the standard treatment as well as to explore whether these procedures maintain the benefits of open surgery without jeopardizing the oncologic and morbidity outcomes. We also examine the use of MIS in special situations such as in elderly, children and young patients, and patients with hereditary renal carcinoma or renal carcinoma with renal vein or inferior vena cava tumour thrombus. Finally, the role of robotic assisted and laparoendoscopic single-site surgery is analyzed.

Surgical removal is the standard of care for RCC. The available evidence supports MIS as an alternative to open surgery and it has demonstrated safety, feasibility and equivalent oncologic outcomes.

* Corresponding author: H. Rodriguez Nuñez MD. Department of Urology, University Hospital of Pontevedra, Mourente Str. s/n, 36071 Pontevedra, Spain. E-mail address: higinio.r@wanadoo.es.

1. Introduction

Over the past 2-3 decades, the incidence of renal cancer has steadily increased in Europe and North America. There has been an annual increase of about 2% in both [1]. Greater access and use of modern medical imaging has contributed not only to this rise in overall incidence but also to a downstage of the disease. Most renal lesions are first detected by abdominal ultrasound but, in the presence of solid or complex cystic lesions a precise assessment of size, shape and tissue enhancement by triphasic computed tomography or magnetic resonance imaging scans is necessary. The gold standard treatment for localized renal cell carcinoma is surgical removal, whenever technically feasible. Recent progress in technology has led to effective minimally invasive surgical approaches for renal tumor excision, including laparoscopy and robotic-assisted surgery. Historically, the curative treatment for RCC has been the radical nephrectomy, that is, the removal of the entire tumour-bearing kidney. However, surgeons have gained expertise in the partial nephrectomy technique, reporting excellent oncologic outcomes and reduced morbidity, which has contributed to a more frequent use of partial nephrectomy for localized renal cell carcinoma. Moreover, recent evidences favoring partial nephrectomy over radical nephrectomy in the prevention of chronic kidney disease, possibly linked to a better overall survival, constitutes a strong argument for a wider use of partial nephrectomy.

The objective of this chapter is to evaluate, based on the published information, the current status of minimal invasive surgery as the standard treatment and whether these procedures retain the benefits of radical surgery without jeopardizing the oncologic and morbidity outcomes.

2. Surgical Treatments

The surgical options for the management of renal cell carcinoma are the radical nephrectomy and the partial nephrectomy. However, based on evidence, the current oncological outcomes suggest that renal tumours are best managed by partial nephrectomy rather than by radical nephrectomy. In some patients with localized renal carcinoma, the nephron-sparing surgery (partial nephrectomy) is not suitable because of locally advanced tumour growth, partial resection is not technically feasible or there is a significant deterioration of the patient`s general health. In these situations, radical nephrectomy can be used as curative therapy.

2.1. Laparoscopic Radical Nephrectomy

Laparoscopic renal surgery is well established and adapted routinely technique for the treatment of clinical T1 and T2 kidney tumors. At present, because more than 20 years experience, the perioperative advantages of laparoscopy with respect to open surgery are widely known [2]. Data from randomized controlled trials have shown a shorter hospital stay, significantly decreased convalescence time, blood loss, less analgesic requirement and improved cosmetic results [3-8].

Benefits in terms of overall costs and quality of life have also been established. Moreover, retrospective database reviews have demonstrated similar oncologic outcomes between open and laparoscopic radical nephrectomy.

The indications for laparoscopic radical nephrectomy are similar to that of open surgery: patients with locally advanced tumors (clinical T3a tumors) and with renal vein or low-level vena caval tumor thrombus (clinical T3b tumors) or whether partial nephrectomy is not feasible, although it depends on the surgeon´s laparoscopic skills [9-11]. The indications also encompass patients with metastatic disease when cytoreductive or palliative nephrectomy is necessary [12, 13].

2.1.1. Surgical Approaches

There are two laparoscopic approaches to perform radical nephrectomy (retroperitoneal and transperitoneal). Both have similar oncological outcomes and no significant difference in terms of quality of life. However, the retroperitoneal approach is used significantly less often than the transperitoneal approach.

For the transperitoneal approach, the patient is positioned in a modified flank position with the operative side elevated 30-45 degrees. Four or five incisions are made in abdominal wall for insertion the trocars. Right laparoscopic nephrectomy begins with a peritoneal incision along the white line of Toldt to the hepatic flexure. This incision medially deviates the right colon and duodenum, and allows the visualization of the lateral border of the vena cava. To complete the hilum and upper pole of kidney exposure, a Kocher maneuver is performed with sharp dissection to mobilize the duodenum. The next step is the location of the gonadal vessels and the identification of the ureter, which typically lies just posterior to the gonadal vein with a similar course.

Then, an instrument is passed underneath the ureter to provide anterior traction on the kidney and ureter, leaving the gonadal vein down to minimize the risk of avulsion. The plane between the posterior Gerota´s fascia and psoas muscle is developed bluntly, moving from the lower to the upper pole. Dissection of the renal hilum is facilitated by medial retraction of the viscera and simultaneous elevation of the kidney from the renal fossa. The hilar vessels are dissectioned and ligated, dividing first the main renal artery followed by the vein. Dissection continues to the upper pole, and the lateral and posterior renal attachments are divided. Then, the ureter can be clipped and divided, allowing the whole kidney with Gerota´s fascia and perirenal fat to be free. Finally, the specimen is placed in an endoscopic retrieval bag and removed through a 4-5 centimeter muscle splitting flank incision.

The left laparoscopic nephrectomy begins with medial mobilization of the descending colon by incising the white line of Toldt, developing the plane between the bowel mesentery and Gerota´s fascia. The superior extent of the dissection involves division of the lienocolic and lienorrenal ligaments to allow the spleen to be mobilized medially with the colon and tail of the pancreas. This mobilization facilitates the exposure of the upper pole of the kidney and its hilum. Then, the next steps are similar to right nephrectomy.

For a retroperitoneal approach, the patient is placed in a full flank position. A skin incision is made and the aponeurosis is bluntly perforated under safe control. Then the retroperitoneal space is bluntly dissected and a dissection balloon is introduced into the space. After that 800 cc. of saline solution or gas is injected into the dissection balloon. After a blunt dissection, the balloon is removed and four trocars are inserted.

Important landmarks in the retroperitoneal space, such as Zuckerland´s line or psoas muscle are easily identifiable. Gerota´s fascia is incised parallel to the psoas muscle and the hilum renal is recognized. The renal artery is identified first, ligated and transected. Then, the renal vein is also ligated and transected in the same way. After ligation of the vessels, the ureter can be identified, clipped and divided. Mobilization of the kidney is started from the lower pole and continued to the upper pole. The whole kidney is freed from attachments between Gerota´s fascia and peritoneum and finally, the specimen is inserted in an endoscopic retrieval bag and removed. The minimally invasive approach, performed retroperitoneal or transperitoneal, duplicates established oncological principles of open surgery, namely early control of the renal vessels before tumor manipulation, wide specimen mobilization outside Gerota´s fascia, avoidance of specimen trauma or rupture, and intact specimen extraction. In the hands of experienced laparoscopic urological surgeons and respecting the above mentioned principles of open radical nephrectomy, outcome data indicate equivalent cancer-free survival rates when compared with open radical nephrectomy [14].

2.1.2. Complications

Vascular injuries are the most common complication of urologic laparoscopy and inadequate hilar dissection and bleeding are the most common causes for open conversion. The potential for venous bleeding exists from avulsion injuries or inadequate ligation of venous branches during this step. The renal vein has an anterior layer of connective tissue that must often be incised to gain proper exposure. If a vessel wall defect or inadequately ligated vessels are visualized, clips or sutures may be used. Alternatively, direct pressure with gauze is often adequate to control venous bleeding and minimizes blood loss. Appropriate use of the Hem-o-lock polymer clips is critical to avoiding complications while dividing the renal artery and vein. The Hem-o-lock should be placed perpendicularly across the vessel to allow visualization; this ensures that the entire vessel is being divided without incorporating other structures. When bleeding is adequately controlled, laparoscopic management of the injury can be attempted with free hand suturing or clips, if a sufficient portion of the transected vessel is accessible. Conversion to open surgery may be indicated for exploration and control of major vascular injuries and therefore, a laparotomy set with vascular instruments should be always available in the operating table.

Bowel injury can be one of the most overwhelming complications of laparoscopic surgery. It is of paramount importance to dissect at a safe distance away from the bowel to avoid injury or even unintended transmission of thermal energy to the bowel wall.

Laparoscopic bowel injury occurs in approximately 0.65% of abdominal urologic procedures, and blunt, sharp, and thermal dissection account for the vast majority of cases. The transperitoneal approach results in a higher incidence of bowel injury in comparison with the retroperitoneal approach, but intraoperative recognition and management are the pivotal factors in determining outcome. Continuous vigilance in field inspection on the part of the surgeon will help to maximize recognition, and particular attention should be given to cases of nephrectomy. When bowel injury does occur, superficial or small transmural injuries should be overseen while more significant injuries may require bowel resection.

Addressing the injury may be accomplished laparoscopically or converted to an open procedure if necessary. Postoperatively, the patient's diet should be advanced after the return of bowel function.

Diaphragmatic injury can occur during dissection of the spleen or upper pole and can most often be identified visually or indirectly due to billowing of the diaphragm. In the case of inconspicuous injury, an acute rise in ventilation pressures may be the only indication. To avoid a tension pneumothorax, a central line catheter may be placed in the second intercostal space while the injury is located and repaired. The pneumothorax can be evacuated by placing a suction tip in the defect during closure, with the addition of a thoracostomy tube if necessary. Chest X-ray should be performed following surgery and serially thereafter if a chest tube is placed.

2.1.3. Associated Procedures

2.1.3.1. Adrenalectomy

The decision whether to routinely remove of the ipsilateral adrenal gland during radical nephrectomy has been subject to debate for over 25 years. Routine removal carries potential morbidity during and after surgery for the patient [15].

The situation is particularly relevant in cases of bilateral renal tumours or in patients with a solitary adrenal gland, because chronic glucocorticoid and mineralcorticoid replacement might be necessary if the adrenal gland is resected.

Data of recent analyses have shown that there was no difference in overall survival with or without adrenalectomy in high risk tumours, such as upper pole localization or size tumour > 7 centimeters, high nuclear grade, and locally advanced tumours. The ipsilateral adrenalectomy should be done during radical nephrectomy in patients with an abnormal radiographic appearance of the adrenal gland or suspicious intraoperative findings.

Therefore, routine ipsilateral adrenalectomy does not appear to offer any oncologic benefit [16].

2.1.3.2. Lymph Node Dissection (LND)

In the surgical management of renal carcinoma, the role of lymph node dissection (LND) remains controversial [17]. To date, there is no definitive data which indicates an overall survival advantage by performing lymph node dissection in patients with renal carcinoma. Data from a EORTC prospective randomized trial have provided a basis for concluding that LND is not advantageous in the routine management of renal carcinoma for patients with clinical N0 M0 disease (no metastases), because in these cases only 4% of patients shown positive lymph nodes at final pathology, suggesting that LND represented an overtreatment in the majority of cases [18].

However, in patients who present with clinical nodal disease (>1 cm diameter), the LND should be performed to verify the presence of metastatic nodes at pathology analysis (pN+). Nevertheless, pN+ findings are relatively infrequent in patients without distant metastases and isolated positive nodes in the imaging studies, being estimated to occur in 3% to 10% of cases. Therefore, whether suspects of lymph node involvement exist, it is particularly relevant to accurately rule out distant metastatic in the extension studies. Survival of these patients improves when LND is performed compared to nephrectomy alone [19, 20].

Further, the overall survival of patients who undergo LND associated to radical nephrectomy is far superior to those of patients with distant metastases, and in fact, more closely approximates to the survival of patients with T3, No, Mo disease.

2.2. Laparoscopic Partial Nephrectomy (Nephron Sparing Surgery)

Classically, radical nephrectomy (RN) was established as standard treatment for localized renal carcinoma. The overall survival for early-stage following RN is good, with a low rate of local recurrence. Thus, partial nephrectomy (PN) had been reserved for patients with a tumor in a solitary kidney, bilateral renal tumors or renal function impairment. Nevertheless, in recent years the greater access and use of modern medical imaging has contributed not only to an increase in overall incidence, but also to a downstage migration of the disease as the tumors that tend to be smaller and probably lower grade.

In these cases the RN seems likely to be an excessively aggressive therapeutic option, opening the opportunity for the elective PN. The accumulating evidence derived from clinical research has led to an increased use of PN over RN in the prevention of chronic kidney disease and possibly a better overall survival [21].

2.2.1. Surgical Approach

Laparoscopic partial nephrectomy can be performed either with transperitoneal or retroperitoneal access. The choice of approach is based on tumor location and the surgeon´s experience. The transperitoneal approach is preferred in most cases because it offers a larger working space and it allows managing larger and more endophytic renal masses. However, evidence based on clinical randomized trials that compared both approaches observed similar results in terms of analgesic use, blood loss and postoperative complications.

Preoperatively, patients should be consented for the possibility of radical nephrectomy or open surgery. The patient is placed in a flank position with all pressure points carefully padded. The abdomen is insufflated and ports are placed. For patients with prior abdominal surgery and suspected abdominal adhesions, placement of the initial trocar may be performed using an open Hasson technique or by a direct vision technique using an optical trocar. Wide exposure is important to provide adequate exposure of the renal hilum for vascular control. For right-sided tumors, the right colon is reflected medially, the liver is retracted superiorly and the duodenum is mobilized medially.

On the left side, lateral attachments to the spleen are divided and the spleen, pancreas and colon are reflected medially. If an opening in the bowel mesentery is made during mobilization, this should be closed to decrease the risk of internal hernia formation. The ureter is isolated, and the lower pole of the kidney is retracted anteriorly. All posterior attachments to the kidney are dissected. The renal artery and vein are sufficiently dissected for complete en-bloc or individual control of vessels. All vessels should be accessible for clamping as incomplete clamping can lead to severe hemorrhage. Perirenal fat is removed to obtain wide exposure of the real capsule surrounding the tumor to enable complete resection and reconstruction. Prior to clamping, it is important to ensure that all necessary stitches and instruments are available to prevent unnecessary prolongation of warm ischemia time. Hilar clamping is done through the 12 mm port using either laparoscopic bulldog clamps or en-block clamping using a Satinsky clamp. The renal artery is clamped first, followed by the renal vein. For small or exophytic tumors, the renal artery alone may be clamped.

For hilar or endophytic tumors, both the renal artery and renal vein may be clamped to improve visualization to help achieve a negative surgical margin. Small, exophytic tumors may be resected without hilar clamping. However, the renal hilum should be exposed in case clamping is required.

The tumor may be excised using cold excision to help avoid positive margins. The renal defect is then closed with larger absorbable sutures. Hemostatic agents may also be placed in the renal defect, but may not be necessary if the renal defect can be closed without them. Following reconstruction of the renal defect, the hilar clamps are removed. If bulldog clamps are used, the venous clamp is removed first, followed by flashing of the arterial clamp to confirm hemostasis.

The arterial clamp is removed typically after the renal capsule is closed, but may be removed before closure of the renal capsule to ensure specific vessels are overseen and to reduce warm ischemia time [22]. Confirmation of adequate hemostasis with the insufflation pressure decreased to 5 mm Hg and the mean arterial pressure increased to > 90 mm Hg should be performed prior to completing the procedure to help prevent postoperative bleeding. Finally, all the ports are removed under direct vision

2.2.2. Nephrometry Scores: P.A.D.U.A. and R.E.N.A.L.

Table 1. The PADUA score is based on five preoperative anatomic features as well as the maximum tumor diameter to predict the risk and the grade of complications of partial nephrectomy

ANATOMICAL FEATURES	SCORE
Longitudinal(polar) location	
Superior/Inferior	1
Middle	2
Exophytic rate	
$\geq$50%	1
<50%	2
Endophytic	3
Renal rim	
Lateral	1
Medial	2
Renal sinus	
Not involted	1
Involved	2
Urinary collecting system	
Not involved	1
Dislocated/infiltrated	2
Tumor size (cm)	
$\leq$4	1
4,1-7	2
>7	3

*Anterior or posterior face can be indicated with a letter ("a" or "p") following the score.

The scoring systems have been recently developed to provide a better anatomic description and classification of renal tumors that are candidates for PN [23, 24]. P.A.D.U.A. score (Preoperative Aspects and Dimensions Used for an Anatomical classification) uses five preoperative anatomic features and maximum tumor diameter to predict the risk and the grade of complications to perform the partial nephrectomy (Table 1), which is classified as being:

- Score 6-7: Low complexity
- Score 8-9: Intermediate complexity
- Score >10: High complexity

The RENAL score (Radius, Exophytic or endophytic, Nearness, Anterior, Location) is based on five anatomical features of the renal masses. Of five components, four are scored on 1,2,3- point scale with the fifth indicating the anterior or posterior location of the mass relative to the coronal plane of kidney (Table 2).

Table 2. The RENAL score is based on five anatomical features of the renal masses. Of five components, four are scored on 1,2,3- point scale with the fifth indicating the anterior or posterior location of the mass relative to the coronal plane of kidney

	1 POINT	2 POINTS	3 POINTS
Radius Maximal diameter in cm	<4	4,1-7	>7
Exophytic/endophytic properties	>50%	>50%	Entirely endophytic
Nearness of the tumor to the collecting system or sinus(mm)	>7	>4 but < 7	<4
Anterior / Posterior	No points given	No points given	No points given
Location relative to the polar lines	Entirely above the upper or below the lower polar line	Lesion crosses polar line	>50% of mass is across polar line or mass crosses the axial renal midline or mass is entirely between the polar lines

In this classification, the cases are divided in three categories:

- Score 4-6: Low complexity
- Score 7-9: Intermediate complexity
- Score >10: High complexity

These scoring systems are useful tools to classify the complexity of renal tumors and to predict the complications. Additionally, they have potential for patient counseling and treatment decision making.

2.2.3. Complications

The complications rates of the laparoscopic PN (LPN) are slightly higher than RN. Among the most frequent complication of LPN are the following.

2.2.3.1. Hemorrhage

Hemorrhage can occur at different points during the surgery, such as hilar dissection, tumor resection or clamp removal and also immediate or delayed postoperative period.

Immediate postoperative hemorrhage is usually identified clinically by hemodynamic instability and a decreasing hematocrit. This hemorrhage can usually be managed conservatively with close monitoring and transfusions. Delayed postoperative hemorrhage is usually due to the formation of a pseudoaneurysm or arteriovenosus fistula. Hematuria is the most common clinical presentation, and triphasic CT is the initial study of choice to identify these vascular complications. If bleeding is substantial (i.e., gross hematuria, decreasing hematocrit) a renal angiography with supraselective embolization is the chosen procedure [25]. If bleeding still cannot be controlled surgical exploration is indicated and nephrectomy may be necessary.

2.2.3.2. Urine Leakage

Urine leakage is one of the most common complications of laparoscopic partial nephrectomy (LPN). Excision into the collecting system can be performed with increased experience, although there is a higher risk of bleeding and urinary leakage. Preoperatively, careful review of imaging may suggest tumor proximity to the collecting system which might be needed to entry for a complete resection with negative margins.

Intraoperatively, various techniques have been described to recognize the collecting system entry. Thus, close inspection of the resection bed may reveal gross evidence of collecting system entry. Another technique is previous retrograde placement of a ureteral catheter and then use an intraoperative irrigation with methylene blue solution to identify the collecting system and test the integrity after repair.

After surgery, in cases of persistent high output urine drainage, a CT urogram may be performed to determine whether the urinoma needs to be drained. Retrograde placement of ureteral stent will resolve the leakage in most cases. Sometimes, reexploration is necessary to repair the collecting system and rarely nephrectomy may be indicated [26].

2.2.3.3. Renal Failure

Renal hilar clamping is often necessary during the LPN. Renal ischemia may result in postoperative transient renal insufficiency by acute tubular necrosis. Minimizing ischemia time is important to maximize postoperative renal function. Data prospective studies have observed that significant kidney damage occurs with a warm ischemia time (WIT) of more than 30 minutes; and this damage is partially reversible. Therefore, all efforts should be made to reduce WIT to less than 30 minutes to reduce the risk of significant injury [27]. To achieve this goal, several modifications to the LPN technique have been proposed [28-30]:

- Early unclamping technique, which uses clamping during the tumor excision and the placement of the initial running suture on the renal medulla. All subsequent running sutures are done in the perfused and revascularized kidney. This technique allows a significantly shorter WIT and a significantly lower overall rate of postoperative complications.
- Zero ischemia LPN is a technique without hilar clamping. This method is based on anatomic microdissection to isolate and control tumor specific renal artery branches

with neurosurgical bulldog clamps and controlled reduction of blood pressure. Accordingly, WIT is zero and therefore, no decrease in glomerular filtration rate exists with excellent renal functional outcomes.

2.2.4. Preservation of Renal Function

According to the US National Kidney Foundation, chronic kidney disease is defined as either kidney damage for more than 3 months as confirmed by renal biopsy or makers of kidney damage with or without a decrease in glomerular filtration rate (GFR) or GFR less than 60 ml/min per 1,73 m2 for more than 3 months with or without kidney damage [31]. Patients who are commonly diagnosed with a renal tumor have baseline renal dysfunction. Retrospective studies comparing partial nephrectomy to radical nephrectomy with a normal contralateral kidney have shown a higher likelihood of renal function impairment after radical nephrectomy. The mechanism by which PN offers an advantage over RN in preventing chronic kidney disease is certainly the result of a greater preservation of the nephron reserve [32]. Subsequently, we may deduce that PN is the chosen technique to prevent chronic kidney disease.

2.2.5. Oncologic Outcomes

Retrospective non-randomized studies have shown comparable cancer specific outcomes for PN and RN in low stage renal tumors [33]. In a EORTC study, patients with small solitary tumors suspicious of renal carcinoma and normal contralateral kidney were randomized to PN or RN. Over a mean follow-up of 9 years, few renal cancers related deaths were observed. The estimated risk of cancer specific mortality was not found to be significantly higher in the PN arm. In another retrospective study, comparing survival data of patients treated with PN and RN, with a median follow-up of 64 months, cancer specific survival (CSS) rates were similar. Recent SEER data base analysis have shown that in a matched population of T1a renal carcinoma treated with PN or RN, 5-year CSS was not significantly different for the two surgical approaches [34]. Although a longer follow-up is needed, data from these studies suggest that rates of recurrence free survival, CSS and overall survival are similar in both procedures.

3. Special Situations

3.1. Minimally Invasive Surgery in Elderly Patients

Minimally invasive surgery (MIS) is associated with less postoperative discomfort and improved recovery and, moreover, outcome data for cancer specific survival is comparable with open surgery. In this way, laparoscopic radical nephrectomy is an attractive technique in the elderly patients due to the decreased convalescence and pain associated. The requirement of analgesia is diminished and this benefit has shown to result in improved pulmonary function among patients treated by laparoscopic radical nephrectomy compared to open radical nephrectomy. This may be particularly useful in these patients because they have frequently fewer pulmonary reserves.

The most postoperative morbidity of radical nephrectomy is renal dysfunction. This dysfunction leads to changes in the renal tissue (diabetic nephropathy, glomerular hypertrophy and diffuse glomeruloesclerosis) that can be reflected in the renal function. Besides, data of retrospective studies show that incidence of chronic kidney disease is much higher in patients who undergo radical nephrectomy than partial nephrectomy [35].

Therefore, in elderly patients, the partial nephrectomy is an accepted surgical approach to avoid chronic renal disease. However, in the setting of a normal contralateral kidney, one must weigh the additional risk of complications such as increased bleeding, urinary fistula, local recurrence, arteriovenous fistula or non-functional kidney remaining [36].

3.2. Minimally Invasive Surgery in Childhood and Youth

Renal carcinoma accounts for 2% to 6% of paediatric renal malignancies [37]. At this age, renal carcinoma is different from typical adult renal carcinoma in its tumor biology and behavior [38]. Renal carcinoma in this population is often associated to genetic alterations and hereditary syndromes, such as Von-Hippel-Lindau, Birt-Hogg-Dube or tuberous sclerosis. These patients must undergo genetic screening and counseling.

Another feature of renal carcinoma in these patients is the higher incidence of regional lymph node involvement. Fortunately, this lymph node involvement does not appear to portend a serious prognosis as it does in adults [39]. This high incidence of lymph node involvement and the lack of curative adjuvant medical therapy for metastasis from renal carcinoma combined with some data suggesting a therapeutic benefit, suggest that nephrectomy associated to surgical resection of regional lymph node might be a reasonable approach. A review of the surgical experience with renal carcinoma in the Children Oncology Group determined that the majority of children are treated with radical nephrectomy compared to nephron sparing surgery, but only two thirds of these patients had lymph nodes sampled at time of surgery. Given the high rate of lymph node positivity in this population, it is important to educate surgeons that nodal sampling must not be omitted [40]. Surgical approach can be done with minimally invasive surgery or standard open surgery. However, the most important therapeutic consideration is the oncologic outcome. Thus, it is recommended that minimally invasive approaches (LRN and LPN) in this population should be reserved for surgeons experienced in these oncologic techniques.

In conclusion, it is important to know that renal carcinoma is different, starting with the approach to diagnosis and staging. Currently, the management of renal carcinoma focuses on surgery. Minimally invasive surgery has an emerging role and this approach probably is a great hope for increased survival with reduced morbidity.

3.3. Renal Carcinoma in Hereditary Diseases

Renal carcinoma represents 2-3 % of all cancers and approximately 4% of renal carcinomas are hereditary origin. Although hereditary cancer syndromes can be difficult to identify, early recognition is important, because it facilitates a correct management of the patients as well as screening of their relatives. Main genetic changes found are the loss of function mutations in tumor suppressor genes and a gain of function mutations in protooncogenes, which are then called oncogenes. Research regarding hereditary renal carcinoma has led to the identification of a relevant gene locus on the short arm of chromosome 3 [41] (see chapter 1). Von-Hippel-Lindau (VHL) disease is the most frequent hereditary renal cancer syndrome and renal cell carcinoma is the most common malignant neoplasm.

These tumors are seen in 24-45% of patients, they are multicentric and bilateral in at least 75% of patients with VHL disease. The mean age at clinical presentation is 39 ± 10 years, which is 10-20 years earlier than that reported for sporadic renal disease. Although small renal tumors tend to be low grade and minimally invasive in this disease, their growth rate varies widely. Besides, these tumors are capable to progress, developing metastases which represent a frequent cause of death in these patients. The surgical options have evolved during the last 3 decades. Staged bilateral nephrectomy and hemodialysis have progressed to partial nephrectomy and nephron sparing surgery. The best management balances the goals of minimizing risk of renal carcinoma metastasis and preserving renal function, attempting to minimize the total number of surgeries a patient will require over a lifetime.

The indications for nephron sparing surgery are malignancies located in solitary kidneys, bilateral synchronous renal lesions, and renal tumors in patients whose contralateral kidney is threatened by local, systemic or genetic risk factors. Although early results have been promising, subsequent studies have suggested a high incidence of postoperative tumor recurrence in the remaining portion of the kidney. It is likely that most of these local recurrences are a manifestation of residual microscopic cancer that was not removed at the time of the original partial nephrectomy.

A study from the National Institute of Health [42] has shown that tumors less than 3 cms in size are not considered an indication for surgery. These patients are followed expectantly until the renal masses are longer than 3 cms in diameter. Follow up of this study has revealed that metastasis does not develop in any patients who had tumors smaller than 3 cms. Other studies suggest that partial nephrectomy can provide effective initial treatment of patients with renal cancer and VHL disease, but should be withheld until tumor size reaches or eclipses 3 cms. These authors have shown that up to 85% of patients experience de novo renal tumor recurrence at 10 years. After PN, these patients must be observed closely because most will develop recurrent renal carcinoma. In this setting, salvage partial nephrectomy can be challenging, because there is a high risk of complications by severe fibrosis, scaring and the obliteration of normal anatomic planes. Although performed by the laparoscopic approach, the failure to achieve reliable hypothermia along with prolonged ischemia times and increased complication rates have limited in its widespread application. This approach should be performed in selected centers with experienced teams.

3.4. Minimally Invasive Surgery in Renal Cancer with Renal Vein or Inferior Vena Cava Tumour Thrombus

Renal carcinoma with renal vein or inferior vena cava tumor thrombus (IVCTT) is found about 4-10 % of all cases. Surgical removal of the thrombus and the kidney should be sought and this procedure is extremely challenging and technically demanding. The surgical procedure must be scheduled depending on the extent of the thrombus (Figure 1):

- Level I: Infiltration of renal vein
- Level II: Infiltration of the infrahepatic vena cava
- Level III: Infiltration of the intrahepatic vena cava
- Level IV: Infiltration of the suprahepatic vena cava or atrial

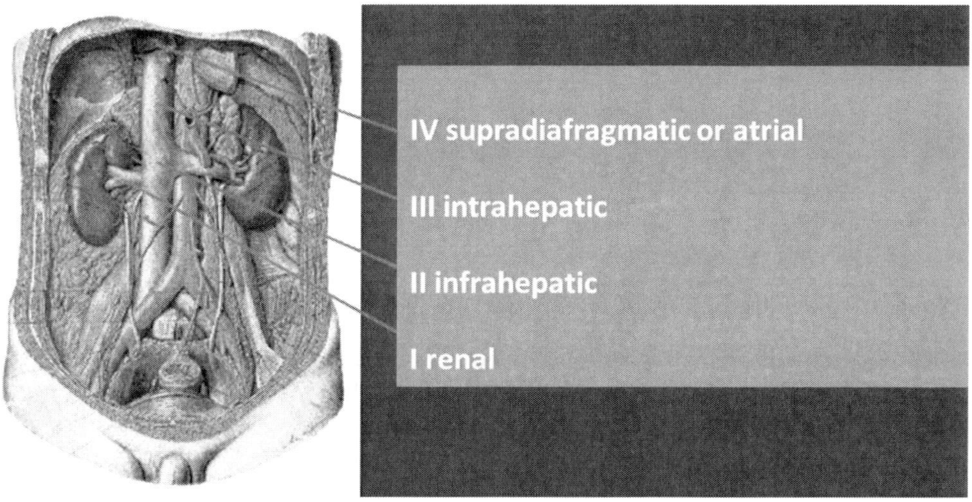

Figure 1. Mayo clinic: Levels of vena cava tumor thrombus.

Although open surgery is still the chosen approach to manage renal cancer with inferior vena caval tumor thrombus [43], the continued advances in laparoscopic surgery and increased experience of urologists have expanded the indications of the laparoscopic techniques to more complex renal tumors. Similar to open surgery, laparoscopic radical nephrectomy with thrombectomy has several important steps:

- Dissection and ligation of renal artery
- Vena cava, contralateral and ipsilateral vein exposure
- Occlusion of the IVC under the thrombus, contralateral renal vein and IVC above the thrombus
- Opening of the vena cava and thrombectomy
- Suturing the IVC and release of the vascular clamps
- Nephrectomy

Generally, the prognosis of patients with a tumor thrombus after a successfully carried out surgery is not related to the size or the extent of the thrombus; but it mainly depends on the metastasis stage. Retrospective cohort studies have shown 5 year cancer specific survival rates up to 70% after this surgery in non-metastasis stage. Current studies report the feasibility and safety of the laparoscopic approach to perform renal cancer with IVCTT, but these have several shortcomings such as retrospective design, short number of cases and relative short length of follow up [44]. Finally, we need long term oncologic outcomes to elucidate the efficiency of this approach.

3.5. Emerging Techniques: Robot Assisted Laparoscopic Surgery and Laparoscopic Single-Site Surgery (LESS)

The use of the robotics in minimally invasive surgery is well established. The six degrees of freedom at the distal end of the instruments, the tridimensional stereoscopic vision, movement scale-down and tremor filters enhance the performance of the most experienced laparoscopic surgeons and make the laparoscopy available to inexperienced surgeons. Some studies have demonstrated that a decreased hospital stay and quicker convalescence is observed with robotic assisted laparoscopic radical nephrectomy compared to open radical nephrectomy [45]. Despite these advantages, data on the direct comparison of robot assisted radical nephrectomy and laparoscopic radical nephrectomy reported similar complication rates and postoperative outcomes. Based on this data and the considerably higher cost per procedure, robot assistance may be considered a technical overtreatment for radical nephrectomy [46]. While radical nephrectomy is mainly an extirpative procedure, partial nephrectomy requires complex dissection and intracorporeal reconstruction and here in this procedure, the robotic renal surgery has demonstrated additional advantages. The largest multi-institutional comparison of the two approaches (LPN versus RAPN) has revealed no significant differences in overall operative time, collecting system entry and positive margin rate for RAPN and LPN. Intraoperative blood loss was less for RAPN compared to LPN as was length of hospital stay.

Warm ischemia time was significantly shorter in the RAPN series [47]. These data confirm that RAPN has a potential advantage by reducing the technical difficulty of the most challenging steps of this procedure. For surgeons with robotic experience, RAPN has shown a warm ischemia time lower than 20 minutes, console times lower than 100 minutes, limited blood loss and acceptable overall complication rates. There are currently no intermediate or long-term oncologic outcomes reported in the literature for RAPN, but short term outcomes from several robotic series seem to be equivalent to those reported for LPN series.

Therefore, oncologic outcomes are still immature and larger series with longer follow up are awaited to confirm these results [48, 49] (Table 3).

LESS is the general term for all surgical procedures performed by one single skin incision for the introduction of a camera and instruments, with or without an additional maximum port of 5 mms. The advantages offered by this approach are still in discussion. The superior cosmetic outcome offered by LESS seems to be the main advantage and the primary reason for using this technology.

LESS radical nephrectomy is the most frequent procedure. The feasibility and safety have been well documented. A recent metaanalysis compared LESS versus conventional laparoscopic nephrectomy, and LESS nephrectomy was associated with less postoperative pain, lower analgesic requirement, shorter hospital stay, shorter recovery time and better cosmetic outcome. However a longer operative time and a higher conversion rate was found compared with laparoscopic nephrectomy [50].

The surgical experience with LESS partial nephrectomy (LESS-PN) is limited because only a few centers are using this challenging procedure.

Most reported outcomes of LESS-PN are similar to the laparoscopic approaches. However, there is a lack of intermediate and long-term follow up data on LESS-PN to prove the benefits of this procedure.

Table 3. Conclusions and recommendations from EAU guidelines on robotic and single-site surgery in urology [49]

Conclusions on RRN and RPN	LE
Conclusive long-term data are not available.	-
RRN and RPN are technically feasible.	-
No comparable long-term data on oncologic, safety, and functional outcomes are available. However, based on short-term data and guidelines panel expertise, no significant differences are expected	4
In ablative surgery, robotics will produce no better outcomes compared with laparoscopy	-
Posible benefit exist in reconstructive surgery (i.e., partial nephrectomy/pyelopasty).	
Recommendations	
Use laparoscopy for simple or radical nephrectomy	C
Use robot-assisted or laparoscopic surgery for partial or reconstructive renal surgery if technically feasible.	C
Use of minimal invasive techniques should not compromise nephron-sparing surgery	C

GR=grade of recommendation; LE=level of evidence; RPN=robot-assisted partial nephrectomy; RRN=robotassisted radical nephrectomy.

In conclusion, LESS surgical procedures are technically feasible with a cosmetic advantage, but long-term oncologic outcomes are not yet available and have no proven documented benefits over the laparoscopic approach.

Conclusion

Radical nephrectomy is the standard of care for renal carcinoma. Nevertheless, in recent years minimally invasive surgery (laparoscopic nephrectomy and laparoscopic partial nephrectomy) has become an established surgical procedure worldwide as an alternative to open surgery which has demonstrated safety, feasibility and equivalent oncologic outcomes.

References

[1] Mathew, A., Devesa, S. S., Frameni, Jr J. F., Chow, W. H. Global increases in kidney cancer incidence 1973-1992. *Eur. J. Cancer Prev.* 2002, 11: 171-8.

[2] Robson, C. J., Churchill, B. M., Anderson, W. The results of radical nephrectomy for renal cell carcinoma. *J. Urol.* 1969, 101: 297-301.

[3] Burgess, N. A., Koo, B. C., Calvert, R. C., Hindmarsh, A., Donaldson, P. J., Rhodes, M. Randomized trial of laparoscopic v open nephrectomy. *J. Endourol.* 2007; 21(6): 610-613.

[4] Dunn, M. D., Portis, A. J., Shalhav, A. L., et al. Laparoscopic versus open radical nephrectomy: a 9-year experience. *J. Urol.* 2000 164 (4): 1153-1159.

[5] Hemal, A. K., Kumar, A., Kumar, R., Wadhwa, P., Seth, A., Gupta, N. P. Laparoscopic versus open radical nephrectomy for large renal tumours: a long-term prospective comparison. *J. Urol.* 2007, 177 (3): 862-866.

[6] Kerbl, K., Clayman, R. V., McDougall, E. M., Kavoussi, L. R. Laparoscopic nephrectomy: the Washington University Experience. *Br. J. Urol.* 1994, 73(3): 231-236.

[7] McDougall, E., Clayman, R. V., Elashry, O. M. Laparoscopic radical nephrectomy for renal tumour: the Washington University Experience. *J. Urol.* 1996; 155(4): 1180-1185.

[8] Ono, Y., Kinukawa, T., Hattori, R., et al. Laparoscopic radical nephrectomy for renal cell carcinoma: a five year experience. *Urology* 1999, 53(2): 280-286.

[9] Desai, M. M., Gill, I. S., Ramani, A. P., Matin, S. F., Kaouk, J. H., Campero, J. M. Laparoscopic radical nephrectomy for cancer with level I renal vein involvement. *J. Urol.* 2003; 169(2) 487-491.

[10] Guzzo, T. S., Schaeffer, E. M., McNeil, B. K., Pollock, R. A., Pavlovich, C. P., Allaf, M. E. Laparoscopic radical nephrectomy for patients with pathologic T3b renal cell carcinoma: the Johns Hopkins experience. *J. Endourol.* 2009; 23(11):63-67.

[11] Steinnerd, L. E., Vardi, I. Y., Bhayassi, S. B. Laparoscopic radical nephrectomy for renal carcinoma with known level I renal vein tumour thrombus. *Urology* 2007; 69(4): 662-665.

[12] Eisenberg, M. S., Meng, M. V., Master, V. A., et al. Laparoscopic versus open cytoreductive nephrectomy in advanced renal-cell carcinoma. *J. Endourol.* 2006; 20(7): 504-508.

[13] Matin, S. F., Madsen, L. T., Wood, C. G. Laparoscopic cytoreductive nephrectomy: the M.D. Anderson Cancer Center experience. *Urology* 2006; 68(3):528-532.

[14] Desai, M. M., Strzempkowski, B., Matin, S. F., et al. Prospective randomized comparison of transperitoneal versus retroperitoneal laparoscopic radical nephrectomy. *J. Urol.* 2005; 173: 38-41.

[15] O´Malley, R. L., Godoy, G., Kanofsky, J. A., Taneja, S. S. The necessity of adrenalectomy at the time of radical nephrectomy: a systematic review. *J. Urol.* 2009; 181: 2009-2017.

[16] Ljunberg, B., Cowan, N. C., Hanbury, D. C., et al. EUA guidelines on renal cell carcinoma; the 2010 update. *Eur. Urol.* 2010; 58: 398-406.

[17] Bekema, H. J., MacCleman, S., Imanura, M., et al. Systematic review of adrenalectomy and lymph node dissection in locally advanced renal cell carcinoma. *Eur. Urol.* 2013 Nov., 64(5):799-810.

[18] Blom, J. H., Van Poppel, H., Mavechal, J. M., et al. Radical Nephrectomy with and without lymph-node dissection: Final Results of European Organization for Research and treatment of Cancer (EORTC) Randomized Phase 3 Trial 30881. *Eur. Urol.* 2009 Jan; 55(1): 28-34.

[19] Freeland, S. J. and Dekernion, J. B. Role of lymphadenectomy for patients undergoing radical nephrectomy for renal cell carcinoma. *Reviews Urology* Vol. 5; pp. 191-195. 2003.

[20] Peters, P. C. and Brown, G. L. The role of lymphadenectomy in the management of renal cell carcinoma. *Urologic Clinics of North America.* Vol. 7, nº 3, pp. 705-709 1980.

[21] Huang, W. C., Levy, A. S., Serio, A. M., et al. Chronic kidney disease after nephrectomy in patients with renal cortical tumours: a retrospective cohort study. *Lancet Oncol.* 2006; 7: 735-40.

[22] Nguyen, M. M., Gill, I. S. Halving ischemia time during laparoscopic partial nephrectomy. *BJU Int.* 2009; 103(9): 1296-1311.
[23] Ficarra, V., Novara, G., Secco, S., et al. Preoperative aspects and dimensions used for an anatomical (PADUA) classification of renal tumours in patients who are candidates for nephron-sparing surgery. *Eur. Urol.* 2009; 56: 786-93.
[24] Kutikov, A., Uzzo, R. G. The RENAL. Nephrometry score: a comprehensive standardized system for quantitating renal tumor size, location and depth. *J. Urol.* 2009 182: 844-53.
[25] Cohenpour, M., Strauss, S., Gottlieb, P., et al. Pseudoaneurysm of the renal artery following partial nephrectomy: imaging findings and coil embolization. *Clin. Radiol.* Nov. 2007: 62(11): 1104-1109.
[26] Meeks, J. J., Zhao, L. C., Navai, N., Perry, K. T., Jr, Nadler, R. B., Smith, N. D. Risk factors and management of urine leak after partial nephrectomy. *J. Urol.* Dec. 2008; 180(6): 2375-2378.
[27] Porpiglia, F., Renard, J., Billia, M., et al. Is renal warm ischemia over 30 minutes during laparoscopic partial nephrectomy posible?. One year results of a prospective study. *Eur. Urol.* 2007: 52 1170-1178.
[28] Baumert, H., Ballaro, A., Shah, N., et al. Reducing warm ischemia time during laparoscopic partial nephrectomy: a prospective comparison of two renal closure techniques. *Eur. Urol.* 2007; 52: 1164-1169.
[29] Bollens, R., Rosenblatt, A., Espinoza, B. P., et al. Laparoscopic partial nephrectomy with "on-demand" clamping reduces warm ischemia time. *Eur. Urol.* 2007; 52: 804-810.
[30] Gill, I. S., Kamoi, K., Aron, M., Desai, M. M. 800 Laparoscopic partial nephrectomies: a single surgeon series. *J. Urol.* 2010; 183: 34-41.
[31] National Kidney Foundation. K/DOQI clinical practice guidelines for chronic kidney disease: evaluation, classification and stratification. *Am. J. Kidney Dis.* 2002; 39 (suppl. 1): S1-266.
[32] Lane, B. R., Babineau, D. C., Poggio, E. D., et al. Factors predicting renal functional outcome after partial nephrectomy. *J. Urol.* 2008; 180: 2363-2368, discussion 2368-9.
[33] Van Poppel, H., Da Pozzo, L., Albrecht, W., et al. A prospective randomized EORTC intergroup phase 3 study comparing the oncologic outcome of elective nephron-sparing surgery and radical nephrectomy for low-stage renal cell carcinoma. *Eur. Urol.* 2011; 59: 543-552.
[34] Crepel, M., Jeldres, C., Sun, M., et al. A population based comparison of cáncer control rates between radical and partial nephrectomy for T1a renal cell carcinoma. *Urology* 2010; 76: 883-8.
[35] Huang, W. C., Levey, A. S., Serio, A. M., et al. Chronic kidney disease after nephrectomy in patients with renal cortical tumours: a retrospective cohort study. *Lancet Oncol.* 2006, 7: 735-40.
[36] Gill, I. S., Matin, S. F., Desai, M. M., Kaouk, J. H., Steinberg, A., Mascha, E., et al. Comparative analysis of laparoscopic versus open partial nephrectomy for renal tumors in 200 patients. *J. Urol.* 2003,170 (1): 64-68.
[37] Horner, M. J., Ries, L. A. G., Krapcho, M., et al.: *SEER Cancer Statistics Review, 1975-2006*. Bethesda, Maryland: National Cancer Institute 2009.

[38] Sausville, J. E., Hernandez, D. J., Argani, P., et al.: Pediatric renal cell carcinoma. *J. Pediatr. Urol.* 2009, 5; 308-314.

[39] Geller, J. I. and Dome, J. S. Local lymph node involvement does not predict por outcome in pediatric renal cell carcinoma. *Cancer* 2004; 101 (7): 1575-83.

[40] Ehrlich, P. F., Cost, N. G., Khanna, G., et al. A description of the surgical experience in children, adolescents and young adults with renal cell carcinoma: A report from the Children´s Oncology Group Study AREN 03B2. *BJU Int. suppl.* 2012; 110:18, Abstract 39.

[41] Pavlovich, C. P., Schmidt, L. S. Searching for the hereditary causes of renal cell carcinoma. *Nat. Rev. Cancer* 2004; 4: 381-393.

[42] Walther, M. M., Choyke, P. L., Glenn, G., et al. Renal cancer in families with hereditary renal cancer: Prospective analysis of a tumor size threshold for renal parenchymal sparing surgery. *J. Urol.* 1999, 161(5): 1475-1479.

[43] Eisenberg, M. S., Meng, M. V., Master, V. A., et al. Laparoscopic versus open cytoreductive nephrectomy in advanced renal cell carcinoma. *J. Endourol.* 2006, 20: 504-508.

[44] Martin, G. L., Castle, E. P., Martin, A. D., et al. Outcomes of laparoscopic radical nephrectomy in the setting of vena caval and renal vein thrombus: seven year experience. *J. Endourol.* 2008; 22(8): 1681-1686.

[45] Horgan, S., Vanuno, D. Robots in laparoscopic surgery. *J. Laparoendosc. Adv. Surg. Tech. A* 2001 11: 415-419.

[46] Nazemi, T., Galich, A., Sterrett, S., et al. Radical nephrectomy performed by open, laparoscopy with or without hand-assistance or robotic methods by the same surgeon produces comparable perioperative results. *Int. Braz. J. Urol.* 2006; 32: 15-22.

[47] Benway, B. M., Bhayani, S. B., Rogers, C. G., et al. Robot assisted partial nephrectomy versus laparoscopic partial nephrectomy for renal tumours: a multi-institutional analysis of perioperative outcomes. *J. Urol.* 2009; 182: 866-872.

[48] Box, G., Averch, T., Cadeddu, J., et al. Nomenclature of natural orifice transluminal endoscopic surgery (NOTES) and laparoendoscopic single site surgery (LESS) procedures. *J. Endourol.* 2008; 22: 2575-2581.

[49] Merseburger, A. S. 1., Herrmann, T. R., Shariat, S. F., Kyriazis, I., Nagele, U., Traxer, O., Liatsikos, E. N., European Association of Urology. EAU guidelines on robotic and single-site surgery in urology. *Eur. Urol.* 2013; 64 (2): 277-91.

[50] Fan, X., Lin, T., Xu, K., et al. Laparoendoscopic single site nephrectomy compared with conventional laparoscopic nephrectomy: a systematic review and meta-analysis of comparative studies. *Eur. Urol.* 2012; 62: 601-612.

In: Renal Cell Carcinoma ISBN: 978-1-63482-495-8
Editors: J. M. Fernández-Gomez, J. García-Rodríguez

Chapter 7

Ablative Therapies for the Treatment of Renal Cell Carcinoma

A. Plata Bello,** *PhD and T. Concepción Masip, PhD
University Hospital of Canary Islands, La Laguna. Spain

Abstract

Introduction: Partial nephrectomy is the standard treatment of choice for small renal masses (cT1). However, presently, thermal ablation is an alternative option that is increasingly used with less morbidity than surgical treatment. The most popular ablative techniques are radiofrequency ablation (RFA) and cryotherapy.

Material and methods: We conducted a systematic review using databases such as MEDLINE and EMBASE by entering keywords such as "Laparoscopy renal radiofrequency", "ablation radiofrequency" (RF), "cryoablation", "cryosurgery", "microwave", "hifu", "electroporation", "cryotherapy", "ablation", "renal", "kidney", and renal cell carcinoma "RCC". We reviewed the clinical guidelines of the European Association of Urology (EAU) and American Urology Association (AUA). We considered the indications of the Cochrane Library, Up to Date and The Centre for Reviews and Dissemination of National Institute for Health Research. We explored the websites of different companies that offer radiofrequency technology, cryotherapy, microwave and high-intensity focused ultrasound. We analyzed the epidemiology, oncological results, survival and safety of the major ablative techniques available today.

Results: Ablative therapies are a safe alternative with higher recurrence rates than standard surgical treatment. Metastasis-free survival is higher for partial nephrectomy and cryotherapy than for RFA. Overall survival is greater after partial nephrectomy, most likely due to a selection bias of patients. The rate of complications is low, and the ambulatory procedure allows the reduction of costs associated with the treatment of renal cancer.

Conclusion: Partial nephrectomy is the standard treatment for cT1 renal tumors. In the absence of randomized clinical trials that validate published results in this respect,

* Correspondence to: Ana Plata Bello. anaplatabello@hotmail.com. Urology Department. C/Ofra sn 38320 La Laguna, Tenerife. Spain.

ablative therapies are a valid option for selected patients with a high surgical risk that offers recurrence-free survival rates exceeding 85% and metastasis-free rates in over 95% of cases.

Introduction

In 2014, it is estimated that 63,920 new cases of renal cancer were diagnosed in the United States, and 13,860 people have died from this cause [1]. In Europe, the incidence values are higher with 84,000 new cases and 34,700 deaths from renal cancer [2]. Renal parenchymal tumors are most commonly observed (85%) compared with kidney tumors of the urinary tract (12%).

Because imaging tests are presently increasingly used to assess other abdominal clinical entities, the incidence of renal tumors discovered incidentally in asymptomatic patients is 48-66% [3]. The latter finding has indicated that, in recent decades, there has been an annual 2-3% increase in the incidence of renal cancer at the expense of increased detection of stage 1 (<7 cm) tumors [4,5]. This trend has caused a stage migration at the diagnosis of renal cancer and a change in the contemporary management of patients with renal cancer in early stages, resulting in an increased rate of surgery performed [6]. Partial nephrectomy, in any of its technical variants (open, laparoscopic or robotic) has replaced classical radical nephrectomy in the treatment of T1a tumors and some T1b tumors whenever technically possible, thus preserving the healthy renal parenchyma. Several authors have shown that, in selected patients, conservative surgical treatment (partial nephrectomy) is equivalent to radical treatment (radical nephrectomy) in terms of cancer control [7-12]. In addition, a greater incidence of chronic kidney disease has been demonstrated in patients undergoing radical nephrectomy, particularly in those with comorbidities such as diabetes or hypertension. Therefore, partial nephrectomy has demonstrated a lower incidence of chronic kidney disease (CKD) (GFR≤60 mL per min/1.73 m^2) after surgery. CKD is a significant factor to consider given that it is associated with a greater risk of cardiovascular events that cause a decreased quality of life of patients and increased morbidity and mortality [8, 10-12]. Capitanio et al. have demonstrated that partial nephrectomy reduces the risk of cardiovascular events 1, 5 and 10 years after treatment compared with radical nephrectomy [13].

Thus, partial nephrectomy is considered the standard treatment for T1a tumors and T1b tumors whenever technically feasible [1, 2]. Despite all the advantages offered by this paradigm shift in the treatment of renal cancer, partial nephrectomy is a technically complex procedure not free from complications. Van Popel et al., in a prospective randomized study of patients with stage 1 renal cancer in which complications of partial nephrectomy were compared against radical nephrectomy, noted that patients undergoing partial nephrectomy had an increase in perioperative bleeding (3.1% vs 1.2%), 4.4% urinary fistulas, a greater incidence of pleural lesions (11.5% vs 9.3%) and a higher rate of reoperation (4.4% vs 2.4%) [14]. The experience and skill of the surgeon are critical in reducing morbidity and warm ischemia time.

To offer treatment to frail patients and minimize the morbidity and mortality associated with the surgical treatment of these tumors, ablative therapies appear as an alternative. These have developed rapidly and extensively in the last decade. They combine the advantages of vision, direct (laparoscopy) or by imaging tests in situ, and the preservation of non-tumor renal parenchyma. Lane et al. showed an increase from 3% to 69% for the use of conservative therapies versus radical surgery, primarily for T1a and T1b tumors [4].

Currently, the indications of ablative techniques common to all renal tumors [2, 4]:

- Tumors less than 4 cm (T1)
- Cortico-exophytic tumors (technically easier and fewer complications)
- Elderly patients
- Patients with multiple comorbidities who are not candidates for surgery
- Patients with chronic kidney failure requiring nephron-sparing surgery to avoid dialysis
- Single kidney and renal transplant patients with some degree of chronic kidney failure
- Multiple hereditary tumor syndromes (Von Hippel-Lindau syndrome)
- Rescue technique in the recurrences of partial nephrectomies
- Control of cancer pain and hematuria

The contraindications include:

- Tumors larger than 5 cm
- Locations close to the renal vascular hilum, ureter, spleen, liver or intestinal loops; in these situations, neighboring structures can be separated by injecting different substances (water, saline, dextrose, CO_2)
- Coagulopathies
- Clinical instability of the patient (recent myocardial infarction)
- Metastatic disease
- Active infection
- Life expectancy of less than a year
- Very young patients

The most popular ablative techniques that have passed the experimental stage are cryotherapy and radiofrequency ablation (RFA). However, studies published in this regard are limited to case series, and there are no prospective randomized clinical trials comparing ablative therapies with standard surgical treatment. Other forms of ablative therapy that are still considered experimental are HIFU (high-intensity focused ultrasound), microwave ablation (microwave thermotherapy), interstitial laser ablation (laser interstitial thermal therapy-LITT), irreversible electroporation, and ablation by ultrasonic cavitational pulses (pulse cavitational ultrasound-PCU).

Cryotherapy

a. Fundamentals of Cryotherapy

Cryotherapy is based on the Joule-Thompson principle that describes temperature changes accompanying the expansion of a gas without heat exchange with the environment. Cryoprobes use liquid nitrogen or argon during freezing and helium during the heating phase.

The pathophysiological mechanisms responsible for tissue ablation produced from cryotherapy have been extensively studied both in vitro and in vivo. Argon or nitrogen gas is used during the freezing phase, which results in an initial acute phase of direct mechanical cell damage. Additionally, inducing crystallization of the extracellular space favors the creation of a concentration gradient (increased osmotic pressure) that causes changes in the composition of the intracellular compartment and its pH, leading to protein denaturation and enzymatic damage. This leads to permanent damage of the cell membrane. If the freezing rate reaches -20°C/min, crystallization is produced both in the extracellular and intracellular space. During defrosting, crystals aggregate, resulting in a disrupted cell membrane without the aforementioned pressure gradient [15-18]. Additionally, microcirculatory impairment occurs, and the damage appears to be delayed (hours or days after freezing). Intracellular crystallization produces endothelial damage, causing platelet aggregation, vascular stasis and intravascular thrombus formation and resulting in coagulative necrosis and tissue ischemia [15, 16, 19, 20]. During the thawing process, reperfusion injury occurs, releasing toxic-free radicals that damage cell lipids constituting the cell membrane [15]. This appears to be the most significant mechanism by which cryotherapy induces cell death. Another proposed pathophysiological mechanism is immunological in nature [15]. Matin demonstrated in vivo an increase in the inflammatory response at the expense of neutrophils, macrophages, T cells and interferon in partially exposed cells. This intense inflammatory response is proposed as an antitumor effect [21].

Subjecting cells to multiple freeze-thaw cycles exacerbates necrotic tissue damage [22], and conducting passive or slow thawing appears to be more effective than rapid and active thawing [23,24]. Exposing renal tumor cells to temperatures of -10°C for 60 min only causes the death of 5% of cells; however, if the temperature is -20°C, death occurs in 85% of the cells [25]. Coyller et al. have studied the optimal freezing time that produces the least associated morbidity, encrypting it in 10 min [26]. Thus, for complete cell destruction, it is recommended to subject cells to two freeze/thaw cycles. It is recommended that fast freezing is carried out with a temperature below 20°C, and relatively slow thawing with helium is performed [27].

b. Cryotherapy Devices

Currently, there are four cryotherapy equipment suppliers: Endocare (Irvine, CA, USA), Galil Medical (Yokneam, Isreal), Oncura (Arlington Heights, IL, USA), and Cryomedical Sciences (Rockville, MD, USA). The first three use argon gas during freezing, and the last one uses nitrogen and is not suitable for use in renal masses but rather is limited to the liver and prostate [24,28]. Additionally, the number, size and arrangement of cryoprobes depend on the tumor size and location.

c. Cryotherapy in Renal Cell Cancer Treatment

Ablative therapy with cryotherapy began its path in urology focusing on the prostate gland. The first two generations of cryotherapy machines achieved freezing using liquid nitrogen. Uchida et al. made the first publication referring to the use of cryotherapy in the treatment of renal masses in 1995 using liquid nitrogen [29]. Since 2000, third-generation cryotherapy machines have been developed based on the release of argon and helium gases through fine-puncture needles whose diameter and length are individually adjusted to ensure complete ablation of tumor tissue.

Renal cryotherapy can be performed using a percutaneous approach guided by images or laparoscopy (transperitoneal or retroperitoneal). Traditionally, percutaneous cryotherapy has been carried out mainly by radiologists. It is an effective and less invasive procedure than laparoscopic assisted cryotherapy and allows rapid recovery with short hospitalization. By contrast, direct visualization of the renal mass that laparoscopy provides has reduced iatrogenic injuries produced during the puncture of the cryoprobes and use of hemostatic material in the case of bleeding, greatly reducing complications associated with cryoablation [29].

- Percutaneous vs laparoscopic approach

As previously mentioned, the shortage of prospective randomized studies leads us to cautiously collect data obtained from published case series. The results are contradictory both in terms of local or distant recurrence and the complication rate. Some authors have indicated that, despite the lower morbidity of the percutaneous approach, recurrence rates are greater than in laparoscopy [30-32]. However, another study concluded that there were no differences in the overall and cancer-specific survival or tumor recurrence rate. Numerous publications have indicated no difference in complication rates or oncologic results.

One of the main problems in assessing the effectiveness of ablative therapies is the lack of uniform criteria for local recurrence. Most authors consider recurrence or persistence as the presence of contrast enhancement on computed tomography (CT) or magnetic resonance imaging (MRI), in which case recurrence will be confirmed by biopsy.

In most published series, posterior tumors are treated percutaneously, while medial and anterior tumors are more frequent in the series of laparoscopic cryoablation. In Tables 1 and 2, the main percutaneous and laparoscopic cryotherapy series and their characteristics are presented.

Table 1. Percutaneous criotherapy series

Authors	Number patients/ tumors	Mean tumor size (mm)	Image guidance	Mean FU* (months)	Image FU*	Outcome (CSS) (%)	Complication	Reablation rate
Shingleton 2001 [34]	20 /22	30	MRI	9.1	MRI-CT	100%	Abscess (5%) Residual disease (5%)	5%
Silverman 2005 [35]	23/27	26	MRI	14	MRI	100%	Transfusion (4.3%) Perinephric abscess (3.7%)	11.1% 1 salvage nephrectomy
Bassignani 2004 [36]	4 /4	38	US	7.5	MRI-CT	100%	0%	0
Gupta 2006 [37]	20 /27	25	CT	5.9	CT	100%	Transfusion 5%	0
Littrup 2007 [38]	48 / 49	53	CT	19.2	CT	88.9%	Bleeding (3%), Minor complications (11%)	8.3%

Table 1. (Continued)

Authors	Number patients/ tumors	Mean tumor size (mm)	Image guidance	Mean FU* (months)	Image FU*	Outcome (CSS) (%)	Complication	Reablation rate
Hinshaw 2008 [39]	30 /30	21	MRI-CT	14.5	MRI-CT	100%	13.3	10%
Atwell 2008 [40]	110 /115	33	MRI-CT	13.3	MRI-CT	100%	6%	3%
Derweesh 2008 [41]	26	29	CT	25		100%	26.9%	11.5%
Finley 2008 [42]	18 / 19	27	CT	11.4	MRI-CT	100%	22.2%	5.3%
Mues 2010 [43]	90/ 99		CT-MRI		MRI-CT	100%	2%	9.1% 1 salvage nephrectomy

* FU = Follow-up; CT: Computerized scanner; MRI: magnetic resonance imaging.

Table 2. Laparoscopic criotherapy series

Authors	Number patients/ number lesions	Mean tumor size (mm)	Mean FU (months)	Outcome Success treatment (%)	Image FU	Complication	Recurrence
Lee 2003 [44]	20 /20	37	36	97	MRI-CT	Pancreatic injury 5%	0
Nadler 2003 [45]	15 /15	21.5	15.1	80	MRI-CT	13.33%	2 salvage nephrectomy
Cestari 2004 [46]	37 / 37	25.7	6	100	MRI	11%	1 salvage nephrectomy
Moon 2004 [47]	16 / 16	26	9.6	100	MRI-CT	-	0
Bachmann 2005 [48]	7	26	13.6	100	MRI-CT	28%	0
Gill 2005 [49]	56	23	36	94%	MRI-CT	8%	2 salvage nephrectomy
Desai 2005 [50]	78	21	24.6	97%	MRI-CT	2.2%	3%
Schwartz 2006 [51]	85 / 85	26	10	97.3%	MRI-CT	Bleeding (2.3%)	2 nephrectomy
Lawatsch 2006 [52]	59 /65	25	26.8	95	MRI-CT	Bleeding 3% Pneumothorax 3%	2 salvage nephrectomy
Bandi 2007 [53]	58/58	26	19	98.7%	MRI-CT	Bleeding (3.8%) Bowel injury 1.3%	6.8%
Weld 2007 [54]	31 /36	21	45.7	98.7%	MRI-CT	10%	2.77% (conservative management)
Hinshaw 2008 [39]	46/60	21	14.6	100	MRI-CT	7%	6.7%
Derweesh 2008 [41]	34		25	97.1%	MRI-CT	14.7%	2.9%

Authors	Number patients/ number lesions	Mean tumor size (mm)	Mean FU (months)	Outcome Success treatment (%)	Image FU	Complication	Recurrence
Lehman 2008 [55]	44 / 51	18	11	98%	MRI-CT	9.8% 2 patients died	4.8%
Finley 2008 [42]	37/43	30	13.4	100%	MRI-CT	40%	4.2%
DeCastro 2010 [56]	7 / 15	20	23.3	100	CT	Bleeding (14.3%) Ureteric injury (14.3)	0%
Mues 2010 [43]	81 /97			100	MRI-CT	3.7%	3.1%

* FU = Follow-up; CT: Computerized scanner; MRI: magnetic resonance imaging.

- Cryotherapy vs partial nephrectomy

Several authors have compared oncological results and complications of partial nephrectomy and cryotherapy in T1N0M0 renal tumors. However, there are several inherent limitations in these comparisons. First, the selection of patients is neither homogeneous nor random; younger and healthier patients are mostly the candidates for partial nephrectomy, while older patients with more comorbidities make up most of the cryotherapy group. Second, the follow-up to which patients are subjected is not homogeneous between both techniques in most studies, a finding that may affect the results obtained. Third, most published studies are retrospective reviews of the experience in high-level centers without strong scientific evidence derived from them.

Desai et al. compared laparoscopic partial nephrectomy with laparoscopic cryotherapy. They found no differences in the overall rate of complications, length of hospitalization and transfusion rate between the two treatment modalities. The only differences observed were higher rates of bleeding and surgical time in patients undergoing partial nephrectomy [50]. O'Malley et al. also showed no significant differences between both groups in the rate of complications or recurrence, but the follow-up period was short and limited to 12 months [57]. Linn et al. compared both laparoscopically assisted techniques; although there was a higher rate of bleeding in partial nephrectomy, there were no differences in the overall complication rate, renal function or survival rates [58]. Haber et al. compared laparoscopic partial nephrectomy and laparoscopic cryotherapy. They could not demonstrate statistically significant differences in the overall survival; however, they showed discrepancies in cancer-specific survival, where partial nephrectomy was 100% after 7 years versus 82% in the cryoablation group. Partial nephrectomy also proved to be associated more with recurrence-free and metastasis-free survival [59]. Ko et al. compared laparoscopic cryoablation with open nephrectomy without being able to demonstrate differences between both techniques in overall survival, development of metastasis or complications [60]. Guillotreau et al. indicated the superiority of robotic partial nephrectomy versus laparoscopic cryotherapy in terms of recurrence-free and metastasis-free survival [61]. In contrast, Klatte et al., in a systematic review of more than 10,906 procedures, concluded that there is a greater risk of local progression in patients treated with laparoscopic renal cryotherapy versus laparoscopic partial nephrectomy [62]. Whitson et al. published a comparative study in patients with localized renal cancer (stage T1) who underwent partial nephrectomy and ablative therapies (RFA or cryotherapy) that demonstrated superiority in terms of cancer-specific survival at 5 and 10 years for partial nephrectomy versus ablative therapies (combining RFA and cryotherapy) [63].

Recently, the experience with a large cohort of patients with stage T1N0M0 kidney cancer at the Mayo Clinic was published comparing the rates of complications, survival and local recurrence of partial nephrectomy and percutaneous ablative therapies (RFA and cryotherapy). In this case, they evaluated results from RFA and cryotherapy separately. In the group of T1a tumors, 1,057 partial nephrectomies and 187 percutaneous cryoablations were included. There were no differences in local recurrence (p=0.49), but metastasis-free survival was higher in the group that underwent partial nephrectomy (p=0.005) and cryotherapy (p=0.021) compared with percutaneous RFA. In a second group of T1bN0M0 tumors, there were no differences in local recurrences or metastasis-free survival when comparing partial nephrectomy and laparoscopic cryoablation [64].

- Cryotherapy vs radiofrequency

A meta-analysis conducted by Kunkle et al. [65] showed a lower rate of local recurrence in favor of cryoablation (4.6% vs 11.7%). When both techniques were compared with partial nephrectomy, ablative therapies showed an increased risk of local progression (1.2% for cryoablation and 2.3% for RFA), and there were no differences in metastasis-free survival.

Hegarty et al. compared laparoscopic cryoablation vs percutaneous RFA and showed a higher rate of recurrence or persistence of disease in RFA (11.1% vs 1.8%). In both ablative techniques, cancer-specific survival was greater than 98% [66].

Weight et al. also compared their series of laparoscopic assisted renal cryotherapy and percutaneous renal RFA. The success rate of laparoscopic cryotherapy was higher than that for RFA (93.8% vs 64.8%) [67].

Thompson et al. analyzed the Mayo Clinic series, a total of 1,424 patients with cT1aN0M0 renal masses (1,057 undergoing partial nephrectomy, 180 undergoing RFA and 187 undergoing cryoablation) [64]. Local recurrence-free survival was similar among the three groups of treatment (p=0.49), while metastasis-free survival was significant better for partial nephrectomy (p=0.005) and cryoablation (p=0.021) compared with RFA. When analyzing cT1bN0M0 tumors (379 patients: 326 patients underwent partial nephrectomy and 53 patients were treated with cryoablation), local recurrence-free survival (p=0.81) and metastasis-free survival (p=0.45) were similar between partial nephrectomy and cryoablation. In both groups, there was selection bias of patients because partial nephrectomy patients were significantly younger with lower Charlson scores and better overall survival rates (p<0.001).

Renal cryotherapy in any of its forms is a viable and safe option for the treatment of stage cT1 renal tumors. Despite the aforementioned limitations of the studies published to date, cryotherapy has not robustly demonstrated superiority over the gold standard treatment, partial nephrectomy. Thus, cryotherapy is an alternative to surgical treatment in highly select patients, always balancing the morbidity, oncological outcomes and preferences of each patient.

Radiofrequency Ablation (RFA) on Small Renal Masses

a. Technical Fundamentals of RFA

RFA is a minimally invasive ablative technique of cell destruction that consists of introducing an electrode or antenna within the tumor to raise the temperature of tumor cells until they are destroyed (apoptosis) without affecting healthy surrounding kidney tissue; the treatment area should be controlled by the medical operator. The principles of ablation have been described by Leveille and Hoey [68]. Ablation, unlike random diathermic destruction, depends on the thermodynamic equilibrium of temperatures controlled by the speed of the energy supply and the heat dissipation capacity of surrounding tissues. If heat entry exceeds the heat dissipation capacity of the tissues, they carbonize, producing a suboptimal ablation zone.

In 1997, Zlotta et al. [69] published the first RFA experiences both in vivo and ex vivo in the treatment of renal masses. RFA consists of applying an alternating electric current of high monopolar or bipolar frequency (375-500 kHz) that causes coagulation necrosis of the tumor tissue by frictional heating due to ionic oscillation. The RFA antenna (needle-electrode) transforms RFA waves into heat, which denatures cellular proteins and DNA, interrupts RNA chains, and produces vascular congestion and disintegration of cell membranes. To generate irreversible changes incompatible with life, it is necessary to reach temperatures between 50°C and 120°C for 4-6 min. Effective ablation and cell damage are a binomial time and temperature-dependent process. Temperatures of 55°C for 15 seconds produce reliable destruction [70]; at temperatures between 60°C and 100°C, irreversible damage is immediate. Above 100°C, vaporization and carbonization of tissues are produced that increases intercellular impedance, preventing the transmission of energy and limiting radio tissue destruction [71]. Exophytic tumors are the best candidates for RFA because they have lower heat dispersion; perirenal fat acts as an oven, isolating the tumor. Intra-renal blood circulation dissipates energy through renal vessels [72] and is less effective in intrarenal locations; these are what are known as "skip areas", where post ablation histological studies have demonstrated viable tumor areas in 23% of cases [73]. The volume of necrotic tissue depends on several factors: characteristics of the treated tissue, treatment time, intensity of applied energy, needle-electrode type (gauge-configuration) used for treatment, number of needles, type of energy measurement at the tip of the needle (for temperature or impedance) and type of power station platform used.

b. Technique

The ablative technique starts with a renal mass biopsy to establish malignancy of the lesion and tumor grade. Biopsies are taken by fine needle aspiration (FNA) or, more commonly, by extracting a specimen by automatic needle puncture. It is more common to take a biopsy of the lesion in laparoscopic cryotherapy procedures than in percutaneous RFA (82.3% vs 62.2%; $p<0.0001$) [74]. Kidney biopsies typically have a high incidence of false negatives [75]. There are currently key clinical findings that require the completion of a previous renal biopsy before subjecting a patient to an ablative technique to avoid over-treatment. Approximately 15-20% of renal masses in clinical stage T1 diagnosed by imaging tests are benign [76], not requiring curative invasive treatment, where active monitoring is more logical. Only 17% of lesions are defined correctly as benign using imaging tests.

Additionally, 26% of renal tumors are more aggressive (grade 3) [77], needing higher intensity treatment and follow-up.

- Radiofrequency approaches

Similar to cryotherapy, RFA can be performed percutaneously (by radiologists and urologists trained in interventional techniques) or laparoscopically (exclusively by urologists). The latter can be carried out transperitoneally or retroperitoneally and is preferable in renal tumors on the anterior side, medial location or close to adjacent organs (colon, liver or spleen) because it allows direct visualization of the ablative process. In the percutaneous approach, puncture control and monitoring of the ablation are performed mainly by ultrasound and less frequently by computed axial topography (CT), magnetic resonance (MRI) or contrast enhanced ultrasound (CEUS). There are no clinical trials comparing the different techniques. The technique chosen depends on the availability of equipment and preferences and skills of the intervening radiologist [78]. Ultrasound allows guiding the needle to the center of the lesion but does not control the volume of ablation. The main drawbacks of ultrasound are obesity, interference from intestinal gas and bubbles produced during ablation that distort the quality of the ultrasound image [79]. The results are comparable to CT [80]. MRI is one of the techniques that best guides the ablation electrode into the lesion. It allows real-time monitoring of the tumor ablation and repositioning of the electrode [81]. Use of contrast ultrasound allows real-time improvement of the results obtained with conventional ultrasound using both percutaneous and laparoscopic techniques [82, 83]. Percutaneous techniques in selected patients may be performed under sedoanalgesia [84], as a short-stay regimen or in an outpatient setting. The ambulatory character of the process makes percutaneous techniques more cost-effective using the Markov model adjusted for quality-adjusted life years (QALYs) compared with surgical techniques [85].

In some patients, complementary techniques are required such as injecting water or saline to displace the pancreas, colon or spleen and prevent injuries to these neighboring organs [86]. Hydrodissection with electrolyte solution and 5% dextrose [87] helps to protect neighboring organs by creating an insulating barrier that prevents the perforation of hollow intestinal structures. CO_2 pneumodissection [88] was also reported to be successful. Other maneuvers involve twisting the ablation needle to avoid adjacent organs or introducing an angioplasty balloon to separate the structures adjacent to the tumor [89].

- Energy sources

Currently, we have three RFA generators (see Table 3). Power control at the tip, and thus the ability to destroy tissues, can be performed by measuring the tissue temperature at the tip of the electrode or by measuring tissue impedance.

Experimental studies in animal kidneys have shown that kidney lesions produced by temperature-based systems produce more irreversible damage than those based on impedance, where incomplete necrosis and cellular thermal lesions are observed that are capable of recovery [90].

Table 3. Radiofrequency devices

GENERATOR	ELECTRODE	NEEDLES	POWER CONTROL	POTENTIAL	LESION TYPE
TYCO-COVIDIEN	Cool-tipTM Internal water cooling	Two single 17-gauge needles Five triple electrodes	impedance	200 W	Ovoid 2.3-6.7 cm
ANGIODYNAMICS 1500X RF Generator (formerly RITA Medical systems)	Star Burst XL RFA device Needle opening in various antennas as an umbrella Internal water cooling	Nine models Different sizes Flexible models Support MRI	Temperature	250 W	Spherical 2-5 cm
Boston Scientific RF 3000 Radiofrequency Generator	LeVeen Umbrella opening	Two types of needles with 14 different models	Impedance	200 W	Spherical 2-5 cm

c. Functional and Oncological Results of RFA

The first critical issue is the lack of consensus on the timetable of surveillance. Renal function is controlled by clinical history, physical examination of the patient and determination of the creatinine and estimated glomerular filtration rate. CT during the first month post-RFA should show a minor increase of 10 [91] or 20 [72] Hounsfield units after contrast administration to indicate complete ablation or the absence of lesion growth and the absence of viable tissue. However, the latter observation is questionable because the presence of cancerous viable tissue that does not show enhancement in CT has been shown in anatomo-pathological studies [67]. According to the recommendations of the Working Group of Tumor Ablation, image-guided persistence of viable tumor tissue is considered recurrence [92]. Sterrett has documented post-ablation recurrences up to 31 months after RFA [72]. The incidence of tumor recurrence in the surgical bed is 2.9% [93]. Recurrence in the contralateral kidney is 1.2% and is related to positive margins and a high tumor grade [94]. Post-ablation recurrences can be treated effectively with new repeated cycles of RFA or salvage surgery [95]. The most recommended timing of clinical controls with CT should be at 6, 12, and 24 months post-ablation and annually thereafter [2,4].

Follow-up with post-ablation tissue biopsy is controversial with respect to cell viability criteria and cell staining techniques, with results obtained not recommending this technique with follow-up discretion in tumor recurrence. Park et al. [96] conducted a histological sampling with fine needle aspiration in 37 patients 6 months after percutaneous RFA and compared these results with biopsy after laparoscopic cryoablation in 97 patients. At 6 months, success in the RFA cohort (absence of malignant or atypical cells) was 64.8% and 93.8% in cryoablation.

The weakness of this technique is that there are no prospective randomized clinical trials comparing it with other ablative techniques or with the gold standard of surgery (radical or partial nephrectomy) with follow-up periods of at least 10 years. Furthermore, the technique is not standardized; there are different radiofrequency generators, different types of needles and different application protocols with respect to the exposure time and energy.

- Functional outcomes

Preservation of renal function is maximal in these types of therapies. Lucas et al. [97] published a series of 242 patients with T1a tumors undergoing RFA (86 patients), partial nephrectomy (85 patients) and radical nephrectomy (71 patients). Stage 3 chronic kidney failure at the 3-year follow-up was present in 4.8% of the RFA group, 29.3% of the partial nephrectomy group and 60.1% of the radical nephrectomy group ($p<0.001$). Turna et al. [98] presented a series of renal preservation in renal tumors in patients with a single kidney. Of the 101 single-kidney patients, 36 underwent laparoscopic partial nephrectomy, 36 cryoablation, and 29 RFA. The mean estimated glomerular filtration decreased 26% after the treatment for laparoscopic partial nephrectomy, 6% after the treatment for cryoablation and 13% after the treatment for RFA with statistical significance ($p=0.0016$). Altunrende et al. [99] retrospectively evaluated the functional results of a series of renal tumor ablations in single-kidney patients with cryotherapy and RFA guided by CT. Of the 65 patients included, 29 (44.5%) underwent cryotherapy and 36 (55.4%) underwent RFA. The median follow-up was 15.1 months. No significant differences were found in the glomerular filtration rate between the pre- and post-operative results. Zhang et al. [100] analyzed 12 patients with bilateral synchronous renal carcinomas treated with RFA. Three patients received unilateral RFA and contralateral radical nephrectomy, and nine underwent bilateral RFA. The mean follow-up was 33 months. The mean glomerular filtration rate after RFA did not decrease compared with the preoperative rates (93.7 ± 13.0 mL/min/1.73 m^2 vs 96.9 ± 13.3 mL/min/1.73 m^2; $p>0.05$). Additionally, Arnoux et al. [101] compared a series of 50 patients who underwent RFA (14 patients) or laparoscopic partial nephrectomy (36 patients) for renal carcinomas and observed no differences in the changes in renal function in both groups.

- Oncological outcomes

Matsumoto et al. [102] presented 109 tumors in 91 patients treated with percutaneous RFA guided by CT (63 patients) versus laparoscopy (46 patients) with a mean tumor volume of 2.4 cm. In 107 tumors, complete ablation was obtained in a single session. After 12 months of follow-up, only one local recurrence was observed (1.7%). Levinson et al. [103] showed an initial success rate of 97%, a 90.3% recurrence-free survival rate and 100% metastasis-free survival in 34 patients who underwent primary ablation with RFA, with a mean follow-up of 2.4 months. Zagoria et al. [104] analyzed a series of 125 renal tumors with percutaneous RFA. They concluded that when the tumor was greater than 3.7 cm, treatment was incomplete in 30% of the cases. Breen et al. [105] analyzed a cohort of 105 renal tumors; 79% were fully treated in a single session, and 12 of the remaining tumors required a second ablation. Technical success was achieved in 90.5% of patients, a result that was maintained for a mean follow-up of 16.7 months (range, 1-76 months). In the multivariate analysis, tumor size <3 cm was the only predictor of the outcomes of the total ablation procedure. Gervais et al. [106] published a series of 100 tumors in 85 patients and compared the success rates by size and location; they obtained 100% success in all exophytic tumors, 78% in central locations and 61% in mixed tumors (with peripheral and central component). Ablation was completed in 100% of tumors less than 3 cm, 53% of tumors between 3 and 5 cm and 28% of tumors over 5 cm. Only one recurrence was detected after treatment, which was treated with another session of RFA (See Table 4).

Table 4. Radiofrequency series

Author	Patients / Tumors	Follow-up (months)	Mean tumor size (mm)	Approach	Success rate (%)	CSS (%)	Local Recur-rence (%)	Compli-cations (%)
Su 2003 [107]	35-29	9	2,2	Perc* (CT)	94%	85%	15%	
Mayo 2003 [108]	32-32	9 (1-36)	2,6	Perc (CT-US)	97%			6,25 %
Farrel 2003 [91]	35-20	9 (1-23)	1,7	Perc (CT-US)	100%	100%	0	0
Gervais 2005 [106]	100-85	27 (3-72)	3,2	Perc (CT-US)	100 %(3 cm) 92% (3-5 cm) 25% (5 cm)	96%	0	10%
Zagoria 2007 [104]	125-104	13,8	2,6	Perc (CT)	100% (3,6 cm) 70%(3,7 cm)	88%	12%	8%
Breen 2007 [105]	105-97	16 (1-76)	3,2	Perc (CT-US)	79%	92,7%	2%	4,2 %
Levinso 2008 [109]	18--18	57,4 (41-80)	2,1	Perc	97%	79,9%	20,1%	
Mylona 2009 [110]	18-18	31,2 (12-72)	3,5	Perc	70%	89,9%	10,1%	
Ferakis 2010 [111]	31-39	61,2 (36-84)	3,1	Perc	90%	89%	11%	
Tracy 2010 [84]	208-243	27 (1,5-90)	2,4	Perc (CT) Lap**	97%	90%	10%	
Olweny 2012 [112]	37-37	78 (69-85)	2,1	Perc Lap	94,6%	97,2%	10,8%	
Kim 2012 [113]	48-47	49,6 (12-81)	2,3	Perc (CT-US) Lap	86,1% (perc) 100% (lap)	91,7%	8,3%	35.8%
Zhao 2012 [114]	73	22 (12-42)	3,4	Perc (CEUS)	90,4%	100%	0	
Psutka (2013) [115]	185	77 (6-160)	3	Perc (CEUS-CT)	87%	88,6%	6,5%	

Perc= percutaneous; Lap= laparoscopy; US: ultrasonography; CT: Computerized scanner.

d. RFA vs Cryotherapy vs Nephrectomy

Hegarty et al. [116] compared a laparoscopic cryotherapy ablation group and another treated with percutaneous RFA. In the RFA group, there was greater persistence and radiological recurrence of the tumor; recurrences were treated with a second session.

The index of major complications is higher with laparoscopic cryotherapy and does not allow retreating patients in the event of relapse with another new session of cryotherapy. Stern el al. [117] compared a series of patients treated with partial nephrectomy (open or laparoscopic). At 3 years of follow-up, there weren't significant differences in oncological outcomes. Hui et al. [118] published a meta-analysis that compared 46 series of renal tumor ablations (28 percutaneous and 18 laparoscopic): 1,055 patients and 1,180 tumors were included. Most of the percutaneous series used RFA (28 series), and 7 used cryotherapy. Regarding the laparoscopic techniques, 15 series used cryotherapy, and 3 used RFA. However, they needed additional re-treatments. The better results in the laparoscopic series can be explained by the following: smaller tumors, a larger number of benign tumors, and laparoscopic patients who underwent general anesthesia. Thus, control during treatment was better. Kunkle et al. [74] performed a meta-analysis that compared two ablation techniques (cryotherapy vs RFA), including 47 series that recruited 1,375 kidney lesions. Local progression was greater with RFA (12.9% vs 5.2%), with a higher number of re-treatments (8.5% vs 1.3%) and statistical significance ($p<0.001$). The meta-analysis included very small, low-quality and non-randomized series; the results could not be extrapolated.

Dib et al. [119] performed another meta-analysis on RFA and cryotherapy. Thirty-one series (20 cryotherapy and 11 RFA) were included. The clinical efficacy of cryotherapy was 89% in 457 cases. The clinical efficacy of the RFA series was 90% in 426 cases. The series showed no significant differences and were very homogeneous. There were no significant differences between the complications of RFA and the cryotherapy series.

Miller et al. [120] described a series of 105 tumors in which RFA (44 patients) or cryotherapy (61 patients) was performed. The success rate was 98.4% for cryotherapy and 97.7% for RFA. The rates of progression-free survival estimated at 1, 3 and 5 years were 99%, 97% and 97%, respectively (similar in both groups). The complication rate was higher in cryotherapy (8.6%) versus RFA (0%).

Reiterating the work of Thompson [64], it was previously discussed in the cryotherapy paragraph that percutaneous cryotherapy showed superiority versus percutaneous RFA in terms of metastasis-free survival, but no differences in the rate of local recurrence were shown between both treatment modalities.

e. Percutaneous vs Laparoscopic Radiofrequency Approach

Tracy et al. [84] analyzed 243 small renal masses treated with RFA for 7.5 years, with a median follow-up of 27 months: 71% underwent percutaneous RFA, 28% underwent laparoscopically assisted RFA, and 1% underwent open RFA. They reported the metastasis-free and cancer specific survival rates at 5 years to be 95% and 99%, respectively.

Ji et al. [121] analyzed their experience in laparoscopic RFA with 106 patients with renal tumors between 0.9 and 5.5 cm. A biopsy was taken of the pre-ablation renal mass in all patients with confirmed renal carcinoma (90 patients, 84.9%). Local tumor control was confirmed in 98.1% of the patients. Disease-free survival of the patients diagnosed with cancer was 97.8%. Overall and cancer-specific survival of the entire series was 100%.

Young et al. [122] analyzed their series of 316 renal tumors treated by CT-guided RFA versus laparoscopic RFA (122 laparoscopy and 194 percutaneous). There were no significant differences in demographic variables, complications and post-ablation renal function. Cancer-specific survival at 3 years (21-month median follow-up) was 100% for laparoscopy-assisted RFA and 94% for percutaneous RFA (See Table 4).

A very attractive idea is combining laparoscopic RFA with post-ablation partial nephrectomy. This technique allows, with zero ischemia, the performance of renal tumor enucleation using an avascular plane, avoiding positive margins. Zhao et al. [123] performed this technique in 42 patients with T1 renal tumors. The mean rate of bleeding was 92.5 mL, and there were complications in 16.6% of cases (postoperative fever in four cases and prolonged urinary leakage in three cases). No patients had positive surgical margins, and no changes were recorded in the glomerular filtration rate before and after treatment. The cancer-specific survival, overall survival and absence of cancer progression at 3 years were 100%, 97.3% and 96.4%, respectively. In addition, RFA did not affect the anatomo-pathological study.

f. Complications

They are rare, with the following being the most frequently reported:

- Flu-like syndrome with a 37.5°C to 38.5°C fever, self-limited to 10 days, that appears in 33% of patients with pain, nausea, vomiting, malaise, and myalgia and that yields with paracetamol [124]
- Post ablation peri-renal abscess [124]
- Hematuria <24 h that is not anemic
- Postoperative intestinal ileus (laparoscopic surgery)
- Urinary leakage (urinoma), ureteral lesions (stenosis), hydronephrosis [106]
- Vascular lesions
- Post-ablation hemorrhage-hematoma requiring transfusion (2.3%) [106]
- Pain of the genitofemoral lumbar plexus (neuropraxia) of the thigh psoas [126] resulting in sensitivity and chronic pain in the ipsilateral groin [127] and limitation in flexion of the hip
- Inflammation of the ablation path
- Skin burn
- Reno-colonic fistula [128]
- Reno-duodenal fistula [129]

Other Treatment Modalities

- Microwave

This technique refers to the use of electromagnetic probes to induce cell destruction. These waves have frequencies between 900 and 2450 MHz and can induce high levels of ion oscillation. The latter causes an increase in the temperature proportional to the agitation of water molecules around the tissue, producing friction and heat and inducing cell death by coagulative necrosis [130]. Its advantages are as follows [130, 131]:

1) It can reach higher intratumoral temperatures
2) It allows ablation of larger volume tumors
3) The ablation time is faster

4) There is less pain post-ablation
5) It can be conducted from a percutaneous, laparoscopic or open surgery approach

The percutaneous approach is mostly performed under conscious sedation guided by ultrasound or CT. A 14.5-gauge fine needle (antenna) is used to directly puncture the tumor. An electromagnetic wave generator is connected to the antenna via a coaxial cable, and tumor ablation is achieved [130, 132]. This technology has found its maximum field expansion in the treatment of liver and lung tumors. Experience in the field of renal cancer is scarce and very recent, with only a short-medium term follow-up.

Yu et al. [132] conducted a retrospective review of 46 patients with renal cancer who underwent ultrasound-guided percutaneous ablation with microwaves with a mean follow-up of 20.1 months. The mean diameter of the lesions was 3.3 cm (range: 0.6-7 cm). They used a single antenna if the tumor was <2 cm and two antennas for tumors ≥2 cm. They did not describe any major complications. Follow-up was carried out with CT, MRI or contrast ultrasound. One month after treatment, the success rate was 98%, and metastasis-free survival was 100%. The progression rates at 1, 2 and 3 years were 4.6%, 7.7% and 7.7%, respectively. Cancer-specific survival the first two years after treatment was 100%; at three years, it was 97.8%. The rates of disease-free survival at 1, 2 and 3 years were 95.4%, 92.3% and 92.3%, respectively. Castle et al. [133] published a series of 10 cases of single-kidney patients with a mean follow-up of 18 months; patients underwent ablation with percutaneous or laparoscopic microwaves with 38% local recurrence, 20% intraoperative complications and 40% postoperative complications.

Guan et al. [134] conducted a prospective clinical trial comparing the efficacy of microwave ablation and partial nephrectomy. A total of 102 patients were included (54 partial nephrectomy and 48 open or laparoscopic microwave ablation procedures). They found no differences in the length of hospitalization or surgical time. There was a low rate of complications. The decline in glomerular filtration was similar in both groups, and recurrence-free survival after 3 years of treatment was higher in the partial nephrectomy group (96% vs 91.3%) with no statistical significance.

Moreland et al. [135] evaluated a cohort of 53 patients who underwent ablation of T1a renal tumors with microwaves using a percutaneous approach. Follow-up was with MRI or CT, and the average size was 2.6 cm. The complication rate was 11.3%, all grade 1 or 2 of the Clavien-Dindo classification. After a mean follow-up of 8 months, there was no recurrence in any case or the appearance of metastatic disease.

Finally Lin et al. [136] published their results of percutaneous microwave ablation in 16 single-kidney patients. Complete ablation was achieved in 93.8% after one or two treatment sessions; however, two patients (14.3%) died from metastatic involvement.

The lack of scientific evidence for percutaneous microwave ablation is reflected in the consideration of this therapy as experimental; however, the physical properties of the energy source make it ideal for tumor ablation. Randomized controlled clinical trials are necessary to evaluate the safety and oncological outcomes of this treatment.

- HIFU

HIFU is an experimental ablative therapy that uses ultrasonic energy to produce heat and tissue destruction. During the propagation of ultrasonic waves through biological tissue, they are gradually absorbed and dissipate energy as heat. If the ultrasound beam is precisely focused at the selected depth, the high intensity of energy generated produces sufficient heat to cause coagulative necrosis and cellular apoptosis [137]. In theory, the energy decreases sharply outside the treatment zone so that it has no effect on surrounding tissues. The amount of coagulative necrosis depends on the absorption coefficient of the tissues it crosses, energy intensity at the focal point, time it takes to pass through the tissue and ultrasonic properties of the absorbing structures. At first, tumor ablation is initiated from outside the body without direct contact with the suspected area. These devices use wavelengths from 0.5 to 10 MHz. As a general rule, high frequencies are used when the zone acted on is more accurate, but it requires a small distance between the wave generating probe and ablation zone (such as transrectal HIFU application for the treatment of prostate tumors).

However, for intraabdominal or retroperitoneal structures such as the kidneys, the distance between the skin and organ is considerably greater; thus, wavelengths shorter than 0.5 to 1.5 MHz are required, where the treatment area is less accurate, with the consequent risk of damaging surrounding healthy tissue [137,138]. Follow-up of these patients is performed by CT, MRI, positron emission tomography or ultrasound with microbubble contrast. It seems that the latter enhances the efficiency of the visualization of ablated tissue.

There is not much experience with extracorporeal HIFU. A clinical trial was conducted by Illing et al. [139] with 30 patients who underwent HIFU for liver or kidney tumors. The procedure was performed under general anesthesia. Only in 67% of renal tumors was complete ablation achieved. There were no differences in complications with other ablative techniques such as RFA or cryotherapy. Most of the complications were skin-related (swelling and irritation). In no case was grade 2 skin toxicity exceeded. Körhman et al. [140] published three cases of patients with renal tumors with a 6-month follow-up by MRI. The procedure was also performed under general anesthesia. They managed tumor ablation in two of the three patients. Another study on extracorporeal HIFU application prior to surgical resection [141] conducted at the University of Vienna in which 16 renal tumors were included showed coagulative necrosis confirmed histopathologically in only nine cases, and further tissue damage caused only 15-35% of the tissue to be destroyed. Consistent with these results, Hacker et al. [142] published a cohort of 19 patients with renal cancer who underwent HIFU ablation prior to surgical resection of the tissue. In 15 of the 19 specimens, thermal damage caused by the treatment was observed. The energy used was insufficient to produce complete necrosis in the lesion to be treated.

The laparoscopic approach arises to overcome the aforementioned problems of distance from the transducer to the renal tumor area. The transducer is placed directly over the area to be treated. It is also possible to simultaneously monitor through ultrasound using a laparoscopic ultrasound transducer [137]. This approach allows ablative therapy without the need for clamping renal vessels or puncturing the renal tumor. Klinger et al. [141] published preliminary results of laparoscopic HIFU ablation in 10 patients with renal tumors. The mean tumor size was 2.2 cm. Partial nephrectomy was subsequently performed on seven patients for tumor excision. The mean treatment duration was 19 minutes. Histopathological analyses showed complete necrosis in four cases (57%). In those not receiving surgical treatment after biopsy at 6 months, there was coagulative necrosis. Subsequently, in a series update, this author noted that after treating 31 patients, predictors of successful laparoscopically assisted HIFU ablation are tumors <3 cm, peripheral tumors, and tumors located in the middle- and lower-third of the kidney. The author noted the lower success rate and oncological control with respect to partial nephrectomy [137].

- Irreversible electroporation (IRE)

The Irreversible electroporation ablation (IRE) uses non-thermal short electrical pulses to destroy a volume of tumor target tissue without damaging and respecting adjacent structures such as blood vessels or ureters in clinical situations where is contraindicated surgical resection or thermal ablation by its collateral effects on blood vessels or urinary tract when they are near the tumor. The Irreversible electroporation ablation offers a conservative specific approach of nephrons in the treatment of renal tumors [143,144]. The distribution of electrical impulses through the tissues can be planned with mathematical models which have been studied in animals and extrapolated to human kidney tissue. Numerical simulations are used to treatment planning in clinical applications of irreversible electroporation, to determine the size and shape of the ablation [145,146]. To assess the reliability of the simulations results of the simulation have been compared with the empirical findings of irreversible renal electroporation using computed tomography (CT) and histology in an animal model post-ablation. Both numerical simulations of the IRE and the results of CT renal post-IRE may overestimate the size of the ablation area compared to histology since the effects of ablation are incomplete in the periphery of the treated tissue presenting a transition perimeter in the viability of the tissue [147]. We still await the test of time and the translation from the laboratory to clinical practice with well-designed clinical trials that reveal the scope of this new technique in focal cancer therapy.

References

[1] Siegel R., Ma J., Zou Z., et al. Cancer statistics, 2014. CA *Cancer J. Clin.* 2014;64(1):9-29.

[2] Ljungberg B., Bensalah K., Bex A., et al. *EAU Guidelines on Renal Cell Carcinoma.* Update April 2014. http://www.uroweb.org/gls/pdf/10% 20Renal%20Cell% 20Carcinoma_LR.pdf

[3] Volpe A., Panzarella T. Rendon R.A., et al. The natural history of incidentally detected small renal masses. *Cancer.* 2004; 100(4):738-45.

[4] Lane BR., Campbell SC. Management of small renal masses. *AUA Update Series* 2009.

[5] Campbell SC., Novick AC., Belldegrun A., et al. Guideline for management of the clinical T1 renal mass. J Urol 2009;182:1271-9.

[6] Hollingsworth JM., Miller DC., Daignault S, et al. Rising incidence of sall renal masses: a need to reassess treatment effect. *J. Natl. Cancer Inst.* 2006;98:1331-24.

[7] Lee CT, Katz J, Shi W et al. Surgical management of renal tumors 4 cm. or less in a contemporary cohort. *J. Urol.* 2000; 163: 730-6.

[8] Huang WC, Elkin EB, Levey AS et al. Partial nephrectomy versus radical nephrectomy in patients with small renal tumors is there a difference in mortality and cardiovascular outcomes? *J. Urol.* 2009; 181: 55-61.

[9] Thompson RH, Siddiqui S, Lohse CM et al. Partial versus radical nephrectomy for 4 to 7 cm renal cortical tumors. *J. Urol.* 2009; 182: 2601-6.
[10] Weight CJ, Larson BT, Fergany AF et al. Nephrectomy induced chronic renal insufficiency is associated with increased risk of cardiovascular death and death from any cause in patients with localized ct1b renal masses. *J. Urol.* 2010; 183: 1317-23.
[11] Huang WC, Levey AS, Serio AM et al. Chronic kidney disease after nephrectomy in patients with renal cortical tumours: a retrospective cohort study. *Lancet Oncol.* 2006; 7: 735-40.
[12] Go AS., Chertow GM., Fan D., et al. Chronic kidney disease and the risk of death, cardiovascular events and hospitalisations. *N. Engl. J. Med.* 2004;351: 1296-305.
[13] Capitanio U., Terrone C., Antonelli A., et al. Nephron-sparing techniques independently decrease the risk of cardiovascular events relative to radical nephrectomy in patients with a T1a-T1b renal mass and normal preoperative renal function. *Eur. Urol.* 2014-in press.
[14] Van Poppel H., Da Pozzo L. Albrecht , et al. A prospective randomized EORTC intergroup phase 3 study comparing the complications of elective nephron-sparing surgery and radical nephrectomy for low-stahe renal cell carcinoma. *Eur. Urol.* 2007;51:1606-15.
[15] Mohammed A. , Miller S., Douglas-Moore J., et al. Cryotherapy and its applications in the management of urologic malignancies: A review of its use in prostate and renal cancer. *Urol. Oncol.* 2014;32(1): 39.
[16] Hoffmann NE, Bischof JC. The cryobiology of cryosurgical injury. *Urology* 2002;60:40–9.
[17] Bischof JC, Smith D, Pazhayannur PV, Manivel C, Hulbert J, Roberts K.P. Cryosurgery of dunning AT-1 rat prostate tumor: Thermal, biophysical, and viability response at the cellular and tissue level. *Cryobiology.* 1997; 34:42-69.
[18] Acker JP, Larese A, Yang H, Petrenko A, McGann LE. Intracellular ice formation is affected by cell interactions. *Cryobiology.* 1999; 38:363-71.
[19] Daum PS, Bowers WD, Tejada J, Morehouse D, Hamlet MP. Vascular casts demonstrate microcirculatory insufficiency in acute frostbite. *Cryobiology.* 1987; 24:65-73.
[20] Rioja J., Tzortzis V., Mamoulakis C., et al. Cryotherapy for renal tumors: Current status and contemporary developments. Actas Urol Esp 2010; 34(4): 309-317.
[21] Matin SF, Sharma P, Gill IS, et al. Immunological response to renal cryoablation in an in vivo orthotopic renal cell carcinoma murine model. *J. Urol.* 2010;183:333–8.
[22] Auge BK., Santa-Cruz RW., Polascik TJ. Effect of freeze time during renal cryoablation: a swine model. *J. Endourol.* 2006;20(12):1101-5.
[23] Berger A., Crouzet S., Canes D., et al. Minimally invasive nephron-sparing surgery. *Curr. Opin. Urol.* 2008;18: 462–466.
[24] Ramanathan R., Leveillee RJ. Ablative therapies for renal tumors. *Ther. Adv. Urol.* 2010;2:51-68.
[25] Stephenson RA., King DK., Rohr LR. Renal cryoablation in a canine model. *Urology* 1996;47:772-776.
[26] Collyer W., Venkatesh R., Vanlangendonck R., et al. Enhanced renal cryoablation with hilar clamping and intrarenal cooling in a porcine model. *Urology* 2004; 63(6): 1209–1212.

[27] Woolley ML., Schulsinger DA., Durand DB., et al. Effect of freezing parameters (freeze cycle and thaw process) on tissue destruction following renal cryoablation. *J. Endourol.* 2002; 16:519-22.

[28] Matin SF., Ahrar K. Nephron-sparing probe ablative therapy: long-term outcomes. *Curr. Opin. Urol.* 2008;18:150-56.

[29] Uchida M., Imaide Y., Sugimoto K., et al. Percutaneous cryosurgery for renal tumours. *Br. J. Urol.* 1995;75: 132–6.

[30] Bandi G., Hedican S., Moon T., et al. Comparison of postoperative pain, convalescence, and patient satisfaction after laparoscopic and percutaneous ablation of small renal masses. *J. Endourol.* 2008;22:963–7.

[31] Mues AC., Okhunov Z., Haramis G., et al. Comparison of percutaneous and laparoscopic renal cryoablation for small (<3.0cm) renal masses. *J. Endourol.* 2010;24:1097–100.

[32] Volpe A., Cadeddu J., Cestari A. Contemporary Management of Small Renal Masses. *Eur. Urol.* 2011 (60); 501-515.

[33] Kim EH, Tanagho YS, Bhayani SB, et al. Outcomes of laparoscopic and percutaneous cryoablation for renal masses. *J. Urol.* 2013;189(4S):492.

[34] Shingleton WB., Sewell PE Jr. Percutaneous renal tumor cryoablation with magnetic resonance imaging guidance. *J. Urol.* 2001;165(3):773-6.

[35] Silverman SG., Tuncali K., vanSonnenberg E. et al. Renal tumors: MR imaging-guided percutaneous cryotherapy--initial experience in 23 patients. *Radiology.* 2005;236(2):716-24.

[36] Bassignani M., Moore Y., Watson L., et al. Pilot experience with real-time ultrasound guided percutaneous renal mass cryoablation. *J. Urol.* 2004;171(4):1620-3.

[37] Gupta A., Allaf ME., Kavoussi LR., et al. Computerized tomography guided percutaneous renal cryoablation with the patient under conscious sedation: initial clinical experience. *J. Urol.* 2006;175(2):447-52.

[38] Littrup PJ., Ahmed A., Aoun HD., et al. CT-guided percutaneous cryotherapy of renal masses. *J. Vasc. Interv. Radiol.* 2007;18(3):383-92.

[39] Hinshaw JL., Shadid AM., Nakada SY. et al. Comparison of percutaneous and laparoscopic cryoablation for the treatment of solid renal masses. *AJR Am. J. Roentgenol.* 2008;191(4):1159-68.

[40] Atwell TD., Farrell MA., Leibovich BC., et al. Percutaneous renal cryoablation: experience treating 115 tumors. *J. Urol.* 2008;179(6):2136-40.

[41] Derweesh IH., Malcolm JB., Diblasio CJ. et al. Single center comparison of laparoscopic cryoablation and CT-guided percutaneous cryoablation for renal tumors. *J. Endourol.* 2008;22(11):2461-7.

[42] Finley DS., Beck S., Box G., et al. Percutaneous and laparoscopic cryoablation of small renal masses. *J. Urol.* 2008;180(2):492-8.

[43] Mues AC., Landman J. Results of kidney tumor cryoablation: renal function preservation and oncologic efficacy. *World J. Urol.* 2010;28(5):565-70.

[44] Lee DI., McGinnis DE., Feld R., et al. Retroperitoneal laparoscopic cryoablation of small renal tumors: intermediate results. *Urology.* 2003;61(1):83-8.

[45] Nadler RB., Kim SC., Rubenstein JN., et al. Laparoscopic renal cryosurgery: the Northwestern experience. *J. Urol.* 2003;170(4 Pt 1):1121-5.

[46] Cestari A., Guazzoni G., dell'Acqua V., et al. Laparoscopic cryoablation of solid renal masses: intermediate term followup. *J. Urol.* 2004;172(4 Pt 1):1267-70.
[47] Moon TD., Lee FT.Jr, Hedican SP., et al. Laparoscopic cryoablation under sonographic guidance for the treatment of small renal tumors. *J. Endourol.* 2004;18(5):436-40.
[48] Bachmann A., Sulser T., Jayet C., et al. Retroperitoneoscopy-assisted cryoablation of renal tumors using multiple 1.5 mm ultrathin cryoprobes: a preliminary report. *Eur. Urol.* 2005;47(4):474-9.
[49] Gill IS., Remer EM., Hasan WA. et al. Renal cryoablation: outcome at 3 years. *J. Urol.* 2005;173(6):1903-7.
[50] Desai MM., Aron M., Gill IS. Laparoscopic partial nephrectomy versus laparoscopic cryoablation for the small renal tumor. *Urology.* 2005;66(5 Suppl):23-8.
[51] Schwartz BF., Rewcastle JC., Powell T., et al. Cryoablation of small peripheral renal masses: a retrospective analysis. *Urology.* 2006;68(1 Suppl):14-8.
[52] Lawatsch EJ., Langenstroer P., Byrd GF., et al. Intermediate results of laparoscopic cryoablation in 59 patients at the Medical College of Wisconsin. *J. Urol.* 2006;175(4):1225-9.
[53] Bandi G., Wen CC., Hedican SP., et al. Cryoablation of small renal masses: assessment of the outcome at one institution. *BJU Int.* 2007;100(4):798-801.
[54] Weld KJ., Figenshau RS., Venkatesh R., et al. Laparoscopic cryoablation for small renal masses: three-year follow-up. *Urology.* 2007;69(3):448-51.
[55] Lehman DS., Hruby GW., Phillips CK., et al. First Prize (tie): Laparoscopic renal cryoablation: efficacy and complications for larger renal masses. *J. Endourol.* 2008;22(6):1123-7.
[56] DeCastro GJ., Gupta M., Badani K., et al. Synchronous cryoablation of multiple renal lesions: short-term follow-up of patient outcomes. *Urology.* 2010;75(2):303-6.
[57] O'Malley RL., Berger AD., Kanofsky JA., et al. A matched-cohort comparison of laparoscopic cryoablation and laparoscopic partial nephrectomy for treating renal masses. *BJU Int.* 2007; 99(2):395-8.
[58] Lin YC., Turna B., Frota R,. et al. Laparoscopic partial nephrectomy versus laparoscopic cryoablation for multiple ipsilateral renal tumors. *Eur. Urol.* 2008;53:1210–6.
[59] Haber GP., Lee MC., Crouzet S., et al. Tumour in solitary kidney: laparoscopic partial nephrectomy vs laparoscopic cryoablation. *BJU Int.* 2012;109(1):118-24.
[60] Ko YH., Park HS., Moon du G., et al. A matched-cohort comparison of laparoscopic renal cryoablation using ultra-thin cryoprobes with open partial nephrectomy for the treatment of small renal cell carcinoma. *Cancer Res. Treat.* 2008;40(4):184-9.
[61] Guillotreau J., Haber GP., Autorino R., et al. Robotic partial nephrectomy vs. laparoscopic cryoablation for the small renal mass. *Eur. Urol.* 2012;61(5):899-904.
[62] Klatte T., Mauermann J., Heinz-Peer G., et al. Perioperative, oncologic, and functional outcomes of laparoscopic renal cryoablation and open partial nephrectomy: a matched pair analysis. *J. Endourol.* 2011;25(6):991-7.
[63] Whitson JM., Harris CR., Meng MV. Population-based comparative effectiveness of nephron-sparing surgery vs ablation for small renal masses. *BJU Int.* 2012;110(10):1438-43;discussion 1443.

[64] Thompson RH., Atwell T., Schmit G., et al. Comparison of partial nephrectomy and percutaneous ablation for cT1 renal masses. *Eur. Urol.* 2014: IN PRESS.
[65] Kunkle DA., Egleston BL., Uzzo RG. Excise, ablate or observe: the small renal mass dilemma—a meta-analysis and review. *J. Urol.* 2008;179:1227–33.
[66] Hegarty NJ., Gill IS., Desai MM., et al. Kaouk JH. Probe-ablative nephron-sparing surgery: cryoablation versus radiofrequency ablation. *Urology* 2006;68:7–13.
[67] Weight CJ., Kaouk JH., Hegarty NJ., et al. Correlation of radiographic imaging and histopathology following cryoablation and radio frequency ablation for renal tumors. *J. Urol.* 2008;179:1277–81.
[68] Leveillee R.J., Hoey M.F. Radiofrequency interstitial tissue ablation: wet electrode. *J. Endourol.* 2003 Oct;17: 563–577.
[69] Zlotta AR, Wildschutz T, Raviv G, Peny MO, et al. Radiofrequency interstitial tumor ablation (RITA) is a possible new modality for treatment of renal cancer: ex vivo and in vivo experience. *J. Endourol.* 1997 Aug;11(4):251-8
[70] Bhowmick S, Swanlund DJ, Coad JE, et al. Evaluation of thermal therapy in a prostate cancer model using a wet electrode radiofrequency probe. *J. Endourol.* 2001 Aug;15(6):629-40.
[71] Estebanez Zarranz J1, Artozki Morras E, Aguirreazaldegui García L, et al. Radiofrequency ablation of renal cell carcinoma. *Actas Urol. Esp.* 2009 May;33(5):514-21.
[72] Sterrett SP, Nakada SY, Wingo MS, et al. Renal thermal ablative therapy. *Urol. Clin. North Am.* 2008 Aug;35(3):397-414.
[73] Fernández Rosado E, Sánchez Rodríguez-Losada J, Chantada Abal V, et al. Nephron sparing renal surgery as salvage treatment after failure of radiofrequency thermal ablation in a patient with a single kidney and renal adenocarcinoma. *Arch. Esp. Urol.* 2006 Jul-Aug;59(6):577-82.
[74] Kunkle DA, Uzzo RG. Cryoablation or radiofrequency ablation of the small renal mass: a meta- analysis. *Cancer* 2008; 113:2671-2680.
[75] Dechet CB, Zincke H, Sebo TJ, et al. Prospective analysis of computerized tomography and needle biopsy with permanent sectioning to determine the nature of solid renal masses in adults. *J. Urol.* 2003 Jan;169(1):71-4.
[76] Schmidbauer J, Remzi M, Memarsadeghi M, et al. Diagnostic accuracy of computed tomography-guided percutaneous biopsy of renal masses. *Eur. Urol.* 2008 May;53(5):1003-11.
[77] Remzi M, Ozsoy M, Klingler HC, et al. Are small renal tumors harmless? Analysis of histopathological features according to tumors 4 cm or less in diameter. *J. Urol.* 2006 Sep;176(3):896-9.
[78] Venkatesan AM, Wood BJ, Gervais DA. Percutaneous ablation in the kidney. *Radiology*. 2011 Nov;261(2):375-91.
[79] Boss A, Clasen S, Kuczyk M, et al. Image-guided radiofrequency ablation of renal cell carcinoma. *Eur. Radiol.* 2007;17(3):725–733.
[80] McGahan JP, Loh S, Fitzgerald E, et al. Pretreatment imaging can be used to select imaging guidance, ultrasound alone versus CT plus ultrasound, for percutaneous renal radiofrequency ablation. *AJR Am. J. Roentgenol.* 2011 Nov;197(5):1244-50.

[81] Boss A, Rempp H, Martirosian P, et al. Wide-bore 1.5 Tesla MR imagers for guidance and monitoring of radiofrequency ablation of renal cell carcinoma: initial experience on feasibility. *Eur. Radiol.* 2008 Jul;18(7):1449-55.

[82] Zhao X, Wang W, Zhang S, et al. Improved outcome of percutaneous radiofrequency ablation in renal cell carcinoma: a retrospective study of intraoperative contrast-enhanced ultrasonography in 73 patients. *Abdom. Imaging.* 2012 Oct;37(5):885-91.

[83] Yang R, Lian H, Zhang G, et al. Laparoscopic radiofrequency ablation with intraoperative contrast-enhanced ultrasonography for T1bN0M0 renal tumors: initial functional and oncologic outcomes. *J. Endourol.* 2014 Jan;28(1):4-9.

[84] Tracy CR, Raman JD, Donnally C, et al. Durable Oncologic Outcomes after radiofrequency ablation. *Cancer* 2010; 116:3135- 3142.

[85] Pandharipande PV, Gervais DA, Mueller PR,, et al. Radiofrequency ablation versus nephron-sparing surgery for small unilateral renal cell carcinoma: cost-effectiveness analysis. *Radiology.* 2008 Jul;248(1):169-78.

[86] Clark TW, Malkowicz B, Stavropoulos SW, et al. Radiofrequency ablation of small renal cell carcinomas using multitined expandable electrodes: preliminary experience. *J. Vasc. Interv. Radiol.* 2006 Mar;17(3):513-9.

[87] Gupta A, Raman JD, Leveillee RJ, et al. General anesthesia and contrast-enhanced computed tomography to optimize renal percutaneous radiofrequency ablation: multi-institutional intermediate-term results. *J. Endourol.* 2009 Jul;23(7):1099-105.

[88] Kariya S, Tanigawa N, Kojima H, et al. Radiofrequency ablation combined with CO2 injection for treatment of retroperitoneal tumor: protecting surrounding organs against thermal injury. *AJR Am. J. Roentgenol.* 2005 Oct;185(4):890-3.

[89] Ginat DT, Saad W, Davies M, et al. Bowel displacement for CT-guided tumor radiofrequency ablation: techniques and anatomic considerations. *J. Endourol.* 2009 Aug;23(8):1259-64.

[90] Rehman J, Landman J, Lee D, et al. Needle-based ablation of renal parenchyma using microwave, cryoablation, impedance and temperatura based monopolar and bipolar radiofrequency, and liquid and gel chemoablation: laboratorystudies and review of the literature. *J. Endourol.* 2004;18:83-104.

[91] Farrell MA, Charboneau WJ, DiMarco DS, et al. Imaging-guided radiofrequency ablation of solid renal tumors. *AJR Am. J. Roentgenol.* 2003;180(6):1509–1513.

[92] Goldberg SN, Grassi CJ, Cardella JF, et al. Image-guided tumor ablation: standardization of terminology and reporting criteria. *Radiology.* 2005 Jun;235(3):728-39.

[93] Bruno JJ, Snyder ME, Motzer RJ, et al. Renal cell carcinoma local recurrences, impact of surgical treatment and concomitant metastasis on survival. *BJU Int.* 2006 May;97(5):933-8.

[94] Bani-Hani AH, Leibovich BC, Lohse CM, et al. Associations with contralateral recurrence following nephrectomy for renal cell carcinoma using a cohort of 2,352 patients. *J. Urol.* 2005 Feb;173(2);391-4.

[95] Matin SF, Ahrar K, Cadeddu JA, et al. Residual and recurrent disease following renal energy ablative therapy: a multi-institutional study. *J. Urol.* 2006 Nov;176(5):1973-7.

[96] Park BK, Kim CK, Lee HM. Image-guided radiofrequency ablation of Bosniak category III or IV cystic renal tumors: initial clinical experience. *Eur. Radiol.* 2008;18(7):1519–1525.
[97] Lucas SM, Stern JM, Adibi M, et al. Renal function outcomes in patients treated for renal masses smaller than 4 cm by ablative and extirpative techniques. J Urol. 2008 Jan;179(1):75-9; discussion 79-80. *Epub* 2007 Nov 13.
[98] Turna B, Kaouk JH, Frota R, et al. Minimally invasive nephron sparing management for renal tumors in solitary kidneys. *J. Urol.* 2009 Nov;182(5):2150-7.
[99] Altunrende F, Autorino R, Hillyer S, et al. Image guided percutaneous probe ablation for renal tumors in 65 solitary kidneys: functional and oncological outcomes. *J. Urol.* 2011 Jul;186(1):35-41.
[100] Zhang S, Zhao X, Ji C, et al. Radiofrequency ablation of synchronous bilateral renal cell carcinoma. *Int. J. Urol.* 2012 Mar;19(3):241-7.
[101] Arnoux V, Descotes JL, Sengel C, et al. Perioperative outcomes and mid-term results of radiofrequency ablation and partial nephrectomy in indications of renal tumor treatment and imperative nephron-sparing procedure. *Prog. Urol.* 2013 Feb;23(2):99-104.
[102] Matsumoto ED, Johonson DB, Ogan K, et al. Short-term efficacy of temperature-based radiofrequency ablation of small renal tumors. *Urology.* 2005;65(5):877-881.
[103] Levinson AW, Su LM, Agarwal D, et al. Long-term oncological and overall outcomes of percutaneous radio frequency ablation in high risk surgical patients with a solitary small renal mass. *J. Urol.* 2008;180:499-504
[104] Zagoria RJ, Traver MA, Werle DM, et al. Oncologic efficacy of CT-guided percutaneous radiofrequency ablation of renal cell carcinomas. *AJR Am. J. Roentgenol.* 2007;189(2):429–436.
[105] Breen DJ, Rutherford EE, Stedman B, et al. Management of renal tumors by image-guided radiofrequency ablation: experience in 105 tumors. *Cardiovasc. Intervent. Radiol.* 2007;30(5):936–942.
[106] Gervais DA, McGovern FJ, Arellano RS, et al. Radiofrequency ablation of renal cell carcinoma: part 1, Indications, results, and role in patient management over a 6-year period and ablation of 100 tumors. *AJR Am. J. Roentgenol.* 2005 Jul;185(1):64-71
[107] Su LM, Jarrett TW, Chan DY, et al. Percutaneous computed tomography-guided radiofrequency ablation of renal masses in high surgical risk patients: preliminary results. *Urology* 2003;61(4 Suppl 1):26–33.
[108] Mayo-Smith WW, Dupuy DE, Parikh PM, et al. Imaging-guided percutaneous radiofrequency ablation of solid renal masses: techniques and outcomes of 38 treatment sessions in 32 consecutive patients. *AJR Am. J. Roentgenol.* 2003;180(6):1503–1508.
[109] Levinson AW., Su LM., Agarwal D., et al. Long-term oncological and overall outcomes of percutaneous radio frequency ablation in high risk surgical patients with a solitary small renal mass. *J. Urol.* 2008;180(2): 499-504.
[110] Mylona S., Kokkinaki A., Pomoni M., et al. Percutaneous radiofrequency ablation of renal cell carcinomas in patients with a solitary kidney: 6 years experience. *Eur. J. Rad.* 2009;69(2):351-356.
[111] Ferakis N, Bouropoulos C, Granitsas T, et al. Long-term results after computed-tomography-guided percutaneous radiofrequency ablation for small renal tumors. *J. Endourol.* 2010 Dec;24(12):1909-13.

[112] Olweny EO, Park SK, Tan YK, et al. Radiofrequency ablation versus partial nephrectomy in patients with solitary clinical T1a renal cell carcinoma: comparable oncologic outcomes at a minimum of 5 years of follow-up. *Eur. Urol.* 2012 Jun;61(6):1156-61.

[113] Kim SD, Yoon SG, Sung GT. Radiofrequency ablation of renal tumors: four-year follow-up results in 47 patients. *Korean J. Radiol.* 2012 Sep-Oct;13(5):625-33.

[114] Zhao X, Wang W, Zhang S, et al. Improved outcome of percutaneous radiofrequency ablation in renal cell carcinoma: a retrospective study of intraoperative contrast-enhanced ultrasonography in 73 patients. *Abdom. Imaging*. 2012 Oct;37(5):885-91.

[115] Psutka SP, Feldman AS, McDougal WS, et al. Long-term oncologic outcomes after radiofrequency ablation for T1 renal cell carcinoma. *Eur. Urol.* 2013 Mar;63(3):486-492.

[116] Hegarty NJ, Gill IS, Desai MM, et al. Probe-ablative nephron-sparing surgery: cryoablation versus radiofrequency ablation. *Urology.* 2006;68(1 Suppl):7-13.

[117] Stern JM, Svatec R, Park S, et al. Intermediate comparison of partial nephrectomy and radiofrequency ablation for clinical T1a renal tumours. *BJU Int.* 2007;100(2):287-290.

[118] Hui GC, Tuncali K, Tatli S, et al. Comparison of percutaneous and surgical approaches to renal tumor ablation: meta- analysis of effectiveness and complication rates. *J. Vasc. Interv. Radiol.*, 2008; 19:1311-1320.

[119] El Dib R, Touma NJ, Kapoor A. Cryoablation vs radiofrequency ablation for the treatment of renal cell carcinoma: a meta-analysis of case series studies. *BJU Int.* 2012;10.1111/j.1464- 410X.2011.10885.x.

[120] Miller AJ, Kurup AN, Schmit GD, et al. Percutaneous Clinical T1a Renal Mass Ablation in the Octogenarian and Nonagenarian: Oncologic Outcomes and Morbidity. *J. Endourol.* 2014 Nov 11.

[121] JiC, LiX, ZhangS, GanW, et al. Laparoscopic radiofrequency ablation of renal tumors: 32-month mean follow-up results of 106 patients. *Urology* 2010; 77:798-802.

[122] Young EE, Castle SM, Gorbatiy V, et al. Comparison of safety, renal function outcomes and efficacy of laparoscopic and percutaneous radiofrequency ablation of renal masses. *J. Urol.* 2012; 187:1177-1182.

[123] Zhao X, Zhang S, Liu G, Ji C, et al. Zero ischemia laparoscopic radio frequency ablation assisted enucleation of renal cell carcinoma: experience with 42 patients. *J. Urol.* 2012 Oct;188(4):1095-101.

[124] Wah TM, Arellano RS, Gervais DA, et al. Image guided percutaneous radiofrequency ablation and incidence of post-radiofrequency ablation syndrome: prospective survey. *Radiology* 2005; 237:1097-1102.

[125] Rhim H, Dodd GD, 3rd, Chintapalli KN, et al. Radiofrequency thermal ablation of abdominal tumors: lessons learned from complications. *RadioGraphics* 2004;24(1):41–52.

[126] Baker M, Anderson JK, Jaffer O, et al. Pain after percutaneous radiofrequency ablation of renal tumors. *J. Endourol.* 2007 Jun;21(6):606-9.

[127] Boss A, Clasen S, Kuczyk M, et al. Thermal damage of the genitofemoral nerve due to radiofrequency ablation of renal cell carcinoma: a potentially avoidable complication. *AJR Am. J. Roentgenol.* 2005;185(6):1627–1631.

[128] Uribe PS, Costabile RA, Peterson AC. Progression of renal tumors after laparoscopic radiofrequency ablation. *Urology.* 2006 Nov;68(5):968-71.

[129] De Arruda HO, Goldman S, Andreoni C, et al. Renoduodenal fistula after renal tumor ablation with radiofrequency. *Surg. Laparosc. Endosc. Percutan. Tech.* 2006 Oct;16(5):342-3.

[130] Simon C.J., Dupuy D.E., Mayo-Smith W.W. Microwave ablation: principles and applications. *Radiographics* 2005;25(Suppl 1): S69–S83.

[131] Shock SA, Meredith K, Warner TF, et al. Microwave ablation with loop antenna: in vivo porcine liver model. *Radiology* 2004;231:143–149.

[132] Yu J., Liang P., Yu XL., et al. US-guided percutaneous microwave ablation of renal cell carcinoma: intermediate-term results. *Radiology* 2012;163(3):900-8.

[133] Castle SM, Salas N, Leveillee RJ. Initial experience using microwave ablation therapy for renal tumor treatment: 18-month follow-up. *Urology* 2011;77(4):792–797.

[134] Guan W., Bal J., Liu J., et al. Microwave ablation versus partial nephrectomy for small renal tumors: intermediate-term results. *J. Surg. Oncol.* 2012;106(3):316-21.

[135] Moreland AJ., Ziemlewicz TJ., Best SL., et al. High-powered microwave ablation of T1a renal cell carcinoma: safety and initial clinical evaluation. *J. Endourol.* 2014;28(9)_1046-52.

[136] Lin Y., Liang P., Yu XL., et al. Percutaneous microwave ablation of renal cell carcinoma is safe in patients with solitary kindney. *Urology* 2014;83(2):357-63.

[137] Klingler C., Margreiter M., Marberger M. New ablative treatments for small renal masses: HIFU ablation. *Arch. Esp. Urol.* 2013;66(1):79-89.

[138] Marberger M, Schatzl G, Cranston D, et al. Extracorporeal ablation of r. Renal tumors with high-intensity ultrasound. *BJU Int.* 2005:95,Suppl2,52-5.

[139] Illing RO, Kennedy JE, Wu F, et al. The safety and fea- sibility of extracorporeal high-intensity focused ultrasound (HIFU) for the treatment of liver and kidney tumors in a Western population. *Br. J. Cancer* 2005:93:890-5.

[140] Kohrmann KU, Michel MS, Gaa J, et al. High intensity focused ultrasound as noninvasive therapy for multilocal renal cell carcinoma: Case study and review of the literature. *J. Urol.* 2002;167:2397–403.

[141] Klingler HC, Susani M, Seip R, et al. A novel approach to energy ablative therapy of small renal tumours: Laparoscopic high-intensity focused ultrasound. *Eur. Urol.* 2008;53:810–6. discussion 817-8.

[142] Hacker A, Michel MS, Marlinghaus E, et al. Extracorporeally induced ablation of renal tissue by high-intensity focused ultrasound. *BJU Int.* 2006;97:779–85.

[143] Liehr UB, Wendler JJ, Blaschke S, et al. Irreversible electroporation: the new generation of local ablation techniques for renal cell carcinoma. *Urologe A.* 2012 Dec;51(12):1728-34.

[144] Sommer CM, Fritz S, Wachter MF, et al. Irreversible electroporation of the pig kidney with involvement of the renal pelvis: technical aspects, clinical outcome, and three-dimensional CT rendering for assessment of the treatment zone. *J. Vasc. Interv. Radiol.* 2013 Dec;24(12):1888-97.

[145] Neal RE , Garcia PA, Robertson JL, et al. Experimental characterization and numerical modeling of tissue electrical conductivity during pulsed electric fields for irreversible electroporation treatment planning. *IEEE Trans Biomed Eng.* 2012 Apr;59(4):1076-85.

[146] Ben-David E, Ahmed M, Faroja M, et al. Irreversible electroporation: treatment effect is susceptible to local environment and tissue properties. *Radiology*. 2013 Dec;269(3):738-47.

[147] Wimmer T, Srimathveeravalli G, Gutta N, et al. Planning Irreversible Electroporation in the Porcine Kidney: Are Numerical Simulations Reliable for Predicting Empiric Ablation Outcomes?. *Cardiovasc Intervent Radiol.* 2014 May 17.

In: Renal Cell Carcinoma
Editors: J. M. Fernández-Gomez, J. García-Rodríguez
ISBN: 978-1-63482-495-8

Chapter 8

Follow-up after Treatment of Localized Renal Tumor (Surgery, Surveillance, Ablative Therapies)

F. J. Perez Garcia, PhD*
Department of Urology, Hospital San Agustin, Aviles, Asturias, Spain

Abstract

Renal cell carcinoma (RCC) comprises approximately 2%-3% of all adult malignancies, representing the seventh most common cancer in men and nine commonest cancers in women. Surgical resection (radical or partial nephrectomy) remains the only effective therapy for clinically localized RCC. Other treatment options like Active Surveillance and Ablation therapies can be used in selected patients.

Follow-up after surgery, active surveillance and ablation treatment allows the urologist to monitor for postoperative complications, renal function, local recurrence, recurrence in the contralateral kidney and development of metastasis.

A review of the most important and relevant guidelines was conducted to summarize the necessity and the studies to do for surveillance in these patients.

Introduction

Renal cell carcinoma (RCC) comprises approximately 2%-3% of all adult malignancies, representing the seventh most common cancer in men and nine commonest cancers in women. It is the tenth most common cause of cancer-related deaths among men [1, 2]. Risk factors for RCC include active and passive smoking, obesity, end-stage renal failure, acquired

* Correspondance to:Francisco Javier Perez Garcia; Hospital San Agustin. Camino de Heros 6, 33401. Aviles. Asturias. Spain; E-mail: franjapg@yahoo.es.

renal cystic disease and hereditary conditions associated with a mutation in the von-Hippel-Lindau gene [3,4]. Surgical resection (radical or partial nephrectomy) remains the only effective therapy for clinically localized RCC. Other treatment options like Active Surveillance and Ablation therapies can be used in selected patients.

Surgical management with resection of the primary tumor provides for immediate local control of renal tumors and valuable pathologic data that may aid in understanding prognosis and guide patient follow-up.

Indications for active surveillance include elderly patients, those with decreased life expectancy or those with medical comorbidities that would be associated with increased risk if a therapeutic intervention were to be undertaken. Alternatively, a strategy of observation with delayed intervention as indicated may be elected in order to determine the growth rate or to obtain alternative diagnostic imaging. Ablative techniques may be performed by a variety of approaches (open/laparoscopic/percutaneous) and operators (urologic surgeons/ interventional radiologists). The majority of neoplasms selected for ablative procedures are less than 4 cm and exophytic, as markedly higher incomplete ablation rates have been noted for endophytic, central and larger neoplasms.

Staging

The Union for International Cancer Control tumour–node–metastasis staging system should be used (Table 1).

Table 1. The Union for International Cancer Control tumour–node–metastasis staging system

T	Primary tumour
Tx	Primary tumour cannot be assessed
T0	No evidence of primary tumour
T1 T1a T1b	Tumour of < or = 7cm in greatest dimension limited to the kidney Tumour < or = 4 cm Tumour > 4 cm but < or = 7 cm
T2 T2a T2b	Tumour >7cm in greatest dimension limited to the kidney Tumour > 7 cm but < or = 10 cm Tumour > 10 cm limited to the kidney
T3 T3a T3b T3c	Tumour extends to major veins or perinephric tissues but not into the ipsilateral adrenal gland and not beyond Gerota´s fascia Tumour grossly extends into the renal vein or its segmental (muscle-containing) branches, or tumour invades peri-renal or renal sinus fat (peripelvic) but not beyond Gerota´s fascia Tumour grossly extends into the vena cava below the diaphragm Tumour grossly extends into the vena cava above the diaphragm or invades the

T	Primary tumour
	wall of the vena cava
T4	Tumour invades beyond Gerota´s fascia (including contiguous extension into the ipsilateral adrenal gland)
N	Regional lymph nodes
Nx	Regional lymph nodes cannot be assessed
N0	No regional lymph node metastasis
N1	Metastasis in regional lymph node(s)
M	Distant metastasis
CM0	Clinically no distant metastasis
CM1	Clinically distant metastasis
PM1	Pathologically proven distant metastasis e.g., needle biopsy
Stage Grouping	
Stage I	T1 N0 M0
Stage II	T2 N0 M0 T3 Any N M0
Stage III	T1-3 N1 M0 T4 Any N M0
Stage IV	Any T Any N M1

Risk Assessment

RCC is recognised as having a very variable natural history. Risk assessment models have been developed to provide prognostic information for patients and to inform the eligibility and risk stratification designs of clinical trials. [5]

Localised disease. Two systems can be used to assess the risk of progression in localised tumors: the stage, size grade and necrosis (SSIGN) score [6] and the University of California Los Angeles Integrated Staging System (UISS) [7]. These systems are described in Tables 2 and 3. In SSIGN, risk points are accumulated as noted in Table 2 and added up to provide a risk score.

Table 2. Stage, size grade and necrosis (SSIGN) score for localized RCC

Feature		Score
Pathological T category of primary tumour (TNM 2002)	pT1a	0
	pT1b	2
	pT2	3
	pT3a-4	4
Regional lymph node status	pNx or pN0	0

Table 2. (Continued)

Feature		Score
	pN1 or pN2	2
Tumour size (cm)	<10	0
	>10	1
Nuclear grade	1 or 2	0
	3	1
	4	3
Histological tumour necrosis	No	0
	Yes	1
Scores	Group	5-year metastasis free survival (%)
0-2	Low risk	97.1
3-5	Intermediate risk	73.8
> or = 6	High risk	31.2

Table 3 .University of California Los Angeles Integrated Staging System (UISS) risk groups and 5-year disease-specific survival

Patient group		Pronostic group			
		T stage	Fuhrman´s grade	ECOG status	5-year disease-specific survival (%)
Localised disease (N0, M0)	Low risk	1	1-2	0	91.1
	Intermediate risk	1	1-2	1 or more	80.4
		1	3-4	Any	
		2	Any	Any	
		3	1	Any	
		3	2-4	Any	
	High	3	2-4	1 or more	54.7
		4	Any	Any	
Metastatc disease	Low risk	N1 M0	Any	Any	32
		N2M0/M1	1-2	0	
	Intermediate risk	N2M0/M1	1-2	1 or more	19.5
			3	0, 1 or more	
			4	0	
	High	N2M0/m1	4	1 or more	0

The SSIGN score compared favourably with the UISS score in predictive accuracy in a series of patients who had surgically resected clear-cell RCC. On the other hand, the UISS provides prognostic predictions for both localised and metastatic disease.

Advanced disease. Prognostic models were first built when immunotherapy was the standard therapy. The Memorial Sloane Kettering Cancer Centre (MSKCC) or Motzer score was the standard system. The MSKCC score has now been validated and updated for use in the current era of targeted therapies as the Heng or International Metastatic RCC Database Consortium (IMDC) criteria [8]. Patients are stratified according to the presence of six risk factors:

- Karnofsky performance status (PS) <80%.
- Haemoglobin <lower limit of normal.
- Time from diagnosis to treatment of <1 year.
- Corrected calcium above the upper limit of normal.
- Platelets greater than the upper limit of normal.
- Neutrophils greater than the upper limit of normal.

The number of risk factors present is added up and the risk is sratified as can be seen in table 4.

Table 4. The Memorial Sloane Kettering Cancer Centre (MSKCC) score

Number of Risk factors	Risk group	Median overall Survival (OS) months	2-year OS (%)
0	Favourable	43	75
1-2	Intermediate	27	53
3-6	Poor	8.8	7

Rationale for Surveillance

There is no evidence that any particular follow-up protocol influences the outcome in early RCC. No standard recommendation can be given for the follow-up in advanced RCC either. The follow-up scheme for localized RCC following surgery should be dependent on the therapeutic possibilities upon recurrence. CT scans of thorax and abdomen are routinely performed, with time intervals dependent on risk factors. Long term follow-up is proposed in some institutions, due to the possibility of late relapse, but its benefit has never been demonstrated. [5]

A review of the most important and relevant guidelines was conducted to summarize the necessity and the studies to do for surveillance in these patients.

According to NCCN guidelines, [9] after surgical excision, 20% to 30% of patients with localized tumors experience relapse. Lung metastasis is the most common site of distant recurrence, occurring in 50% to 60% of patients. The median time to relapse after surgery is 1 to 2 years, with most relapses occurring within 3 years. [10]

When it comes to AUA guidelines, [11] follow-up for adult cancer survivors has traditionally focused on the early detection of a cancer recurrence based on the presumption that treatment of a lower tumor burden would result in better patient outcomes, although the evidentiary data supporting this presumption is limited [12]. The recommended essential elements of adult cancer survivorship care now include not only monitoring for cancer recurrence, secondary cancers and treatment effects, but also the prevention of recurrences or new tumors, medical interventions for the consequences of cancer and its treatment effects and the coordination between specialists and primary care physicians to meet survivors' needs [13]. Treatment "effects" include those related to the sequelae of surgery, systemic therapies, ablative therapy and radiation.

There is now an increasing rate of detection and subsequent treatment of small renal masses of uncertain biological potential as well as a widening spectrum of contemporary treatment options with varied treatment related effects. Such options include observation/surveillance, ablative therapies and minimally-invasive as well as open approaches to partial and radical nephrectomy. The advent of a new generation of targeted systematic therapy now holds the promise of prolonged survival of patients with metastatic disease. Additionally, patients with renal cell cancer tend to be older and have a greater incidence of pre-existing kidney disease, which places them at an increased risk for either the development or progression of chronic kidney disease following therapy [14-15]. Since effective treatment strategies are available to slow the progression of chronic kidney disease and reduce cardiovascular risks, it would seem prudent to include renal function monitoring in the follow-up of renal cancer patients to facilitate early interventions or referral to nephrology.

Surveillance after surgery allows the urologist to monitor for postoperative complications, renal function, local recurrence, recurrence in the contralateral kidney and development of metastasis. [16]

Renal function and postoperative complications are commonly assessed by history, physical examination, and measurement of serum creatinine and haemoglobin at 4–6 weeks postsurgery. Long-term monitoring of serum creatinine is recommended particularly in patients with compromised renal function prior to surgery or significant increase in creatinine after surgery.

Early diagnosis of local and contralateral kidney recurrence (incidence < 2%) is useful since the most effective treatment is surgical resection. Recurrence in the kidney is associated with positive surgical margins, multifocality and grade. Tumors that develop in the contralateral kidney can be treated with nephron-sparing surgery when detected at a small size. Patients who underwent surgery when local recurrences became symptomatic have a higher rate of incomplete resection of recurrence, positive surgical margins and poorer survival.

Extensive tumor recurrence reduces the possibility of complete surgical resection, which is standard therapy for patients with local recurrence or resectable solitary metastasis.

Furthermore, an early diagnosis of disease relapse may enhance efficacy of systemic therapy if the tumour burden is low. Hence, this supports the rationale for surveillance of patients to detect recurrences and metastases early.

According to the EAU guidelines, there is no consensus on surveillance after treatment for RCC, and there is no evidence that early vs later diagnosis of recurrences improves survival. [17]

It is reasonable to stratify the follow-up, taking into account the risk of a recurrence or metastases developing. There have been large studies examining prognostic factors with long follow-up periods, from which some conclusions can be drawn:

- The sensitivity of chest radiography for small metastases is poor and US has limitations. [18]
- When the risk of relapse is intermediate or high, CT of the chest and abdomen is the investigation of choice. Findings using CT can clearly reveal metastatic lesions from RCC. [19]
- Surveillance should also include clinical evaluation of renal function and cardiovascular risk factors.
- Positron-emission tomography (PET) and PET-CT as well as bone scintigraphy are not the standard of care in RCC surveillance, due to their limited specificity and sensitivity.
- More strict follow-up schedules may be required after cryotherapy and RFA due to the higher local recurrence rate after these modality of treatment.
- There is controversy over the optimal duration of follow-up. Some argue that follow-up with imaging is not cost-effective after 5 years; however, late metastases are more likely to be solitary and justify more aggressive therapy with curative intent. In addition, patients with tumors that develop in the contralateral kidney can be treated with nephron-sparing surgery if the tumors are detected when small. In addition, for tumors < 4 cm in size, there is no difference between partial and radical nephrectomy with regard to recurrences during the follow-up. [20]

The American Urological Association published in the year 2013 the guideline for follow-up for clinically localized renal neoplasms and established several guideline statements [11]. Patients undergoing follow-up for treated or observed renal masses should undergo a history and physical examination directed at detecting signs and symptoms of metastatic spread or local recurrence. They should undergo basic laboratory testing to include blood urea nitrogen (BUN)/creatinine, urine analysis (UA) and estimated glomerular filtration rate (eGFR). Other laboratory evaluations, including complete blood count (CBC), lactate dehydrogenase (LDH), liver function tests (LFTs), alkaline phosphatase (ALP) and calcium level, may be used at the discretion of the clinician. Patients with progressive renal insufficiency on follow-up laboratory evaluation should be referred to nephrology.

The guideline recommends a bone scan in patients with an elevated alkaline phosphatase (ALP), clinical symptoms such as bone pain, and/or if radiographic findings are suggestive of a bony neoplasm.

Patients with a history of a renal neoplasm presenting with acute neurological signs or symptoms must undergo prompt neurologic cross-sectional CT or MRI scanning of the head or spine based on localization of symptomatology.

Follow Up After Surgical Treatment Based in NCCN and AUA Recommendations (Table 5)

Low Risk Patients (pT1, N0, Nx)

Patients should undergo a baseline abdominal scan (CT or MRI) for nephron sparing surgery and abdominal imaging (US, CT or MRI) for radical nephrectomy within three to twelve months following renal surgery.

Additional abdominal imaging (US, CT or MRI) may be performed in patients with low risk (pT1, N0, Nx) disease following a radical nephrectomy if the initial postoperative baseline image is negative at the discretion of the clinician.

Abdominal imaging (US, CT, or MRI) may be performed yearly for three years in patients with low risk (pT1, N0, Nx) disease following a partial nephrectomy based on individual risk factors if the initial postoperative scan is negative.

Patients with a history of low risk (pT1, N0, Nx) renal cell carcinoma should undergo yearly chest x-ray (CXR) to assess for pulmonary metastases for three years and only as clinically indicated beyond that time period.

Moderate to High Risk Patients (pT2-4N0 Nx or any stage N+)

Moderate to high risk patients should undergo baseline chest and abdominal scan (CT or MRI) within three to six months following surgery with continued imaging (US, CXR, CT or MRI) every six months for at least three years and annually thereafter to year five.

It is recommended site-specific imaging as warranted by clinical symptoms suggestive of recurrence or metastatic spread.

Imaging (US, CXR, CT or MRI) beyond five years may be performed at the discretion of the clinician for moderate to high risk patients.

Routine FDG-PET scan is not indicated in the follow-up for renal cancer.

Follow-Up in Active Surveillance (Table 6)

Indications for active surveillance include elderly patients, those with decreased life expectancy or those with significant medical comorbidities that would be associated with increased risk if a therapeutic intervention were to be undertaken. Alternatively, a strategy of observation with delayed intervention as indicated may be elected in order to determine the growth rate or to obtain alternative diagnostic imaging.

It is assumed that the patient who has been chosen for active surveillance is one who would undergo intervention if, in the course of active surveillance, changes occur in the primary tumor for which intervention would normally be indicated. In the patient for whom no surgical or minimally invasive intervention (i.e., surgery or percutaneous ablative procedure) would ever be considered due to comorbidities, no imaging is necessary.

Table 5. Follow up after surgical treatment. Radical or Partial Nephrectomy

Follow-up Measure	Radical or Partial Nephrectomy	
Physical Exam and History	History and physical examination directed at detecting signs and symptoms of metastatic spread or local recurrence	
Laboratory Testing	– blood urea nitrogen (BUN)/creatinine, urine analysis (UA) and estimated glomerular filtration rate (eGFR). – complete blood count (CBC), lactate dehydrogenase (LDH), liver function tests (LFTs), alkaline phosphatase (ALP) and calcium level, may be used at the discretion of the clinician. – Patients with progressive renal insufficiency on follow-up laboratory evaluation should be referred to nephrology.	
CNS Scan	Acute neurological signs or symptoms must undergo prompt neurologic cross-sectional CT or MRI scanning of the head or spine based on localization of symptomatology	
Bone scan	Elevated alkaline phosphatase (ALP), clinical symptoms such as bone pain, and/or if radiographic findings are suggestive of a bony neoplasm.	
Follow-up Measure	Low Risk	Moderate to High Risk
Abdominal Scan/Imaging	Partial Nephrectomy - Baseline abdominal scan (CT or MRI) within 3 to 12 months following surgery: - If the initial postoperative scan is negative, abdominal imaging (US,CT or MRI) may be performed yearly for 3 years based on individual risk factors Radical Nephrectomy - Patients should undergo abdominal imaging (US,CT,MRI) within 3 to 12 months following renal surgery. - If the initial postoperative imaging is negative , abdominal imaging beyond 12 months may be performed at the discretion of the clinician	– A baseline abdominal scan (CT or MRI) within 3 to 6 months following surgery with continued imaging (US,CT, MRI) every six months for at least three years and annually thereafter to year five – Imaging beyond 5 years may be performed at the discretion of the clinician – Perform site specific imaging as symptoms warrants
Chest Imaging/Scan	Obtain a yearly chest x-ray for 3 years and only as clinical indicated beyond that time period	Obtain a baseline chest scan (CT) within 3 to 6 months following surgery with continued imaging (CXR or CT) every 6 months for at least 3 years and annually thereafter to year five. Imaging beyond 5 years is optional and should be based on individual patient characteristics and tumour risk factors

Follow-up protocols may vary depending on whether the patient has undergone a biopsy of the renal mass. The AUA guidelines considered clinical scenarios including biopsy-proven, untreated, clinically localized renal cancers; biopsies yielding low-malignant potential neoplasms or normal renal parenchyma; and renal lesions radiographically suspicious for neoplasm that either have not been biopsied or have indeterminate biopsy results.

Physicians should counsel patients on their other therapeutic options, as addressed in the AUA Treatment of T1 Renal Mass Guidelines [21]. Specifically, the patient should be counselled about the small but potential risk of cancer progression while on active surveillance, the potential loss of a window of opportunity for nephron-sparing surgery, the lack of curative salvage therapies if metastases develop and the deficiencies of the current data used to support this approach. Potential triggers for intervention while on active surveillance primarily involve absolute tumor size, tumor growth rate or a change in patient preference.

Table 6. Follow-up in Active Surveillance

Follow-up Measure	Active Surveillance
Physical Exam and History	History and physical examination directed at detecting signs and symptoms of metastatic or local progression
Laboratory Testing	Basic laboratory testing to include BUN/creatinine. UA and eGFR; CBC, LDH, LFTs. ALP and calcium level test may be used at the discretion of the physician; Progressive renal insufficiency should prompt a nephrology referral
CNS Scan	Acute neurological signs should undergo prompt cross sectional (CT or MRI) scan of the head or spine based on localized symptomatology
Bone Scan	Elevated ALP, clinical symptoms such as bone pain, and/or radiographic findings suggestive of a bony neoplasm should prompt a bone scan; A bone scan should not be performed in the absence of these symptoms
Percutaneous Biopsy	Percutaneous biopsy may be considered prior to active surveillance
Abdominal Scan/Imaging	Cross-sectional abdominal scanning (CT or MRI) within six months of active surveillance initiation to establish a growth rate with continued imaging (US, CT or MRI) at least annually thereafter
Chest X-ray	Patients with biopsy proven RCC or a tumour with oncocytic features on active surveillance should undergo an annual chest x-ray to assess for pulmonary metastases

The precise growth rate or absolute tumor size that would trigger intervention is controversial given the limited available data. Some would propose that because the normal growth rate is approximately 0.3 cm/year, a persistent tumor growth rate of greater than 0.3-0.5 cm per year, and/or an absolute tumor size of greater than 3cm would justify intervention. The intervention would primarily involve local treatment, although a biopsy (in the case of biopsy-unproven renal masses) or a change to more frequent imaging could also be incorporated.

Percutaneous biopsy may be considered in patients planning to undergo active surveillance.

The Panel of the AUA guidelines recommends that patients undergo cross-sectional abdominal scanning (CT or MRI) within six months of active surveillance initiation to establish a growth rate. They also recommend continued imaging (US, CT or MRI) at least annually thereafter. CT and MRI tend to be used more often for surveillance because they provides higher quality information over US, especially for neoplasms under 3cm; however, there may be benefits in reducing the risks of contrast and radiation exposure by employing alternative imaging. Alternative methods for limiting the amount of radiation and contrast exposure, include limiting CT use to once yearly unless otherwise clinically indicated, using a low dose radiation CT protocol for imaging, using MRI, and/or alternating the use of CT or MRI with US for surveillance. Importantly, with respect to tumor size measurements, differences of < 3.1 mm for inter-observer or < 2.3 mm for intra-observer evaluations are within the variability of measurement and should, therefore, not be attributed to tumor growth [20], unless in the case where there are persistent increases over two or more interval exams. Although it has been shown that the growth rate of a renal mass does not necessarily predict the presence of cancer and no robust method exists for distinguishing benign/indolent versus malignant/aggressive tumors based purely on radiologic features, more rapid rates and larger size trend towards association with true cancer and aggressive disease.

Patients on active surveillance with biopsy proven renal cell carcinoma or a tumor with oncocytic features should undergo an annual chest x-ray (CXR) to assess for pulmonary metastases.

Follow-up after Ablation Therapy (Table 7)

Thermal ablative modalities, specifically cryoablation and radiofrequency ablation (RFA), currently represent accepted minimally invasive treatment options for clinical T1a renal masses in select patients with appropriate informed consent and counselling. Ablative techniques may be performed by a variety of approaches (open/laparoscopic/percutaneous) and operators (urologic surgeons/interventional radiologists). The majority of neoplasms selected for ablative procedures are less than 4 cm and exophytic, as markedly higher incomplete ablation rates have been noted for endophytic, central and larger neoplasms.

A urologist should be involved in the clinical management of all patients undergoing renal ablative procedures including percutaneous ablation. All patients undergoing ablation procedures for a renal mass should undergo a pretreatment diagnostic biopsy.

A standardized definition of treatment failure or local recurrence should be adopted by clinicians. This should be further clarified to include a visually enlarging neoplasm or new nodularity in the same area of treatment whether determined by enhancement of the neoplasm on post-treatment contrast imaging, or failure of regression in size of the treated lesion over time, new satellite or port site soft tissue nodules or biopsy proven recurrence.

Patients should undergo cross-sectional scanning (CT or MRI) with and without intravenous (IV) contrast unless otherwise contraindicated at three and six months following ablative therapy to assess treatment success. This should be followed by annual abdominal scans (CT or MRI) thereafter for five years.

Patients may undergo further scanning (CT or MRI) beyond five years based on individual patient risk factors.

Table 7. Follow-up after Ablation Therapy

Follow-up Measure	Renal Ablation
Physical Exam and History	History and physical examination directed at detecting signs and symptoms of metastatic spread or local recurrence
Laboratory Testing	Basic laboratory testing to include BUN/creatinine. UA and eGFR; CBC, LDH, LFTs. ALP and calcium level test may be used at the discretion of the physician; Progressive renal insufficiency should prompt a nephrology referral
CNS Scan	Acute neurological signs should undergo prompt cross sectional (CT or MRI) scan of the head or spine based on localized symptomatology
Bone Scan	Elevated ALP, clinical symptoms such as bone pain, and/or radiographic findings suggestive of a bony neoplasm should prompt a bone scan; A bone scan should not be performed in the absence of these symptoms
Percutaneous Biopsy	Patients should undergo a pre-treatment diagnosis biopsy
Abdominal Scan	Cross-sectional abdominal scanning (CT or MRI) with and without IV contrast unless otherwise contraindicated at three and six months following ablative therapy with continued scanning annually thereafter for five years; Scanning beyond five years is optional based on individual risk factors
Chest X-ray	Patients who have either biopsy proven low risk RCC, oncocytoma, a tumour with oncocytic features, non-diagnostic biopsies or no prior biopsy should undergo annual chest x-ray to assess for pulmonary metastases for five years; Imaging CXR or CT beyond five years is optional based on individual patient risk factors and the determination of treatment success; Radiologic scanning is not recommended with pathological confirmation of benign disease at or before treatment and post treatment radiographic confirmation of treatment success and no evidence or treatment-related complications.
Repeat Biopsy	New enhancement, a progressive increase in size of an ablated neoplasm with or without contrast enhancement, new nodularity in or around the treated zone, failure of the treated lesion to regress over time, satellite or port side lesions, should prompt a repeat lesion biopsy. Observation, repeat treatment and surgical intervention should be discussed.

Patients undergoing ablative procedures who have either biopsy proven low risk renal cell carcinoma, oncocytoma, a tumor with oncocytic features, non-diagnostic biopsies or no prior biopsy should undergo annual chest x-ray (CXR) to assess for pulmonary metastases for five years. Imaging beyond five years is optional based on individual patient risk factors and the determination of treatment success.

Patients who underwent an ablative procedure with pathological confirmation of benign histology at or before treatment and who have radiographic confirmation of treatment success and no evidence of treatment related complications don't need further imaging studies.

The alternatives of observation, repeat treatment and surgical intervention should be discussed, and repeat biopsy should be performed if there is radiographic evidence of treatment failure within six months if the patient is a treatment candidate. A progressive increase in size of an ablated neoplasm, with or without contrast enhancement, new nodularity in or around the treated zone, failure of the treated lesion to regress in size over time, satellite or port side lesions, should prompt lesion biopsy.

Evaluation of the Guidelines and Future Directions

In November 2014 an evaluation of the National Comprehensive Cancer Network and American Urological Association Renal Cell Carcinoma Surveillance Guidelines was presented at the American Society of Clinical Oncology 2014 Genitourinary Cancers Symposium, San Francisco, CA, January 31-February 1, 2014, and the 2014 Annual Meeting of the American Urological Association, Orlando, FL, May 16-21, 2014, and published in the Journal of Clinical Oncology [22]. 3,651 patients who underwent surgery for M0 RCC between 1970 and 2008 were stratified as AUA low risk (pT1Nx-0) after partial (LR-partial) or radical nephrectomy (LR-radical) or as moderate/high risk (M/HR; pT2-4Nx-0/pTanyN1). Guidelines were assessed by calculating the percentage of recurrences detected when following the 2013 and 2014 NCCN and AUA recommendations, and associated Medicare costs were compared. At a median follow-up of 9.0 years a total of 1,088 patients (29.8%) experienced a recurrence.

Surprisingly, nearly one third of recurrences were missed when following American Urological Association or National Comprehensive Cancer Network guidelines, with a need for significantly longer follow-up (up to 21 years) to capture 95% of these recurrences. In an editorial that accompanied that article, Angela B. Smith, MD, and Matthew I. Milowsky, MD, of the University Of North Carolina Lineberger Comprehensive Cancer Center, called the results striking, but added a few additional points to help put the results in perspective. [23]

First, they noted that the results were taken from a single center making it difficult to generalize more widely. Next, because the researchers found higher recurrence rates among low-risk radical nephrectomy patients, physicians may lack an accurate system for characterizing low- and high-risk RCC.

Gaining a better understanding of tumor biology may improve risk stratification and translate to a surveillance regimen that more accurately captures meaningful recurrences (ie, those that require treatment, affect survival outcomes, or diminish quality of life). Without stronger data associating surveillance with survival and quality of life, justification for extending surveillance guidelines and incurring the additional cost cannot be recommended at this time.

There is a critical need for high quality, prospectively defined cohort studies to better define the prognosis of various renal masses and to establish prognosticators of important patient outcomes, such as overall survival, disease specific survival, cardiovascular and metabolic sequelae and quality of life. Given the potential burden of long-term follow-up of renal masses, randomized trials of different surveillance regimens should be conducted in order to better tailor follow-up to the patients' needs. There is a need for better prospectively designed studies to define the diagnostic accuracy of renal biopsies to define the underlying pathology, natural history and need for treatment, and also renal biopsies following ablative therapies to define the treatment response, natural history and need for further treatment. In light of the expanding use of ablative therapies for renal masses there is need for a uniform definition of treatment success and failure. There is a essential for better prospectively designed studies to examine the utility of tissue, plasma, or tumor markers or existing markers of systemic inflammation/immune response, in predicting survival, recurrence or metabolic sequelae. [11]

Conclusion

Follow-up after surgery, active surveillance and ablation treatment allows the urologist to monitor for postoperative complications, renal function, local recurrence, recurrence in the contralateral kidney and development of metastasis. No single follow-up plan is appropriate for all patients. There is no evidence that any particular follow-up protocol influences the outcome in early RCC. No standard recommendation can be given for the follow-up in advanced RCC either. The follow-up scheme for localised RCC following surgery should be dependent on the therapeutic possibilities upon recurrence. CT scans of thorax and abdomen are routinely performed, with time intervals dependent on risk factors. Long-term follow-up is proposed in some institutions, due to the possibility of late relapse, but its benefit has never been demonstrated. Most follow-up test after ablative therapy are similar to the test included during active surveillance. All the guidelines and recommendations should be modified for the individual patient using clinical judgment.

Current guidelines miss a significant proportion of RCC recurrences. Further research remains necessary to identify an optimal surveillance approach that balances patient benefit and health care costs.

References

[1] Jemal A, Siegel R, Ward E, et al. Cancer statistics, 2006. *CA Cancer J. Clin.* 2006; 56:106-30.

[2] Rini BI, Campbell SC, Escudier B. Renal cell carcinoma. *Lancet* 2009;373:1119-1132.

[3] Bergstrom A, Hsieh CC, Lindblad P, et al. Obesity and renal cell cancer — a quantitative review. *Br. J. Cancer* 2001;85:984-90.

[4] Lindblad P. Epidemiology of renal cell carcinoma. *Scand. J. Surg.* 2004;93:88-96.

[5] Renal cell carcinoma: ESMO Clinical Practice Guidelines for diagnosis, treatment and follow-up. B. Escudier, C. Porta, M. Schmidinger, F. Algaba, J. J. Patard, V. Khoo, T. Eisen & A. Horwich on behalf of the ESMO Guidelines Working Group Annals of Oncology 25 (Supplement 3): iii49–iii56, 2014. doi:10.1093/annonc/mdu25.

[6] Leibovich BC, Blute M, Cheville JC et al. Prediction of progression after radical nephrectomy for patients with clear cell renal cell carcinoma: a stratification tool for prospective clinical trials. *Cancer* 2003; 97: 1663–1671.

[7] Patard JJ, Kim HL, Lam JS et al. Use of the University of California Los Angeles integrated staging system to predict survival in renal cell carcinoma: an international multicenter study. *J. Clin. Oncol.* 2004; 22: 3316–3322.

[8] Heng DY, Xie W, Regan MM et al. Prognostic factors for overall survival in patients with metastatic renal cell carcinoma treated with vascular endothelial growth factor-targeted agents: results from a arge, multicenter study. *J. Clin. Oncol.* 2009; 27: 5794–5799.

[9] NCCN guidelines. http://www.nccn.org/professionals/physiccian_ gls/ pdf/kidney.pdf

[10] Eggener SE, Yossepowitch O, Pettus JA et al. Renal cell carcinoma recurrence after nephrectomy for localized disease: predicting survival from time of recurrence. *J. Clin. Oncol.* 2006;24:3101-3106.

[11] Follow-up for clinically localized renal neoplasms: AUA Guideline. American Urological Association Education and Research, Inc. April 2013.

[12] Brennan MF: Follow up is valuable and effective: true, true and unrelated? *Ann. Surg. Oncol.* 2000; 7: 2.

[13] Jacobs LA, Palmer SC, Schwartz LA et al: Adult cancer survivorship: evolution, research and planning care. *CA Cancer J. Clin.* 2009; 59: 391.

[14] Huang WC, Levey AS, Serio AM et al: Chronic kidney disease after nephrectomy in patients with renal cortical tumors: a retrospective cohort study. *Lancet Oncol.* 2006; 7: 735.

[15] Lane BR, Poggio ED, Herts BR et al: Renal function assessment in the era of chronic kidney disease: renewed emphasis on renal function centered patient care. *J. Urol.* 2009; 182: 435.

[16] Follow-up guidelines after radial or partial nephrectomy for localized and locally advanced renal cell carcinoma. *Can. Urol. Assoc. J.,* 2009;3(1):73.76.

[17] Follow-up after radical or partial nephrectomy or ablative therapies for RCC. EAU guidelines. *Renal Cell Carcinoma*. Update April 2014; 65-68.

[18] Doornweerd BH, de Jong IJ, Bergman LM, et al. Chest X-ray in the follow-up of renal cell carcinoma. *World J. Urol.* 2013 Oct 6. http://www.ncbi.nlm.nih.gov /pubmed/ 24096433.

[19] Coquia SF, Johnson PT, Ahmed S, et al. MDCT imaging following nephrectomy for renal cell carcinoma: Protocol optimization and patterns of tumor recurrence. *World J. Radiol.* 2013 Nov; 5(11):436-45.

[20] Patard JJ, Shvarts O, Lam JS, et al. Safety and efficacy of partial nephrectomy for all T1 tumors based on an international multicenter experience. J Urol 2004 Jun;171(6 Pt 1):2181-5; quiz 2435. http://www. ncbi.nlm.nih.gov/pubmed/15126781.

[21] Novick AC, Campbell SC, Belldegrun A et al: Guideline for Management of the Clinical Stage 1 RenalMass. *American Urological* Association 2009.

[22] Suzanne B. Stewart, R. Houston Thompson, Sarah P. Psutka, John C. Cheville, Christine M. Lohse, Stephen A. Boorjian, and Bradley C. Leibovich Evaluation of the National Comprehensive Cancer Network and American Urological Association Renal Cell Carcinoma Surveillance Guidelines. *J. Clin. Oncol. 32*:4059-4065,2014

[23] Is Extending Surveillance Guidelines for Renal Cell Carcinoma Without Understanding PatientOutcomes Putting the Cart Before the Horse? *Journal of Clinical Oncology*, Vol 32, No 36 (December 20), 2014: pp 4031-4032.

In: Renal Cell Carcinoma
Editors: J. M. Fernández-Gomez, J. García-Rodríguez
ISBN: 978-1-63482-495-8

Chapter 9

Radiotherapy for Renal-Cell Carcinoma

H. González-Suárez, PhD[1,2,*] ***and I. Jimenez-Garcia,***[1] ***MD***
[1]Radiological Oncologist, Department of Radiological Oncology, University Hospital Central of Asturias, Oviedo, Spain
[2]Associate Professor of Radiation Oncology, Medicine School, University of Oviedo, Spain

Abstract

Renal cell carcinoma is a radioresistant tumor. Preoperative radiation therapy yields no survival advantage. Controversies exist concerning postoperative radiation therapy, but it may be considered in patients with perinephric fat extension, adrenal invasion, or involved margins. A dose of 45 Gy is delivered, with consideration of a boost.

In this way, radiation therapy may be considered as primary therapy for palliation in patients whose clinical condition precludes surgery, because of either extensive disease or poor overall condition. In these cases, a dose of 45 gray (Gy) is delivered, with consideration of a boost up to 55 Gy. Moreover, palliative radiation therapy is often used for local or symptomatic metastatic disease, such as painful osseous lesions or brain metastasis, to preclude potential neurologic progression. Surgery should also be considered for solitary brain or spine lesions, followed by postoperative radiotherapy.

About 11% of patients develops brain metastasis during the course of their disease. Patients with untreated brain metastasis have a median survival time of 1 month, which can be improved with glucocorticoid therapy and brain radiation. Radiation treatment of brain metastasis improves quality of life, local control, and overall survival duration. Stereotactic radiosurgery is more effective than surgical extirpation for local control and can be performed on multiple lesions.

Keywords: renal cell carcinoma, preoperative radiation, posoperative radiation, palliative radiation, stereotactic radiation therapy

---

* H. González-Suárez; Department of Radiological Oncology. Hospital Universitario Central of Asturias, Oviedo, Avda de Roma sn. 33011. Oviedo, Asturias, Spain.

Introduction

Kidney cancers represent approximately 2% of all new cancers. [1] The average age at diagnosis is 55 to 60 years. The tumors affect males more commonly than females with a ratio of 1,5:1.

Environmental, occupational, hormonal and genetic factors have been associated with the development of renal cell carcinoma. [2] Long-term cigarette smoking, high body weight and hypertension are associated with a higher relative risk for development of these tumors. [3] Von Hippel Lindau disease has been associated association with renal cell carcinoma. [4]

Primary renal cancer may spread by local infiltration throught the renal capsule to involve the perinephric fat and Gerota´s fascia. The tumor may grow directly to the renal vein or vena cava along the venous channels. Lymph node metastases often involve the renal hiliar, para-aortic and paracaval lymph nodes with an incidence of 9% to 27%. The renal vein is invaded by tumor in 21% of cases and the inferior vena cava is invaded aproximately in 4% of cases. [5] The sites of distribution of metastases among patients presenting with spread disease include lung, soft tissue, bone, liver, skin and central nervous system. Patients with metastatic disease at diagnosis have a poor prognosis with an expected survival less than 5 years. [6, 7]

Classic triad (gross hematuria, palpable flank mass and pain) occurs only in 5%-10% of patients. Most of patients with renal cell carcinoma may present with an occult primary tumor or with signs and symptoms attributable to a local mass or systemic paraneoplastic síndromes. [8, 9]

Standard therapy for nonmetastatic renal cell carcinoma is radical nephrectomy. Adenocarcinoma of the kidney is a variable radiosensitive neoplasm. In *vivo* experiments demonstrated a decrease in the rate of tumor transplantation in nude mice after pretreatment of human renal cell carcinoma cells with radiation therapy. These data support the existence of a theoretical benefit to preoperative radiation in decreasing tumor shedding at the time of an operation. [10] Other data suggest that some renal cell cancer lines are resistant to conventionally radiation therapy schedules. [11] Clinical experiences demonstrated very good response rates in patients receiving palliative radiation for symptomatic metastases from renal cell carcinoma. [12, 13, 14, 15, 16]

Despite the favorable effect that radiation has against this neoplasm in advanced disease, it has not convincingly improved the results of patients treated in an adjuvant setting for early stage disease. Historically several retrospective series suggested a clinical benefit of adjuvant radiation. These reports can be appropiately criticized for inadequate balance between groups of patients treated. [17]

The side effects and complications from radiation therapy for cancer of the kidney are similar to those expected from radiation of the upper abdomen and pelvis. These side effects include nausea, vomiting, diarrea and abdomianl cramping. Patients with right-sided tumors may have significant portions of the liver irradiated, and radiation-induced liver damage is possible.

Preoperative Radiation

Two European prospective randomized studies were undertaken to test the efficacy of preoperative radiation therapy in renal cell carcinoma.

The first study was conducted in Rotterdam and no advantage was demonstrated to overall survival or survival free of distant metastases in patients receiving radiation therapy. The technique used in these patients was 30-Gy midplane dose to the involved kidney and regional lymph nodes, with 2-Gy daily fractions administered over a period of 3 weeks. After completion of radiation therapy the patients underwent radical nephrectomy. Preoperative radiation therapy did appear to increase the rate of complete resectability in patients with locally advanced tumors. No benefit was demonstrated with preoperative radiation. [18] The second study was conducted in Sweden and it was unable to demonstrate an advantage to patients receiving preoperative radiation therapy. [18]

Radiation therapy appears to increase the resectability of locally advanced tumors either in retrospective and prospective series of patients. [19, 20]

Postoperative Radiation

In early retrospective studies postoperative radiation therapy was reported to be beneficial. [21,22] Rafla reported series of patients receiving radiation therapy after nephrectomy had better rates of survival and local control at 5 and 10 years than patients undergoing just nephrectomy . The series were not well characterized in regard to radiation therapy technique or dose used and the method through wich patients were selected to receive or not receive radiation therapy was not described. [22] Other series showed no advantage of postoperative radiation therapy. [23]

Later series testing the value of postoperative radiation did not demonstrate the benefit to patients receiving radiation therapy after surgery. The first study, a prospective randomized study, from New Castle; United Kingdom, demonstrated an inferior survival for patients receiving radiation therapy compared with those treated with surgery alone. Local recurrences were not affected by the postoperative radiation therapy. No stratification of patients by tumor stage or grade was made. [24] The second study, another prospective randomized study, conduced by the Cophenagen Renal Cancer Study Group compared patients with stage II or III renal cell cancer treated with nephrectomy and patients treated with nephrectomy plus radiation therapy to the kidney bed and regional lymph nodes. No difference in relapse rate was found between the two study groups. There were significant complications involving 44% of patients receiving postoperative radiation therapy and 19% of deaths in the irradiated group were attributed to radiation-induced complications. [25]

Randomized trials studying the benefits of postoperative radiotherapy coincide in pointing out that regular use does not seem to be a clinical indication. Just seems to be beneficial in some clinical situations.

The lack of benefit of posoperative radiation in the prospective clinical trials may be explained by poor patient selection and radiation therapy technique. The majority of patients in these series had T1 or T2 tumors. Patients with lymph node metastases or positive margins had a higher local failure rate of 21% compared with 4% in patients without these bad prognostic features. [26] This suggests that a benefit from postoperative radiation exists, but it would be demonstrable only in patients with adverse pathologic features and a higher risk of local failure. Early tumors have good local control rate and, therefore radiation therapy would not be expected to demonstrate a beneficial role in patients with these tumors.

Kao et al., in a retrospective series, reported that patients with high-risk locally advanced tumors with perinephric invasion or surgical positive margins had a 100% local control rate if treated with adjuvant postoperative radiation. The local control rate was 30% at 5-year in comparation to a similar group treated with surgery only, with statistical significance. Sequelae after high doses of radiation were minimal due to the use of CT-based simulation. [27] Another retrospective series revealed that patients with T3 tumors had a statistical significant lower local failure rate when given postoperative radiation, compared with similar patients undergoing just surgery [28]. This series has been updated and actually the risk of local recurrence ocurred exclusively in patients with T3b disease. These autors have now concluded that postoperative radiation therapy is not indicated for patients with renal cell cancer. [29]

In a retrospective series of patients with locally advanced renal cell carcinoma for patients with T3/N0 disease, radiation therapy reduced the rate of local recurrence, although an impact on survival was not shown. No other subgroups benefited from the adjuvant radiation therapy. [30]

Some contemporary retrospective series have suggested a limited benefit of postoperative radiation therapy in selected patients with a high risk of local recurrence. [28, 29, 31]

Based in all these aforementioned prospective and retrospective data, the following indications for radiation therapy should be considered:

- Unresectable nonmetastatic tumors
- Incomplete resection with gross or microscopically positive margins

Althought radiation therapy may decrease the local recurrence rate, an improvement in overall survival may not be demonstrated.

Radiotherapy for Metastatic and Recurrent Disease

Palliative radiation therapy is effective at relieving symptoms from metastatic renal cell cancer. [14, 15, 31, 17] A patient with a solitary bone metastasis may have a long survival and consequently, a sufficient radiation dose should be administered to allow durable pain relief. If surgery is used to remove a metastasis, postoperative radiation therapy is indicated to prevent its recurrence.

Lee et al. showed that a high percentage of patients treated for pain had experienced significant pain relief with 30 Gy radiation delivered in 10 fractions.[32] Palliation of neurologic symptoms from brain metastases, spinal-cord compression or nerve invasión is not as successful as relief of pain from bone metastases. [16, 32]

Radiation Therapy Techniques

CT-based treatment planning contributes to good local control with minimal morbidity. Posoperatively, careful definition of the target volumen to encompass the nephrectomy bed, lymph node drainage sites, and surgical clips on the planning CT scan is important.

Exclusive use of anterior-posterior field arrangements, particularly on the right side is likely to result in radiation of large volumes of bowel and liver beyond tolerance. Multiple-beam arrangements, including anterior, posterior, oblique and lateral projections with beam´s eye-view shaping and differential weighting of dose from each field, can optimize the radiation dose distribution to maximize target volumen coverage while minimizing the dose to bowel or liver. Total radiation doses of 45-50 Gy in 1.8-2 Gy daily fractions to the nephrectomy bed and regional lymph nodes with a boost to small volumes or microscopic or gross residual disease with an additional 10 to 15 Gy to a total dose of 50-60 Gy are appropiate. If the scar is not included in the target volume an additional electron beam field to treat the scar may be considered. The high complication rates reported in the prospective trials of postoperative radiation therapy have taught radiation oncologists an important lesson regarding radiation therapy planning, patient selection and the tolerance of the upper-abdominal viscera. Field projections and shaping should be selected to keep no more than 30% of the liver receiving doses over 36 to 40 Gy. The contralateral kidney dose should not exceed 20 Gy in 2 to 3 weeks. The spinal cord dose should be limited to 45 Gy in conventionally fractionated doses of 1.8 to 2 Gy daily. Intensity-modulated radiation therapy (IMRT) may be a reasonable consideration due the sensivity of adjacent surronding structures. If IMRT is considered, a plan to manage the uncertainties in the target localization such as gating or breathing control needs to be considered.

Multiple-field techniques, similar to those described for postoperative radiation therapy, should be considered in patients receiving preoperative treatment. In unresectable lesions, 40 to 50 Gy preoperative radiation therapy directed to the kidney and regional lymphatics may improve resectability. [18]

Because of the possibility of long survival even in the presence of distant metastases, agressive treatment for palliation must be considered in patients who have limited metastatic disease with good performance status. Treatment fields should encompass metastatic foci with adequate margins, 2-3 cm. Radiation therapy doses of 35-40 Gy provide symptomatic relief in 64%-84% of treated patients. [14, 15, 17]

Some series have reported higher symptomatic response rates with higher radiation doses in renal cancer [17]. A palliative dose of 45-50 Gy in 3-4.5 weeks might be considered in selected patients.

New Technologies in Radiotherapy. Stereotactic Radiation Therapy

Stereotactic radiosurgery (SRS) is a highly precise procedure of radiation therapy initially developed to treat small brain tumors and functional abnormalities of the brain. The principles of cranial SRS, namely high precision radiation whith accurate delivery within one to two millimeters, are now being applied to the treatment of body tumors with a technique called stereotactic body radiotherapy (SBRT).

Despite its name, SRS is a non-surgical procedure that delivers precisely-targeted radiation at much higher doses, in only a single or few treatments, as compared to traditional radiation therapy. This treatment is only possible due to the development of highly advanced radiation technologies that permit maximum dose delivery within the target while minimizing dose to the surrounding healthy tissue. The goal is to deliver doses that will destroy the tumor and achieve permanent local control.

SRS and SBRT rely on several technologies:

- Three-dimensional imaging and localization techniques that determine the exact target coordinates within the body
- Systems to immobilize and carefully place the patient maintaining an adequate position during therapy.
- Highly focused gamma-ray or x-ray beams that converge on a tumor or abnormality
- Image-guided radiation therapy (IGRT) which uses medical imaging to confirm the location of a tumor immediately before, and in some cases, during the delivery of radiation. IGRT improves the precision and accuracy of the treatment.

Three-dimensional imaging, such as CT, MRI and PET/CT is used to locate the tumor within the body and to define its exact size and shape. These images also guide the treatment planning (in which radiation beams are designed to converge on the target area from different angles and planes) as well as the careful positioning of the patient for therapy sessions.

Prospective follow-up of 105 patients with extracranial metastases, using single-fraction stereotactic body radiotherapy (≤ 24 Gy) or hypofractionation (eg, five times 12 Gy), showed a 3-year local relapse-free survival of 88% in the group of single-fraction stereotactic body radiotherapy using 24 Gy, compared with 20% survival (significant difference; p=0.001) in the group of single-fraction stereotactic body radiotherapy with less than 24 Gy or hypofractionation. In multivariate analysis, one dose of at least 24 Gy significantly predicted better local progression-free survival. The treatment was very well tolerated, although the authors included a note of caution about increased fracture risk when spinal or heavily involved vertebral bodies were the sites of treatment. [33]

High local control (88% at 18 months), dose-response relation, and dose-per-fraction-response relation was confirmed by data from a retrospective series of patients with renal-cell carcinoma with oligometastatic disease (13 patients, 25 lesions) [34]. All patients were pretreated with targeted drugs (sorafenib and sunitinib). After a median follow-up of 28 months, median overall survival was still not reached. The authors suggested a dose of at least 48 Gy given in three fractions of 16 Gy to achieve optimum local control. [35]

Teh and colleagues [35] treated 14 patients with oligometastatic renal-cell carcinoma who had 23 lesions in total. All patients were heavily pretreated with interleukin 2, interferon, sorafenib, or sunitinib, or in clinical trials of new systemic drugs. 13 patients had improvement in quality of life. Local control at 1 year was 87%. A similar local control rate was noted in 18 patients with 39 metastatic lesions treated with stereotactic body radiotherapy. Fractionation schedules varied from ten times 4–5 Gy to three times 8–14 Gy. [36]

The largest series reported included 50 patients with 162 metastases using doses per fraction of 5–16 Gy according to the localisation of the metastasis and the treatment era [37]. The local control rate was 98% in the 149 lesions that could be assessed. Patients with one to three synchronous metastases had a median survival of 37 months. The same group of authors started a prospective phase 2 trial including 30 patients with 90 lesions. Most lesions were metastatic, with lung and mediastinum being the most frequently involved sites. The investigators used different fractionation schedules, with three and four times 10 Gy and two times 15 Gy being the most frequent. Daily fraction dose was at least 5 Gy in all patients. Overall response rate was 98%, with a complete response at a fifth of treated sites [38]. In all of the above studies of extracranial metastases, one constant reassuring feature is that late toxicity was very mild, with severe toxicity noted in less than 5% of patients.

On the basis of this information, stereotactic body radiotherapy for extracranial renal-cell carcinoma metastases could be considered (level of evidence three; grade C recommendation). The overall response rate is about 90% and the treatment has very little toxicity. [39]

Moreover, stereotactic body radiotherapy is an excellent alternative to metastasectomy for treatment of extracranial metastases that are technically not operable. The major disadvantage of stereotactic body radiotherapy is absence of histopathological confirmation, which is obvious after metastasectomy; however, this issue is less important for known metastatic disease.

Stereotactic radiotherapy in Nervous Central System has been successful at controlling and palliating symptoms [33]. In 69 patients with brain metastases from renal cell cancer, Sheehan et al. reported that in 63% of cases the lesions had decreased and in 33% they remained stable[40]. In 48 patients with spinal metastases, Gerszten et al. reported that 89% of patients experienced improvement in pain following single stereotactic treatments ranging from 17,5 to 25 Gy in dose [41]. The volume of the spinal cord allowed to exceed 8 Gy was kept lower than 3 cm^3.

Conclusion

Radiation therapy has been used in patients with renal cell carcinoma in a number of circunstances including preoperative radiation therapy, postoperative radiation therapy and palliative radiation therapy for either local disease or distant metastases.

Limited benefit of pre and postoperative radiation therapy has been shown. In this way, radiation could be used in unresectable nonmetastatic tumors and incomplete resection with gross or microscopically positive margins. Althought radiation therapy may decrease the local recurrence rate, an improvement in overall survival may not be demonstrated. However, palliative radiation therapy is effective relieving symptoms from metastatic renal cell cancer in 64%-84% of treated patients. Agressive treatment for palliation must be considered in patients who have limited metastatic disease and good performance status. Stereotactic radiotherapy for renal-cell carcinoma metastases may reach response rates of 90% with very little toxicity. [39] Stereotactic body radiotherapy is an excellent alternative to metastasectomy for treatment of extracranial metastases that are technically not operable.

References

[1] Jemal A, Thomas A, Murray T, et al. Cancer statistics, 2006. CA *Cancer J Clin* 2006;56: 106-130.

[2] Michalsky JM. Kidney, renal pelvis and uréter. In: Halperin EC, Perez CA, Brady LW, eds. *Principles and practice of radiation oncology 5th edition.* Philadelphia: Lippincot WW.

[3] Muscat JE, Hoffmann D, Wynder EL. The epidemiology of renal cell carcinoma. A second look. *Cancer* 1995;75:2552-2557.

[4] Christoferson LA, Gustafson MB, Petersen AG. Von Hippel-Lindau´s disease. *JAMA* 1961;178:280-282.

[5] Waters WB, Richie JP. Aggresive surgical approach to renal cell carcinoma: review of 130 cases. *J Urol* 1979; 122:306-309.

[6] Giuliani L, Giberti C, Martorana G et al. Radical extensive surgery for renal cell carcinoma: long-term results and prognostic factors. *J Urol* 1990; 152: 1082-1085.

[7] Selli C, Hinshaw WM, Woodard BH, et al. Stratification of risk factors in renal cell carcinoma. *Cancer* 1983;52:899-903.

[8] Skinner DG, Colvin RB, Vermillion CD, et al. Diagnosis and management of renal cell carcinoma. A clinical and pathologic study of 309 cases. *Cancer* 1971;28: 1165-1177.

[9] Smith RB, deKernion JB, Ehrich RM, et al. Bilateral renal cell carcinoma and renal cell carcinoma in the solitary kidney. *J Urol* 1984;132:450-454.

[10] Otto U, Huland H, Baisch H, et al. Transplantation of human renal cell carcinoma into NMRI nu/nu mice. III. Effect of radiation on tumor acceptance and tumor growth. *J Urol* 1985;134:170-174.

[11] Ning S, Trisler K, Wessels BW, et al. Radiobiologic studies of radioinmnotherapy and external bem radiotherapy in vitro and in vivo in human renal cell carcinoma xenografts. *Cancer 1997*;80:2519-2528.

[12] Dibiase SJ, Valicenti RK, Schultz D, et al. Palliative radiation for focally symptomatic metastatic renal cell carcinoma: support for dose escalation base don a biological model. *J Urol* 1997;158:746-749.

[13] Fossa SD, Kjolseth I, Lund G. RAdiotherapy of metastases from renal cancer. *Eur Urol* 1982;8:340-342.

[14] Halperin EC, Harisiadis L. The role of radiation therapy in the management of metastatic renal cell carcinoma. *Cancer* 1983;51:614-617.

[15] Huguenin PU, Kieser S, Glanzmann C, et al. Radiotherapy for metastatic carcinomas of the kidney or melanomas: an analysis using palliative end points. *Int J Radiat Oncol Biol Phys* 1998;41:401-405.

[16] Onufrey V, Mohiuddin M. Radioation therapy in the treatment of metastatic renal cell carcinoma. *Int J Radiat Oncol Biol Phys* 1985;11:2007-2009.

[17] Flocks RH, Kadesky MC. Malignant neoplasm of the kidney; an analysis of 353 patients followed five yeras or more. *J Urol* 1958;79:196-201.

[18] Juusela H, Malmio K, Alfthan O et al. Preoperative radiation in the treatment of renal adenocarcinoma. *Scand J Urol Nephrol* 1977;11:277-281.

[19] Riches EW. The natural history of renal tumors. In Riches EW, ed. Tumors of the kidney and uréter. Edinburgh: Williams & Wilkins, 1964.

[20] van der Werf-Messing B, van der Heul RO, Ledeboer RC. Renal cell carcinoma trial. Strahlentherapie (Sonderb) 1981;76:169-715.
[21] Blom JH. Adjuvant therapy for adenocarcinoma of the kidney: present position and prospects. *Br J Urol* 1973;45:237-257.
[22] Rafla S. Renal cell carcinoma. Natural history and results of treatment. *Cancer* 1970;25:26-40.
[23] Peeling WB, Mantell BS, Shepheard BG. Post-operative irradaition in the treatment of renal cell carcinoma. *Br J Urol* 1969;41:23-31.
[24] Fuggit RB, Wu GS, MArtinelli LC. An evaluation of postoperative radiotherapy in hipernefroma treatment. A clinical trial. *Cancer* 1973;32:1332-1340.
[25] Kjaer M, Frederiksen PL, Engrlholm SA. Postoperative radiotherapy in stage II and III renal adenocarcinoma. A randomized trial by the Cophenagen Renal Cancer Study Group. *Int J Radiat Oncol Biol Phys* 1987;13:665-672.
[26] Ravinovitch RA, Zelefsky MJ, Gaynor JJ, et al. Patterns of failure following surgical resection of renal cell carcinoma: implications for adjuvant local and systemic therapy. *J. Cin. Oncol.* 1994;12:206-212.
[27] Kao GD, Malkowicz SB, Whittington R, et al. Locally advanced renal cell carcinoma: low complication rate and efficacy of postnephrectomy radiation therapy planned with CT. *Radiology* 1994;193:725-730.
[28] Stein M, Kuten A, Halpern J et al. The value of postoperative radiation in renal cell cancer. *Radiother. Oncol* .1992;24:41-44.
[29] Gez E, Libes M, Bar-Deroma R, et al. Postoperative radiation in localized renal cell carcinoma: the Rambam Medical Center experience. *Tumori* 2002;88:500-502.
[30] Makarewicz R, Zarycka M, Kulinska G, et al. The value of postoperative radiotherapy in advanced renal cell cancer. *Neoplasma* 1998;45:380-383.
[31] Lee J, Hodgson D, Chow E, et al. A phase II trial of palliative radiotherapy for metastatic renal cell carcinoma. *Cancer* 2005;104:1894-1900.
[32] Wronski M, Maor MH, Davis BJ et al. External radiation of brain metastases from renal carcinoma: a retrospective study of 119 patients from the M.D. Andreson Cancer Center. *Int. J. Radiat. Oncol. Biol. Phys.* 1997;37:753-759.
[33] MJ Zelefsky, C Greco, R Motzer, et al.Tumor control outcomes after hypofractionated and single-dose stereotactic image-guided intensity-modulated radiotherapy for extracranial metastases from renal cell carcinoma. *Int. J. Radiat. Oncol. Bio.l Phys.*, 2012;82:1744–1748.
[34] Stinauer MA, Kavanagh BD, Schefter TE, et al. Stereotactic body radiation therapy for melanoma and renal cell carcinoma: impact of single fraction equivalent dose on local control. *Radiat. Oncol.*, 2011;6:34.
[35] Teh B, Bloch C, Galli-Guevara M, et al. The treatment of primary and metastatic renal cell carcinoma (RCC) with image-guided stereotactic body radiation therapy (SBRT) *Biomed. Imaging Interv. J.*, 2007;3;e6.
[36] Ranck MC, Golden DW, Corbin KS, et al. Stereotactic body radiotherapy for the treatment of oligometastatic renal cell carcinoma. *Am. J. Clin. Oncol.* 2013;36:589–595.
[37] Wersäll PJ, Blomgren H, Lax I, et al. Extracranial stereotactic radiotherapy for primary and metastatic renal cell carcinoma. *Radiother. Oncol.*, 2005;77:88–95.

[38] C Svedman C, Sandström P, Pisa P, et al. A prospective phase II trial of using extracranial stereotactic radiotherapy in primary and metastatic renal cell carcinoma. *Acta Oncol.*, 2006;45:870–875.

[39] de Meeleer G, Khoo V, Escudier B, et al. Radiotherapy for renal-cell carcinoma. *The Lancet Oncology*, 2014;15:170-177.

[40] Sheehan JP, Sun MH, Kondziolka D, et al. Radiosurgery in patients with renal cell carcinoma metástasis to the brain: long-term outcomes and prognostic factors influencing survival and local tumor control. *J. Neurosurg.* 2003;98:342-349.

[41] Gerszten PC, Burton SA, Ozhasoglu C, et al. Stereotactic radiosurgery for spinal metastases from renal cell carcinoma. *J. Neurosurg. Spine* 2005;3:288-295.

In: Renal Cell Carcinoma ISBN: 978-1-63482-495-8
Editors: J. M. Fernández-Gomez, J. García-Rodríguez

Chapter 10

New Strategies for Advanced Renal Cell Carcinoma

E. Esteban González, PhD*, N. Villanueva Palicio, MD, C. Álvarez Fernández, MD, L. Sánchez Lorenzo, MD and P. Solis Hernández, MD

Department of Medical Oncology Hospital Universitario Central de Asturias, Oviedo, Asturias, Spain

Abstract

Renal Cell Carcinoma (RCC) treatment is based on curative surgery in localized stages. For other patients with the baseline-advanced disease, or those with relapse, which account for about 60% of all cases, the therapeutic option of choice had been based on a non-specific systemic immunological treatment with Cytokines (interleukin-2 and/or interferon-alfa) associated or not with primary cyto-reductive surgery. More recently, advances in knowledge of the molecular biology of RCC have allowed understand certain signalling pathways related with the Von Hippel Lindau (VHL) gene. One of its functions is to code for a protein involved in control of the Hypoxia-Inducible Factor and, at the same time, with tyrosine kinase growth factors and receptors associated with angiogenesis and tumour proliferation. The inactivation of the VHL gene leads to an over-expression of these factors and their receptors, thus causing the stimulation of angiogenesis, tumour growth and the activation of the metastatic cascade. Based on that, agents targeting vascular growth factor and mammalian target of rapamycin signalling pathways have been developed showing an improvement in terms of survival and represent the present standard first- and second-line treatment options in advanced RCC. In this chapter details of genetic and molecular biology of RCC, its influence in prognosis and predicting models, and the role of surgery at the present antiangiogenic era as well as new systemic strategies based on more selective immunotherapy are reviewed.

* E-mail: eestebang@seom.org.

Keywords: therapy advanced Renal Cell Carcinoma

Introduction

Renal Cell Carcinoma (RCC) represents about 2% of all tumours occurring in adults and is 12th out of all cancer deaths. [1] Its incidence has been increasing progressively in the Western population over the last three decades by 2% and 4% per year. [2] There are environmental factors, apart from genetic factors, that can have an influence on RCC development. Among them, smoking and obesity are the ones that seem to have the strongest relationship to the development of this tumour. [3, 4] It is estimated that RCC is inherited in ~4% of patients, and is sporadic in origin in 96% of patients with different genetic anomalies identified in most of the patients affected. Hence, RCC is considered to comprise a group of different tumours including clear-cell (75%), papillary (12%) chromophobe (4%), oncocytoma (4%), collecting duct (1%) and other unclassified (3-4%) tumours. [4]

RCC treatment is based on curative surgery in localized stages. For other patients with the baseline-advanced disease or those with relapse, which account for about 60% of all cases, the therapeutic option had been based on a non-specific systemic immunological treatment with cytokines (CK). The small role played by chemotherapy in RCC management is attributed to the intrinsic or primary resistance of this tumour, caused by the expression of a membrane transport protein called glycoprotein P170, which is coded by the multi-resistant MDR-1 genes that are over-expressed in 70% of RCC cases. [5] Advances in knowledge of the molecular biology of RCC have allowed to detect certain signalling pathways that appear to play a relevant role in tumour progression. The most important pathway is associated with the Von Hippel Lindau (VHL) gene, which acts as a tumour suppressor and is located on the 3p chromosome. This gene is inactive in approximately 80% of all clear cell renal carcinomas due to deletion, mutation or methylation. One of its functions is to code for a protein involved in control of the Hypoxia-Inducible Factor (HIF) and, at the same time, with tyrosine kinase (TK) growth factors and receptors associated with angiogenesis and tumour proliferation, such as the vascular endothelial growth factor (VEGF), the platelet-derived growth factor (PDGF) and the transforming growth factor (TGFα). The inactivation of the VHL gene leads to an over-expression of these factors and their receptors, producing the stimulation of angiogenesis, tumour growth and the activation of the metastatic cascade. Thus, these have become therapeutic targets for the development of specific biological antiangiogenic agents. [6-9]

Systemic Therapy for Advanced RCC Based on Immunotherapy

Two decades ago, metastatic RCC patients were treated with non-specific immunotherapy agents such as interferon-alfa (IFN-α) and interleukin-2 (IL-2). In this context, different combinations and dosages of IFN-α and IL-2, both as single agent and in combination, have been tested. Response to high-dose IL-2 were described in up to 20% of patients, of which 5% of them have been considered long-lasting responses. [10] Phase III trials in which high-dose IL-2 was compared with low-dose IL-2 or a combination of IFN-α plus low-dose IL-2, were unable to demonstrate any benefit regarding survival. [11-13] Additionally, higher morbidity was observed in the high-dose of Il-2 arm in special due to the incidence of capillary leak syndrome. [14] In a retrospective analysis of six clinical trials in which patients received IFN-α as first-line systemic therapy, it was concluded that the efficacy outcomes achieved by IFN-α, with a median overall survival (OS) of 13 months, could be used as a baseline for the assessment of new therapies. [15] Based on the acquired experience with IFN-α, five prognostic factors and three risk categories were defined in a retrospective analysis to predict survival (table 1).

The five prognostic factor were related with low Karnofsky status (≤ 70%), high lactate dehydrogenase (LDH), low serum haemoglobin, high corrected serum calcium, and less than one year from diagnosis to IFN-α administration.

Overall, in this retrospective analysis the median survival time was 10 months (95% confidence interval [CI] of 9 to 11 months). Patients were considered as having a favourable risk if they had none of these clinical features (median OS of 20 months). Intermediate risk was assigned to those patients with one or two risk factors (median OS of 10 months) and Poor risk category was assigned to those patients with three or more risk factors (median OS of 4 months). [16]

Table 1. Prognostic Factors Criteria and Overall Survival

	MSKCC Risk Criteria for CK therapy (16)	Median OS (months)	Heng Risk Criteria for antiangiogenic therapy (36)	Median OS (months)
Prognostic Factors	KPS < 80 Diagnosis to therapy < 1 year Anemia Hypercalcaemia Elevated LDH		KPS < 80 Diagnosis to therapy < 1 year Anemia Hypercalcaemia Neutrophilia Thrombocytosis	
Favourable Risk	None factor	20	None factor	38
Intermediate Risk	1-2 factors	10	1-2 factors	27
Poor Risk	> 2 Factors	4	3-6 factors	8.8

Lactate dehydrogenase (LDH)
Memorial Sloan Kettering Cancer Center (MSKCC)
Cytokines (CK)
Overall Survival (OS)

Systemic Therapy for Advanced RCC Based on Angiogenesis Inhibitors

First-Line Treatment

In recent years, several agents inhibiting the VEGF and *m*-TOR pathways have demonstrated activity in RCC. Among these agents, sunitinib an oral multi-targeted inhibitor of several tyrosine kinases (TKIs), including VEGF receptor (VEFGR), PDGFR, c-kit and Flt-3 TK was evaluated as first-line therapy in a large phase III trial. In this study, patients with clear cell RCC and good or intermediate prognosis were randomised to sunitinib (50 mg orally once daily for 4 weeks followed by two weeks' rest) or IFN-α (9 million international units [MIU] subcutaneously three times a week). The median progression free survival (PFS) as the primary objective of this study was statistically longer in the sunitinib arm in comparison with the IFN-α arm (11 vs 5 months; HR: 0.42, p <0.001). In terms of OS, a non-significant strong trend was observed in favour of sunitinib arm (26.4 vs 21.8 months; HR 0.85: p=0.051). Nevertheless, when patients allowed to crossover between both treatment arms were censored, a significant improvement in OS was observed in favour of sunitinib (28.1 vs 14 months; HR 0.64: p=0.0036). [17]

On the other hand, bevacizumab, a humanised recombinant anti-VEGF antibody that binds VEGF-A ligand, has demonstrated its efficacy in two randomised trials carried out in metastatic RCC untreated patients with predominant clear cell histology and good-intermediate prognosis. In a double-blind phase III trial, patients were randomized to receive 10 mg/kg of intravenous bevacizumab every two weeks plus 9 million international units (MIU) of IFN-α three times per week by subcutaneous injection, or placebo plus the same dose of IFN-α. Results of this study, in terms of PFS, were in favour of the bevacizumab plus IFN-α arm (10.2 vs 5.4 months; HR: 0.51 p=0.0001). [18] In a similar second multicenter phase III trial, patients were randomised to bevacizumab (10 mg/kg every two weeks) plus IFN-α (9 million MIU three times per week) or IFN-α monotherapy. [19] Once again, the incorporation of Bevacizumab to IFN-α showed an improvement in terms of PFS with respect to the single agent IFN-α (8.5 months vs 5.2 months; HR; 0.53: p<0.0001) although impact in the OS in both studies was not significant.

On the other hand, temsirolimus an m-TOR selective inhibitor has also been notable due to the improvement described in terms of OS and PFS in a particular group of patients with metastatic RCC. Patients considered as poor prognosis defined if they had at least three factors predictors of short survival (a serum LDH level >1.5 x upper normal limit; a haemoglobin level below the lower normal limit; a corrected serum calcium level >2.5 mmol/L; a time from initial diagnosis to randomisation <1 year, a Karnofsky performance score <60-70; existence of metastases in multiple organs), were randomized to receive treatment with IFN-α (escalated from 3 to 18 MIU three times per week if tolerated), temsirolimus (25 mg as a weekly intravenous infusion), or a combination of both (15 mg of temsirolimus and 3 to 6 MIU). Results of this study confirmed that temsirolimus as single agent was superior to IFN-α in terms of median OS (10.9 vs 7.3 months; HR 0.73: p=0.008), which was the main end-point of the study, and PFS (5.5 vs 3.1 months, p<0.001). The combination of temsirolimus and IFN-α did not improve the results obtained with IFN-α alone. [20] Pazopanib represents a second-generation oral TKI with highly selective activity against VEGFR 1, 2, and 3, PDGFR-α and β, and c-kit. Its efficacy was evaluated initially in a double blind phase III trial (VEG105192; NCT00334282 trial) in which patients with clear-cell advanced RCC, with no prior treatment or one prior CK-based treatment, were randomized to receive pazopanib or placebo. In this study, pazopanib significantly improved PFS, especially in those patients who had not received prior therapy (11.1 vs. 2.8 months with placebo; HR 0.40: $p<0.0000001$). [21] More recently, pazopanib has been compared with sunitinib (COMPARZ study) in a non-inferiority phase III trial. Patients with a good or intermediate prognosis and predominant clear cell were randomized to receive pazopanib (800 mg daily) or sunitinib (50 mg daily 4 week followed by two weeks rest). In that study, Pazopanib was shown to be non-inferior to sunitinib in terms of median PFS (pazopanib 8.4 vs. 9.5 months for sunitinib; HR: 1.047). Additionally, the median OS described was 28.4 months for patients treated with pazopanib and 29.3 months for sunitinib-treated patients. [22]

Based on these data, all these drugs have been approved in first line for the treatment of patients with advanced RCC. Several guidelines in oncology recommend that as first line treatment, patients with favourable or intermediate prognosis and clear cell histology should receive sunitinib or pazopanib or bevacizumab plus IFN-α and those patients with poor prognosis should receive temsirolimus (Table 2). [23, 24]

Second-Line Treatment in Patients Previously Treated with Cytokines

Sorafenib an oral multi-targeted inhibitor of several TK such as Raf-1, B-Raf, VEGFR-2 and PDGFR has been the first TKI showing efficacy on second line treatment. Its efficacy was evaluated through the TARGET study. In this double blind phase III trial, patients with previously CK-treated metastatic clear-cell RCC of low- or intermediate-risk, were randomised to sorafenib (400 mg orally twice a day) or placebo.

The results confirmed that patients treated with sorafenib obtained better results in terms of PFS in comparison with placebo (5.5 vs 2.8 months; HR: 0.44; $P < .00000$). The median OS as primary end-point of this study was comparable between patients treated with sorafenib or placebo (17.8 *v* 15.2 months; HR: 0.88; $p=0.146$). However, when post–cross-over placebo survival data were censored, the difference became significant in favour of those patients who were treated with sorafenib (17.8 *v* 14.3 months, respectively; HR = 0.78; *p:* .029. [25]

Pazopanib has also demonstrated its efficacy in second line treatment in patients previously treated with CK. As was mentioned before, in a phase III trial carried out in patients with advanced clear-cell RCC (VEG105192; NCT00334282 trial), forty-six percent of them had received prior CK-therapy and in this group, pazopanib significantly improved PFS compared to placebo (9.2 months vs. 4.2 months; HR 0.46: $p<0.0001$). [21]

Second-Line Therapy in Anti-VEGF-Refractory Patients

The first agent showing activity in second-line therapy in anti-VEGF refractory patients was everolimus, an mTOR oral inhibitor that affects tumour growth by blocking growth factor stimulation, arresting cell cycle progression and inhibiting angiogenesis.

Table 2. First-Line treatment of advanced Renal Cell Carcinoma. Efficacy overview

Histology and Prognosis	Nº Pts	ORR (%)	Median PFS (months)	Median OS (months)	Guidelines Recommendations	
Clear Cell Favourable-intermediate prognosis					NCCN (23) Category	ESMO (24) Level and grade
Sunitinib vs IFN-α [17]	750	47 vs 12	11 vs 5	26.4 vs 21.8	1 Sunitinib	I,A Sunitinib
Bevacizumab+ IFN-α vs IFN-α [18]	649	31 vs 12	10.1 vs 5.5	23.3 vs 21.3	1 Bevacizumab + IFN	I,A Bevacizumab+ IFN
Bevacizumab+ IFN-α vs IFN-α [19]	732	25.5 vs 13.1	8.4 vs 4.5	18.3 vs 17.4		
Pazopanib vs Placebo [21]	233	32 vs 4	11.1 vs 2.8	22.9 vs 20.5	1 Pazopanib	I,A Pazopanib
Pazopanib vs Sunitinib [22]	1110	33 vs 29	8.4 vs 9.5	28.4 vs 29.3		
Predominant Non-Clear Cell Poor prognosis						
Temsirolimus vs IFN-α [20]	626	8.6 vs 4.8	5.5 vs 3.1	10.9 vs 7.3	1 Temsirolimus	II,A Temsirolimus

Patients (Pts)
Objective Response Rate (ORR)
Progression free Survival (PFS)
Overall Survival (OS)

In a phase III trial named RECORD-1, everolimus (10 mgr a day) was compared to placebo in a double blind design. The median PFS as the primary end-point was in favour of those patients treated with everolimus (4.9 months vs 1.9 months; HR 0.33: $P<.001$). [26] Subsequent analyses of data from this trial showed that everolimus offered similar results in terms of PFS for those patients treated in third-line therapy. These findings support the use of everolimus for patients who do not respond or stop responding to VEGFR TKIs on second and third line (TKI-mTOR sequence). Nevertheless, in this study, the median OS of patients given everolimus was not significant that of patients given placebo (14.7 vs 14.3 months; HR 0.87; *P*=.162), due to patients from the placebo group (76.2%) crossed over to the everolimus group.

The prospective, randomized phase III AXIS trial compared the efficacy of the TKIs axitinib (an oral selective anti-VEGFR TKI) with sorafenib in patients with advanced RCC who developed progressive disease after only one previous systemic therapy with either sunitinib, cytokines, temsirolimus, or a combination of bevacizumab and IFN-α. The median PFS as the primary end-point of this study was statistically longer in the axitinib arm in comparison with the sorafenib arm (6.7 vs 4.7 months; HR: 0.665, $p<0.001$). In a subgroup analysis, patients with axitinib who had been previously treated with CK (30% of population included) had even longer PFS (12.1 months vs 6.5 with sorafenib; HR 0.4, $p=0.0001$) than did patients given axitinib who underwent first-line therapy with sunitinib (55% of population included) (4.8 months vs 3.4 with sorafenib; HR 0.74, $p=0.014$). Additionally, the global analysis of OS in this study did not differ between axitinib and sorafenib (15.2 vs 16.5 months; HR 0.969: $p=0.374$). [27] Either way, the Axis trail can be considered as the first strong evidence supporting the use of another TKI on second line for patients who progress to VEGFR TKIs (TKI-TKI sequence).

The INTORSECT trial has been the third study published in the context of second-line therapy in anti-VEGF-Refractory patients. This is the only a comparing head-to-head an mTOR (temsirolimus) and a VEGFR-TKI (sorafenib) in a pure second line treatment in patients previously treated and in progression to sunitinib. Results did not show superiority of temsirolimus in the median PFS with respect to sorafenib (4.3 vs 3.9 months; HR 0.87, $p=0.19$). However, in terms of median OS as a secondary end-point, patients treated with sorafenib achieved better results with respect to those treated with temsirolimus (16.6 vs 12.3 months) suggesting some advantage in favour of the antiVEGF sequence (TKI-TKI) with respect to the TKI-mTOR sequence. [26]

Based on all these data, either sorafenib, pazopanib or axitinib have been approved for the treatment of patients with advanced RCC previously treated with CK.

At the same time, either everolimus or axitinib have been approved for the treatment on second-line therapy in Anti-VEGF-refractory patients and recommended in several guidelines of oncology (Table 3). [23, 24] At this point, its worthy of mention that axitinib has restricted is indication from the European Medicines Agency (EMA) for adult patients with RCC after failure of prior treatment with sunitinib or a CK.

Third-Line Therapy in Anti-VEGF-Refractory Patients

There exist several randomized studies offering information related with third line therapy in anti-VEGF-Refractory patients. In the RECORD-I study, one hundred and forty-one patients (34% of all population included this trial) who had previously progressed to sunitinib and sorafenib were treated with everolimus or placebo in third line. In this population and in a subgroup analysis, everolimus showed an improvement in the median PFS with respect to placebo (4 vs 1.8 months; HR 0.32: $p< 0.001$) and might be considered the first evidence of activity for a drug in third line of treatment as well as for a TKI-TKI-mTOR sequence. [24]

Table 3. Second-Line treatment of advanced Renal Cell Carcinoma. Efficacy overview

Clear Cell Histology	Nº Pts	ORR (%)	Median PFS (months)	Median OS (months)	Guidelines Recommendations	
Post-CK					NCCN [23] Category	ESMO [24] Level and grade
Sorafenib vs Placebo [25]	903	10 vs 2	5.5 vs 2.8	17.8 vs 15.2	1 Sorafenib	I,A Sorafenib
Pazopanib vs Placebo [21]	202	NR	7.4 vs 4.2	NR	1 Pazopanib	II,A Pazopanib
Axitinib vs Sorafenib [27]	251	19.4 vs 9.4	12 vs 6.5	NR	1 Axitinib	I,A Axitinib
Post-TKI						
Everolimus vs Placebo [26]	89	1.8 vs 0	4.9 vs 1.9	14.8 vs 14.4	1 Everolimus	II,A Everolimus
Axitinib vs Sorafenib [27]	448	NR	4.8 vs 3.4	15.2 vs 16.5	1 Axitinib	I,B Axitinib
Temsirolimus vs Sorafenib [28]	512	8 vs 8	4.3 vs 3.9	12.3 vs 16.6	2B Temsirolimus	NR

Cytokines (CK)
Tirosin Kinase Inhibitor (TKI)
Patients (Pts)
Objective Response Rate (ORR)
Progression free Survival (PFS)
Overall Survival (OS)
No reference (NR)

Later on, the GOLD study has been the first phase III trial comparing two TKIs in the third-line setting following both VEGF and mTOR inhibitor drugs.

This study was based on a hypothetical mechanism for acquired resistance thought activation of the fibroblastic growth factor (FGF) pathway as an antiangiogenic escape from VEGF-targeted therapies. In this way, Dovitinib was selected for comparison with sorafenib based on its targeting profile that includes fibroblastic growth factor receptor (FGFR), in addition to the VEGFR and PDGFR inhibition. Results of this study did not meet its primary endpoint of demonstrating PFS superiority for dovitinib over sorafenib (median 3.7 vs 3.6 months; HR 0.36: p=0.06). [29] Nevertheless, both TKIs showed anti-tumour activity in the third-line setting in comparison with historical control data in terms of PFS and OS (28] Thus, the results of this study support the use of a VEGFR TKI in patients who have already received prior VEGF and mTOR inhibitors as well as a TKI-mTOR-TKI sequence of treatment.

According to these data, guidelines such as ESMO recommend everolimus (level of evidence II, A) for patients already treated with two TKIs (or a TKI and bevacizumab). In the same way, for patients previously treated with VEGF-TKI and mTOR inhibitor, another TKI (in example sorafenib) might be an option of treatment in third line (evidence III, B) (Table 4). [24]

Role of Surgery in Advanced Renal Cell Carcinoma

In contrast to the management of other solid tumours, surgery can be performed in advanced RCC. This approach is justified because of cyto-reductive nephrectomy not only helps to control the symptoms, but also offering a potential benefit in survival. [30] In the era of CK therapy, cyto-reductive nephrectomy before systemic therapy with IFN-α was shown to provide a survival benefit in patients with good PS when compare with only single systemic treatment with IFN-α. In a study performed by the Southwest Oncology Group (SWOG), patients with metastatic RCC were randomised to either IFN-α alone or nephrectomy followed by IFN-α. Patients who underwent surgery plus immunotherapy obtained an advantage in OS over those who received immunotherapy alone (median OS 11.1 vs 8.1 months; p=0.012). [31]

Likewise, the European Organization for Research and Treatment of Cancer (EORTC) carried out a similar study in which patients with metastatic RCC were randomised to either IFN-α alone or nephrectomy followed by IFN-α.

Table 4. Third-Line treatment of advanced Renal Cell Carcinoma. Efficacy overview

Clear Cell Histology	N° Pts	ORR (%)	Median PFS (months)	Median OS (months)	Guidelines Recommendations	
Post-TKI					NCCN[23] Category	ESMO[24] Level and grade
Everolimus vs Placebo [26]	141	NR	4 vs 1.9	NR	NR	II,A Everlolimus
Dovitinib vs Sorafenib [29]	570	4 vs 4	43.7 vs 3.6	11.1 vs 11	NR	I,B Sorafenib

Cytokines (CK)
Tirosin Kinase Inhibitor (TKI)
Patients (Pts)
Objective Response Rate (ORR)
Progression free Survival (PFS)
Overall Survival (OS)
No reference (NR)

The median OS was again significantly higher for patients who underwent surgery plus immunotherapy (17.0 vs 7.0 months; HR: 0.54, p<0.00001). [32] Metastasectomy has also had an important role in advanced RCC with long-term survival described in 30% of patients. In retrospective analysis, favourable predictors of survival for these patients included a single site or limited number (≤ than 4) of lung resectable metastases, and a long disease-free interval. [33]

In the era of antiangiogenic therapy, there exist retrospective information in favor of cyto-reductive nephrectomy for those patients without poor risk and appropriate PS.

Data from 1511 consecutive patients treated at 20 international cancer centers with antiangiogenic targeted therapy (most of them with sunitinib) and with or without nephrectomy for metastatic RCC, have been recently given to know. The results described in this study in terms of median OS were in favour of those patients with reductive nephrectomy (20.6 vs 9.5 months (HR 0.60; p<0.0001). [34] Two prospective phase III clinical trials are currently evaluating cytoreductive nephrectomy and their results should be more definitive than these retrospective analyses. In this way, the SURTIME trial is searching the best sequence between nephrectomy followed by sunitinib or sunitinib at the beginning followed by nephrectomy, and the CARMENA trial is comparing sunitinib associated to nephrectomy versus only sunitinib. On the other hand, metastasectomy can continue being considered for selected patients likewise was mentioned before and especially in patients who have achieved a sufficient decrease in tumour load after antiangiogenic therapy such as sunitinib. [35]

Advances and New Strategies in the Management of Advanced Metastatic Disease

Prognostic and Predictive Factors

Currently, the first and subsequent lines of treatment based on antiangiogenic agents have been able to offer an improvement in the median OS of patients with advanced RCC. In this era of VEGF-targeted therapies, new prognostic variables have been described following the prognostic factor model from the Memorial Sloan-Kettering Cancer Center (MSKCC). [16] In a retrospective analysis Heng and cols, examined 645 patients treated with VEGF-targeted therapies in first line. [36] Their results confirmed that four of the five adverse prognostic factors according to the MSKCC were independent predictors of short survival: hemoglobin less than the lower limit of normal, corrected calcium greater than the upper limit of normal, Karnofsky performance status less than 80%, and time from diagnosis to treatment of less than 1 year. In addition, neutrophils greater than the ULN ($P < .0001$) and platelets greater than the ULN ($P = .01$) were independent adverse prognostic factors. According to this prognostic factors, patients were included into three categories: The Favourable group of prognosis (no prognostic factor) with a median OS of 38 months; the Intermediate group of prognosis (one or two prognostic factors), in which median OS was 27 months; and the Poor group of prognosis (three to six prognostic factors) in which median OS was 8.8 months. [36] Likewise, these results have confirmed the improvement in terms of median OS achieved with the incorporation of VEGF-targeted therapy when compared with historical results described with CK.

On the other hand, the knowledge of biomarkers that predict response to existing agents in RCC should allow targeting of patients expected to derive in an improvement in terms of survival and spare unnecessary drug exposure. Potential biomarkers have been described in plasma (pro-angiogenic and anti-angionenic chemokines, angiogenic factors, and circulating CD34þ/CD35þ cells) or by genetic characteristics (polymorphisms in genes involved in angiogenesis, drug metabolism, or cell differentiation). Among them, polymorphisms of interleukin-8 (IL-8) or VEGFR have been related with VEGF-targeted agents as well as levels of LDH with m-TOR inhibitors. [37-39] On the other hand, some kind of toxicities related with antiantigenic therapy has been described as independent clinical biomarkers of response such as arterial hypertension (AHTN), hand and food syndrome or asthenia/fatigue. [40] Nevertheless, none of these prognostic or predictive plasmatic, genetic or clinical biomarkers have been prospectively validated in multiple independent studies.

Combination and Best Sequence of Treatment

Combination therapy for advanced RCC might be useful because of the possibility of synergistic activity arising from targeting multiple pro-angiogenic pathways limiting escape that are thought to mediate resistance. However, trials of VEGF-targeted agents (bevacizumab or sorafenib) associated with mTOR inhibitors (temsirolimus or everolimus) in advanced RCC such as the INTORAC, RECORD-2 and BEST studies have been disappointing, showing more toxicity and no superior efficacy with respect to standard treatment. [41-43]

Sequential treatment in comparison to combination strategy might be another way to overcome resistance with advantages in terms of cost and minimizing exposure to toxicity. Additional such as was described earlier in this chapter is possible to use a different TKI followed by an mTOR inhibitor or another TKI showing all of these strategies absence of complete cross-resistance. [26-28] Looking at studies investigating the best sequence and their results, to date, only a few of them are available. The large, randomized phase II trial RECORD-3 was designed to compare the sequence of sunitinib in first line followed by everolimus versus everolimus followed by sunitinib at progression disease. The results of this study demonstrated that sunitinib in first line followed by everolimus is the most effective sequential treatment for patients with advanced RCC, given that the reverse combination did not meet the PFS non-inferiority endpoint of a hazard ratio equal or less than 1.1 (median 10.7 months with sunitnib vs 7.8 months with everolimus; HR 1.4; 95% CI, 1.2–1.8). [44]

Additionally, the RECORD-3 study showed that sunitinib in first-line followed by everolimus, (a TKI–mTOR vs mTOR-TKI sequence), offer the best results in terms of patient survival times (median OS up to 32 months). The SWITCH study is another randomized trial (in this case a phase III trial) investigating the best sequence between sorafenib followed by sunitinib vs. the opposite sequence (a TKI-TKI sequence). Once again, that study did not meet the primary endpoint demonstrating superiority of sorafenib-sunitinib over sunitinib-sorafenib for total PFS measured over the two sequential therapies [45]. Additionally, the total PFS duration reached 12.5 months in the sorafenib-sunitinib arm versus 14.9 months in the sunitinib-sorafenib arm (HR: 1.01; p= 0.54) suggest a tendency to better results with this last sequence. The median OS in this study (31.5 months in the sorafenib-sunitinib arm and 30.2 months in the sunitinib-sorafenib arm) is close similar to that described with sunitinib in the RECORD-3 study, encouraging the predominant position of sunitinib in first line sequence treatment for those patients with advanced clear RCC considered as good-intermediate risk prognosis.

Options of Treatment for Patients with Non-Clear Cell Renal Cell Carcinoma

RCC of the non-clear cell histologic subtype are notably less common than clear cell and for that reason there exist limited experience and no standard treatment for advanced stage. [46] Experience with chemotherapy based on gemcitabine associated or not to doxorubicin or capecitabine for RCC with predominantly sarcomatoid features or with cisplatinum for collecting duct carcinoma have been published. [47, 48]

In the era of antiangiogenic therapy, the majority of information available is from retrospective studies or exploratory subgroup analyses of larger phase III trials.

Of the available therapies, mTOR inhibitors, mainly temsirolimus, have shown the greatest efficacy in non-clear cell RCC in a subgroup analysis from a phase III trial in comparison with IFN-α in patients considered as poor prognosis. [20] Anti-VEGFR inhibitors, such as sunitinib and sorafenib, have also proven to be effective in restrictive samples of patients and retrospective analysis. [49]

More recently, a small randomized phase II trial analyzing the best sequence in first and second line treatment between sunitinib and everolimus carried out in 108 patients with non-clear cell histology has shown a tendency to better results with sunitinib in terms of median PFS (6.1 with vs 4.1 months with everolimus $p=0.25$) and OS (not reached vs 10.5 months with everolimus $p=0.01$). [50]

Thus, in the absence of more mature data and confirmative studies, antiangiogenic therapy might represent a therapeutic alternative for advanced non-clear cell subtype RCC.

In this sense, the ESMO guidelines recommend temsirolimus, sunitinib or sorafenib, all with low level of evidence (IIIB) for the treatment of metastatic non-clear cell disease. [24]

Immune Therapy Based on Checkpoint Inhibitors

Immune therapy in advanced RCC has evolved from non-specific agents, mainly IFN-α and IL-2 until more recently the knowledge of Checkpoint inhibition and its relationship with CTLA-4 and PD-1/PDL-1. [51, 52] Their blockades have shown promising results with maintained clinical benefit in a subset of patients previously treated with standard antiangiogenic therapy associated to less toxicity than had been seen with CK. This more specific immune therapy based on CTLA-4 antibodies such as Ipilimumab and tremelimumab has shown activity in patients with several tumours including metastatic RCC and are entering in randomized trials. [53, 54] On the other hand, the PD-1 antibody nivolumab has also demonstrated activity in a group of including patients previously treated with RCC, undergoing confirmatory testing in the phase III trial. [55] Patient selection is going to be the next step of research looking at biomarker development to predict response to these more specific immune therapies. Additionally, combination between agents targeting different immune mechanisms as well as with traditional antiangiogenic therapies are right now being explored.

Conclusion

Traditionally, the therapeutic option of choice for advanced renal cancer has been based on a non-specific systemic immunological treatment with cytokines (interleukin-2 and/or interferon-alfa) associated or not with primary cyto-reductive surgery. Currently, agents targeting vascular growth factor and mammalian target of rapamycin signalling pathways have shown significant improvements in the survival of these patients and represent the present standard first- and second-line treatment options in advanced RCC, mainly whether associated cyto-reductive nephrectomy is possible in those patients without poor risk factors and appropriate performance status. New systemic strategies based on more selective immunotherapy have been developed.

References

[1] Godley P. A., Ataga K. I. Renal cell carcinoma. *Curr. Opin. Oncol.,* 2000 May; 12 (3): 260–264.

[2] Jemal A., Murray T., Ward E., et al. Cancer statistics, 2005. *Cancer J. Clin.*, 2005; 55:10–30.

[3] Vineis P., Alavanja M., Buffer P., et al. Tobacco and cancer: Recent epidemiological evidence. *J. Natl. Cancer Inst.,* 2004 Jan.; 96 (2): 99-106.

[4] Calle E. E., Kaaks R. Overweight, obesity and cancer: epidemiological evidence and proposed mechanisms. *Nat. Rev. Cancer*, 2004 Aug.; 4 (8): 579–591.

[5] Rochlitz C. F., Lobeck H., Peter S., et al. Multiple drug resistance gene expression in human renal cell cancer is associated with the histologic subtype. *Cancer,* 1992 Jun.; 69 (12): 2993–2998.

[6] Gnarra J. R., Tory K., Weng Y., et al. Mutations of the VHL tumour suppressor gene in renal carcinoma. *Nat. Genet.*, 1994 May; 7 (1): 85–90.

[7] Iliopoulos O., Levy A. P., Jiang C., et al. Negative regulation of hypoxia-inducible genes by the von Hippel-Lindau protein. *Proc. Natl. Acad. Sci. USA,* 1996 Oct.; 93 (20): 10595–10599.

[8] Maxwell P. H., Wiesener M. S., Chang G. W., et al. The tumour suppressor protein VHL targets hypoxia-inducible factors for oxygen-dependent proteolysis. *Nature*, 1999 May; 399 (6733): 271–275.

[9] Na X., Wu G., Ryan C. K., et al. Overproduction of vascular endothelial growth factor related to von Hippel-Lindau tumor suppressor gene mutations and hypoxia-inducible factor-1 alpha expression in renal cell carcinomas. *J. Urol.*, 2003 Aug.; 170:588–592.

[10] Fyfe G., Fisher R. I., Rosenberg S. A. et al. Results of treatment of 255 patients with metastatic renal cell carcinoma who received high-dose recombinant interleukin-2 therapy. *J. Clin. Oncol.*, 1995; 13: 688-696.

[11] McDermott D. F., Regan M. M., Clark J. I. et al. Randomized phase III trial of high-dose interleukin-2 versus subcutaneous interleukin-2 and interferon in patients with metastatic renal cell carcinoma. *J. Clin. Oncol.*, 2005; 23: 133-141.

[12] Yang J. C., Sherry R. M., Steinberg S. M. et al. Randomized study of high-dose and low-dose interleukin-2 in patients with metastatic renal cancer. *J. Clin. Oncol.,* 2003; 21: 3127-3132.

[13] Negrier S., Perol D., Ravaud A. et al. Medroxyprogesterone, interferon alfa-2a, interleukin 2, or combination of both cytokines in patients with metastatic renal carcinoma of intermediate prognosis: results of a randomized controlled trial. *Cancer*, 2007; 110: 2468-2477.

[14] Margolin K. A., Rayner A. A., Hawkins M. J. et al. Interleukin-2 and lymphokine-activated killer cell therapy of solid tumors: analysis of toxicity and management guidelines. *J. Clin. Oncol.*, 1989; 7: 486-498.

[15] Motzer R. J., Bacik J., Murphy B. A. et al. Interferon-alfa as a comparative treatment for clinical trials of new therapies against advanced renal cell carcinoma. *J. Clin. Oncol.,* 2002; 20: 289-296.

[16] Motzer R. J., Mazumdar M., Bacik J. et al. Survival and prognostic stratification of 670 patients with advanced renal cell carcinoma. *J. Clin. Oncol.*, 1999; 17: 2530-2540.

[17] Motzer R. J., Hutson T. E., Tomczak P., et al. Sunitinib versus interferon alfa in metastatic renal-cell carcinoma. *N. Engl. J. Med.*, 2007; 356 (2): 115–124.

[18] Escudier B., Pluzanska A., Koralewski P. et al. Bevacizumab plus interferon alfa-2a for treatment of metastatic renal cell carcinoma: a randomised, double-blind phase III trial. *Lancet,* 2007; 370: 2103-2111.

[19] Rini B. I., Halabi S., Rosenberg J., et al. Bevacizumab plus interferon-alpha versus interferon-alpha monotherapy in patients with metastatic renal cell carcinoma: Results of overall survival for CALGB 90206. *J. Clin. Oncol.*, 2009; 27:18s (suppl.; abstr. LBA5019).

[20] Hudes G., Carducci M., Tomczak P., et al. A Phase III, three-arm, randomized, open-label study of interferon alfa alone, CCI-779 alone and the combination of interferon alfa and CCI-779 in fist-line poor-prognosis subjects with advanced renal cell carcinoma. *N. Engl. J. Med.,* 2007; 356 (22): 2271–2281.

[21] Sternberg C. N., Davis I. D., Mardiak J., et al. Pazopanib in locally advanced or metastatic renal cell carcinoma: results of a randomized phase III trial. *J. Clin. Oncol.*, 2010; 28(6): 1061-1068.

[22] Motzer R. J., Hutson T. E., Cella D., et al. Pazopanib versus sunitinib in metastatic renal-cell carcinoma. *N. Engl. J. Med.*, 2013; 369(8): 722-731.

[23] NCCN guidelines kidney Cancer version 2015. www.nccn.org

[24] B. Escudier, C. Porta, M. Schmidinger, et al. Renal cell carcinoma: ESMO Clinical Practice Guidelines for diagnosis, treatment and follow-up. *Ann. Oncol.*, 2014; 25 (suppl. 3): 49-56.

[25] Escudier B., Szezylik C., Eisen T., et al. Sorafenib in advanced clear-cell renal-cell carcinoma. *N. Engl. J. Med.*, 2007; 356 (2): 125–34.

[26] Motzer R. J., Escudier B., Oudard S., et al. Efficacy of everolimus in advanced renal cell carcinoma: a double-blind, randomised, placebo-controlled phase III trial. *Lancet,* 2008; 372(9637): 449-456.

[27] Rini B. I., Escudier B., Tomczak P., et al. Comparative effectiveness of axitinib versus sorafenib in advanced renal cell carcinoma (AXIS): a randomised phase 3 trial. *Lancet,* 2011; 378(9807): 1931-1939.

[28] Hutson T. E., Escudier B., Esteban E., et al. Randomized phase III trial of temsirolimus versus sorafenib as second-line therapy after sunitinib in patients with metastatic renal cell carcinoma. *J. Clin. Oncol.,* 2014; 32 (8): 760-767.

[29] R. J. Motzer, C. Porta, N. J. Vogelzang, E. Esteban et al. Dovitinib versus sorafenib for third-line targeted treatment of patients with metastatic renal cell carcinoma: an open-label, randomised phase 3 trial. *Lancet of Oncology,* 2014, Vol. 15 (3) 286-296.

[30] Guinan P. D., Vogelzang N. J., Fremgen A. M. et al. Renal cell carcinoma: tumor size, stage and survival. Members of the Cancer Incidence and End Results Committee. *J. Urol.*, 1995; 153: 901-903.

[31] Flanigan R. C., Salmon S. E., Blumenstein B. A. et al. Nephrectomy followed by interferon alfa-2b compared with interferon alfa-2b alone for metastatic renal-cell cancer. *N. Engl. J. Med.*, 2001; 345: 1655-1659.

[32] Mickisch G. H., Garin A., van Poppel H. et al. Radical nephrectomy plus interferon-alfa-based immunotherapy compared with interferon alfa alone in metastatic renal-cell carcinoma: a randomized trial. *Lancet,* 2001; 358: 966-970.

[33] Kavolius J. P., Mastorakos D. P., Pavlovich C. et al. Resection of metastatic renal cell carcinoma. *J. Clin. Oncol.*, 1998; 16: 2261-2266.

[34] Heng D. Y. C., Rini B. I., Beuselinck B., et al: Cytoreductive nephrectomy (CN) in patients with synchronous metastases from renal cell carcinoma: Results from the International Metastatatic Renal Cell Carcinoma Database Consortium (IMDC). Genitourinary Cancers Symposium. *J. Clin. Oncol.*, 32, 2014 (suppl. 4; abstr 396).

[35] Karam J. A., Rini B. I., Varella L., et al. Metastasectomy after targeted therapy in patients with advanced renal cell carcinoma. *J. Urol.*, 2011; 185 (2): 439-444.

[36] Heng D. Y., Xie W., Regan M. M., et al. Prognostic factors for overall survival in patients with metastatic renal cell carcinoma treated with vascular endothelial growth factor-targeted agents: results from a large, multicenter study. *J. Clin. Oncol.,* 2009; 27(34): 5794-5799.

[37] Garcia-Donas J., Esteban E., Leandro-Garcia L. J., et al. Single nucleotide polymorphism associations with response and toxic effects in patients with advanced renal-cell carcinoma treated with first-line sunitinib: a multicentre, observational, prospective study. *Lancet Oncol.,* 2011; 12:1143-1150.

[38] Xu C. F., Bing N. X., Ball H. A., Rajagopalan D., Sternberg C. N., Hutson T. E., et al. Pazopanib efficacy in renal cell carcinoma: evidence for predictive genetic markers in angiogenesis-related and exposure-related genes. *J. Clin. Oncol.*, 2011; 29: 2557-2564.

[39] Armstrong A. J., George D. J., Halabi S., et al. Serum lactate dehydrogenase predicts for overall survival benefit in patients with metastatic renal cell carcinoma treated with inhibition of mammalian target of rapamycin. *J. Clin. Oncol.*, 2012; 30:3402–3407.

[40] Rauvaud A. and Schmidinger M. Clinical biomarkers of response in advanced renal cell carcinoma. *Ann. Oncol.*, 2013; 24 (12): 2935-294.

[41] Ravaud A., Barrios C., Anak Ö., et al. Randomized phase II study of first-line everolimus and 840 bevacizumab versus interferon alfa-2A and bevacizumab in patients with metastatic renal cell 841 carcinoma: RECORD-2. *Ann. Oncol.*, 2012; 23 Suppl. 9:258–93. Abstract 783.

[42] Flaherty K., Manola J., Pins M., et al. E2804 The BeST Trial: a randomized phase II study of VEGF, RAF kinase and MTOR combination targeted therapy with bevacizumab, sorafenib and temsirolimus in advanced renal cell carcinoma. 11th annual kidney cancer association symposium. 2012: Oral abstract.

[43] Rini B., Bellmunt J., Clancy J., et al. Randomized phase IIIb trial of846 temsirolimus and bevacizumab versus interferon and bevacizumab in metastatic renal cell 847 carcinoma: results from intoract. *Ann. Oncol.,* 2012; 23 Suppl. 9: Abstract LBA21.

[44] Robert John Motzer, Carlos H. Barrios, Tae Min Kim, et al. Record-3: Phase II randomized trial comparing sequential first-line everolimus (EVE) and second-line sunitinib (SUN) versus first-line SUN and second-line EVE in patients with metastatic renal cell carcinoma (mRCC). *J. Clin. Oncol.*, 2013; 31, (suppl.; abstr. 4504).

[45] Michel M. S., Vervenne W., de Santis M., et al: SWITCH: A randomized sequential open-label study to evaluate efficacy and safety of sorafenib (SO)/sunitinib (SU) versus SU/SO in the treatment of metastatic renal cell cancer (mRCC). *J. Clin. Oncol.*, 2014;32 (suppl. 4) abstr. 393.

[46] Schrader A. J., Olbert P. J., Hegele A., Varga Z., Hofmann R. Metastatic non-clear cell renal cell carcinoma: current therapeutic options. *BJU Int.,* 2008; 101:1343-1345.

[47] Dutcher J. P., Nanus D. Long-term survival of patients with sarcomatoid renal cell cancer treated with chemotherapy. *Med. Oncol.*, 2011; 28(4): 1530–1533.

[48] Oudard S., Banu E., Vieillefond A., et al. Prospective multicenter phase II study of gemcitabine plus platinum salt for metastatic collecting duct carcinoma: results of a getug (Groupe d'Etudes des Tumeurs Uro-Genitales) study. *J. Urol.*, 2007; 177: 1698–1702.

[49] Choueiri T. K., Plantade A., Elson P., et al. Efficacy of sunitinib and sorafenib in metastatic papillary and chromophobe renal cell carcinoma. *J. Clin. Oncol.*, 2008; 26:127-131.

[50] Nizar M. Tannir, Eric Jonasch, Emre Altinmakas, et al. Everolimus versus sunitinib prospective evaluation in metastatic non-clear cell renal cell carcinoma (The ESPN Trial): A multicenter randomized phase 2 trial. *J. Clin. Oncol.*, 2014; 32:5s, (suppl.; abstr. 4505).

[51] Walunas T. L., Lenschow D. J., Bakker C. Y., et al. CTLA-4 can function as a negative regulator of 330 T cell activation. *Immunity,* 1994;1:405–413.

[52] Thompson R. H., Dong H., Lohse C. M., et al. PD-1 is expressed by tumor-infiltrating immune cells and is associated with poor outcome for patients with renal cell carcinoma. *Clin. Cancer Res.*, 2007;13:1757–1761.

[53] Yang J. C., Hughes M., Kammula U., et al. Ipilimumab (anti-CTLA4 antibody) causes regression of metastatic renal cell cancer associated with enteritis and hypophysitis. *J. Immunother.*, 2007;30:825–830.

[54] Rini B. I., Stein M., Shannon P., et al. Phase 1 dose-escalation trial of tremelimumab plus sunitinib in patients with metastatic renal cell carcinoma. *Cancer,* 2011;117:758–767.

[55] Topalian S. L., Hodi S., Brahmer J. R., et al. Safety, activity, and immune correlates of anti–PD-1 antibody in cancer. *N. Engl. J. Med.,* 2012; 366:2443-2454.

Index

A

B

C

D

E

F

G

H

I

M

N

O

P

Q

R

S

T

U

V

W

X

Y